FETAL HEART RATE MONITORING

FETAL HEART RATE MONITORING

Roger K. Freeman, M.D.

Medical Director
Women's Hospital, Memorial Hospital Medical Center
of Long Beach
and
Professor
Department of Obstetrics and Gynecology
University of California, Irvine

Thomas J. Garite, M.D.

Associate Medical Director for Perinatology
Women's Hospital, Memorial Hospital Medical Center
of Long Beach
and
Assistant Professor
Department of Obstetrics and Gynecology
University of California, Irvine

 WILLIAMS & WILKINS
Baltimore • Hong Kong • London • Sydney

Library of Congress Cataloging in Publication Data

Freeman, Roger K
  Fetal heart rate monitoring.

  Includes index.
  1. Fetal heart rate monitoring. I. Garite, Thomas J., joint author. II. Title. [DNLM:
1. Fetal heart. 2. Fetal monitoring. WQ210 F855f]
RG628.3.H42F73   618.3'2   80–14604
ISBN 0–683–03378–6

88 89 90 91   15 14 13 12

DEDICATION

We dedicate this book to
Dr. Edward Hon and
Dr. Ted Quilligan,
our teachers,
and to the hope that
these efforts and theirs
will help to allow all
children to reach their
maximum potential

PREFACE

There is no technology that has had a greater impact on obstetrical care than electronic fetal heart rate monitoring. However, it is really only in the last 10 years that clinicians have begun to use this technique to monitor fetal status and uterine activity. Because of its recent development, most obstetricians practicing today were not trained in the use of electronic fetal heart rate monitoring during their residency. Educational efforts for the physician in practice have been largely limited to brief postgraduate courses and to some workshops. It is because of the great need for comprehensive knowledge in this area that we have written this text.

All of us who practice obstetrics are greatly indebted to the early meticulous and untiring efforts of Doctor Edward Hon who systematized the science of heart rate monitoring and uncoded the language of the fetus as expressed through its heart rate. As a result of his labors we can now offer a great margin of safety to the fetus who comes under surveillance for whatever reason. Although we continue to modify our use of this technique, the basic principles put forth by Doctor Hon more than 20 years ago remain unchanged. Similarly we are indebted to Sir Joseph Barcroft who first began to look at the physiological basis for fetal heart rate changes over 40 years ago. Today, through modern electronic technology, the physiologic studies of Barcroft and the basic work on human fetal heart rate changes by Hon, the fetus can be treated as an individual patient. To a large extent, fetal heart rate monitoring has thus provided the basis for modern fetal medicine.

While there is still a great deal that we do not understand, the major gap in the application of what is known lies in the need for more professional education on the use of fetal heart rate monitoring as a tool in clinical management. Certainly it is incumbent on all physicians practicing obstetrics to familiarize themselves with the clinical use of this technique but it is perhaps equally or more important for the labor and delivery nurse to be skilled in fetal heart rate monitoring. Many labor room nurses today are among the most expert in this field and it is a wise physician who can utilize the expert nurse as an educational resource.

The first section of this text provides basic background information; the history of heart rate monitoring, the physiologic basis of heart rate monitoring and the effects of hypoxia on the fetus. The fourth chapter, we believe, is especially useful in that it explains the necessary technical aspects of instrumentation including artifact detection and recognition of fetal arrhythmias. A lack of understanding of these technical factors is common even among experienced individuals skilled in fetal heart rate monitoring and is a frequent source of confusion in pattern interpretation.

The next section is designed to provide a basic knowledge of intrapartum fetal heart rate pattern recognition with a separate chapter on monitoring uterine activity. This is followed by a brief chapter on fetal acid-base monitoring intended to underline the role of this technique as an adjunct to electronic fetal heart rate monitoring and in preparation for the chapter on the management of intrapartum fetal distress.

The third section is devoted to antepartum fetal heart rate monitoring, including discussion of technique, interpretation, stressed and nonstressed monitoring and case management. As in the intrapartum fetal heart rate section, there are numerous examples of interesting tracings.

The final chapter attempts to analyze the risks and benefits of intrapartum and antepartum fetal heart rate monitoring, an especially timely subject, as government and consumer interest are focusing more heavily on the proliferation of medical technology.

Ultimately we wish to emphasize that while electronic fetal heart rate monitoring is a valuable technique, it is only an adjunct to the competent clinician and obstetrical nurse and cannot replace good clinical judgment. For this reason we have tried to present this technique in a clinical context throughout the book.

We especially would like to thank Mavis Haydon, Donna Gorman, and Catherine Rommal, R.N.C., for their help in the preparation of the manuscript, and to note our sincere appreciation to Shirley Garite, who prepared the original artwork used in this text. We would also like to express our gratitude to the medical and nursing staff and the patients of the Women's Hospital, Memorial Hospital Medical Center, Long Beach, California for providing case examples used in the book.

FETAL HEART RATE MONITORING

CONTENTS

CHAPTER 1

History of Fetal Monitoring

It is somewhat suprising that something as potentially accessible as the fetal heart was not heard or at least described until the 17th century. Phillipe Le-Gaust first described the fetal heart tones in his poetry in an ancient French dialect. LeGaust was a colleague of Marsac, a physician of the province of Limousin, who is credited with having first heard the fetal heart.

This observation apparently went unnoticed until 1818 when Francois Mayor, a Swiss surgeon, reported the presence of the fetal heart sounds which he heard while placing his ear on the maternal abdomen attempting to hear the fetus splash about in its liquor. Three years later, Lejumeau Kergaradec, a French nobleman, apparently unaware of Mayor's report, again described the fetal heart tones. In addition, he described the uterine souffle. He suggested auscultation to be of value in the diagnosis of pregnancy, diagnosis of twins, and determining fetal lie and presentation.

As with many discoveries, the obstetricians of the time were slow to respond to Kergaradec's discoveries and recommendations. In 1833, Evory Kennedy of Dublin published an extensive book entitled *Observations on Obstetric Auscultation*.[1] Kennedy's expressed purpose was to convince clinicians of the value of Kergaradec's discoveries. The book contains many anecdotal examples of cases where auscultation was of clear benefit. In addition, Kennedy described the funic souffle for the first time.

THE FETOSCOPE

Before the development of the fetoscope much attention was paid to whether mediate (stethoscopic) auscultation using Laennec's instrument, or immediate auscultation, using the ear directly on the gravid maternal abdomen, was the more appropriate choice. Rauth and Verardini[2] suggested vaginal stethoscopy to be even more valuable in the early detection of fetal life. The development of the head stethoscope or fetoscope is a story of controversy and professional jealousy. The first report of the head stethoscope was in 1917 in the *JAMA* by David Hillis,[3]

an obstetrican then working in Chicago Lying-In-Hospital (Fig. 1.1). In 1922, J. B. DeLee, the Chief of Staff at the same institution, and a man who became a legend in American obstetrics for his many contributions, published his report of a similar instrument.[4] Although the order of publications is clear, DeLee claimed that he openly talked of this idea for many years preceeding Hillis' publication. The instrument has subsequently come to be known as the DeLee-Hillis stethoscope and has remained largely unchanged since its early development.

DIAGNOSIS OF FETAL DISTRESS

Thirty years after Mayor's description of the fetal heart, Kilian[5] formulated the first proposal that fetal heart rate might be used to diagnose fetal distress in order to intervene on the fetus' behalf. He formulated what is sometimes called "the stethoscopal indication

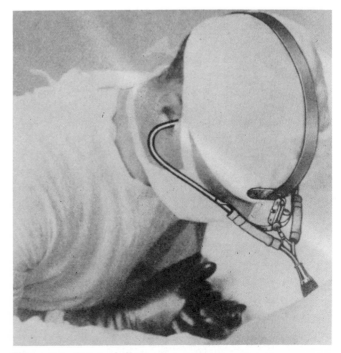

Figure 1.1. Original illustration of the head stethoscope or fetoscope (Reproduced with permission from Reference 3).

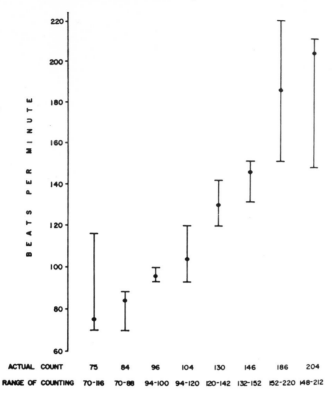

ACTUAL COUNT   75   84   96   104   130   146   186   204

RANGE OF COUNTING 70-116 70-88 94-100 94-120 120-142 132-152 152-220 148-212

Figure 1.2. Range of error in auscultative counting of fetal heart rate by 15 obstetricians asked to count from recorded fetal heart rate. Count as reported by obstetrician on vertical scale vs. actual count on horizontal scale. (Reproduced with permission from Reference 8.)

for forceps delivery," suggesting that heart rates below 100, above 180, those that lost purity of tone, those with distinct intermissions, and when only one tone could be heard, were indications for forceps application without delay where conditions permitted such application. In 1893, Von Winckel[6] described criteria of fetal distress which were to remain essentially unchanged until fetal scalp sampling and electronic heart rate monitoring arrived. These included tachycardia (heart rate more than 160) bradycardia (heart rate less than 100), irregularity of the heart rate, meconium passage, and gross alteration of fetal movement. Few studies challenged or supported the validity of these auscultative and clinical criteria for fetal distress. It was not until 1968 when Benson et al.[7] published the results of the collaborative project, commissioned by the National Institute of Neurologic Diseases and Blindness, that these criteria were seriously questioned. This study reviewed the benefits of fetal heart rate auscultation for the management of intrapartum fetal distress on 24,863 deliveries. Benson concluded that there was "no reliable indicator of fetal distress in terms of fetal heart rate save in extreme degree." Hon[8] had pointed out 10 years earlier how unreliable human counting of fetal heart rate was when he asked 15 obstetricians to count several rates from tape and found a wide divergence in counting (Fig. 1.2).

With these serious doubts and the age of electronic technology fast making its impact on modern medicine, it was inevitable that obstetrical research would turn to more sophisticated methods of fetal evaluation.

THE FETAL ELECTROCARDIOGRAPH (EKG)

In 1906, using abdominal and intravaginal leads, Cremer[9] recorded the fetal EKG for the first time. Until the 1950's the majority of effort using fetal electrocardiography was applied towards the use of this modality to diagnose fetal life. Southern[10] in 1957 suggested that certain fetal EKG changes might correlate with fetal hypoxia. Hon[11] reviewed all the applications fo fetal electrocardiography in 1960 including fetal presentation, diagnosis of twins, antenatal diagnosis of congenital heart disease, diagnosis of fetal maturity, and finally fetal distress. He concluded that the EKG wave form was not of consistent value in any these problems and specifically that in 75 cases of fetal distress "no consistent fetal EKG changes could be detected." Subsequently Pardi et al.,[12] using group averaging techniques, was able to demonstrate ST segment depression with fetal hypoxia (Fig. 1.3). Unfortunately, this technique has not been developed to the point where it has become clinically applicable.

The history of the development of electronic fetal heart rate monitoring or cardiotachometry is a complexity of technologic development and empirical observations of heart rate patterns found to be associated with various causes of fetal distress.

The earliest preliminary report of fetal heart rate monitoring in 1958 came from Doctor Edward Hon,[8] then working at the Yale University School of Medicine. He reported on the continuous instantaneous recording of fetal heart rate via fetal EKG monitor from the maternal abdomen. He further began to elucidate causes of fetal bradycardia and more specifically defined when bradycardia was indicative of fetal distress. In the years that followed, Hon, Caldeyro-Barcia in Uruguay, and Hammacher in Germany and their many coworkers reported their observations on the various heart rate patterns associated with fetal distress. Bradycardia and tachycardia were well-known signs of fetal compromise. Hon[13] defined the type of variable deceleration associated with umbilical cord compression and proposed a mechanism for the hypoxic uteroplacental cause of delayed decelerations in 1959. In 1963, Caldeyro-Barcia et al.[14] reported observations on similar heart rate decelerations which they called Type III and II, respectively, and defined their "prognostic significance." In addition, long- and short-term fetal heart rate variability were defined for the first time. Hammacher[15] subsequently defined this parameter's sig-

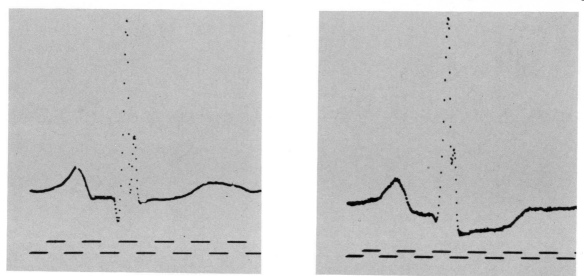

Figure 1.3. *Left*: average of 25 EKG complexes performed before the onset of a contraction: baseline FHR 160 beats/min. *Right*: average of 25 EKG complexes performed immediately after the end of the same contraction, during a late deceleration. Notice the depression of the ST segment. Scalp capillary blood pH 7.34, Apgar score 4/9, umbilical artery pH 7.25. (Reproduced with permission from Crosignani PG, Pardi G: Fetal Evaluation during Pregnancy and Labor. Academic Press New York, p 235, 1971.

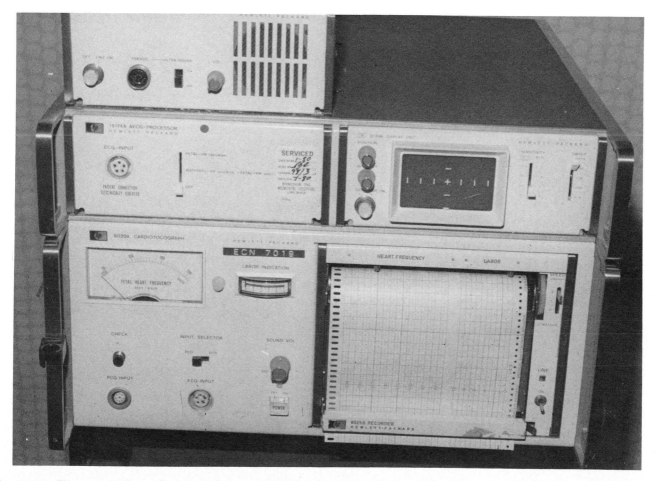

Figure 1.4. First generation of practical commercially available fetal monitors. The original model utilized external monitoring with phonocardiography only. The upper two modules were subsequently added allowing the addition of external ultrasound and internal fetal EKG monitoring (Hewlett-Packard Model 8020A).

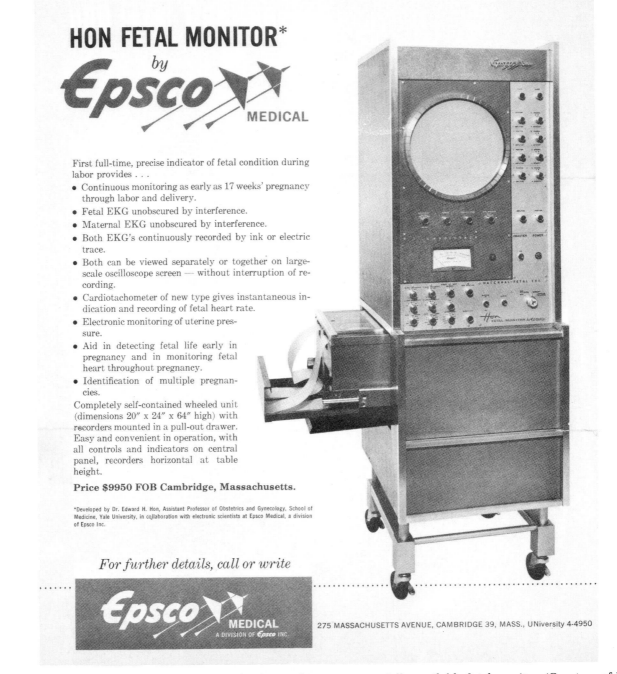

Figure 1.5. This bulky machine was the first attempt at making a commercially available fetal monitor. (Courtesy of Epsco, Inc.)

nificance in terms of loss of heart rate variability in association with fetal distress.

With many investigators throughout the world making similar observations, fetal heart rate terminology became extremely confusing. Hon, Caldeyro-Barcia, and many of their colleagues met at an International Conference on monitoring of the fetal heart in December 1971 in New Jersey and subsequently in Amsterdam in March 1972 to agree on nomenclature and develop standards for fetal heart rate monitoring. They developed and agreed upon a common nomenclature. Efforts were made to agree upon universal scales and paper speed for fetal monitors but these remained variable. Much of the subsequent history has been one of the technologic development for the clinical application of electronic fetal heart rate monitoring. The first monitor practically available for clinical use was produced by Hammacher and Hewlett-Packard in 1968 using external tocography and phonocardiography (Fig. 1.4). Before this time equipment was bulky and generally limited to research equipment although attempts were made to market some equipment for general use earlier (Fig. 1.5). Technologic advances since that first generation of fetal monitors have allowed further and more accurate definition of fetal heart rate patterns and have provided the clinician with a practical tool. Direct EKG monitoring became practical with Hon's introduction of an electrode that could be directly applied to the fetal scalp.[16] This was originally a modification of a surgical skin clip (Fig. 1.6). Subsequently, Hon developed a more convenient disposable spiral electrode (Fig. 1.7) that is widely used in this country today. Doppler ultrasound and external EKG and logic systems that provide adequate approximations of the real beat to beat heart rate have been the final developments which bring us to date.

ERA OF QUESTIONING

Benson's report on the collaborative project data set the stage for rejection of auscultation and the boom in electronic cardiotachometry. By 1978, it was estimated that fetal monitoring was in routine use in over half of labors.[18] Enthusiasm for its use came without clear documentation of its efficacy and safety. There were, however, many reports that came retrospectively analyzing fetal monitoring and nearly all agreed to a beneficial effect, including reduction of intrapartum stillbirth rate and perinatal mortality as well as improved Apgar scores.[19] Randomized control trials have recently been reported.[20-23] While mixed, they do not uniformly show electronic monitoring to be beneficial and indeed suggest that such monitoring may substantially increase the cesarean section rate. Details of all these studies and analysis of the risks and benefits of fetal monitoring are reviewed in Chapter 11. The area of consumer demand for obstetrics in particular, coupled with a

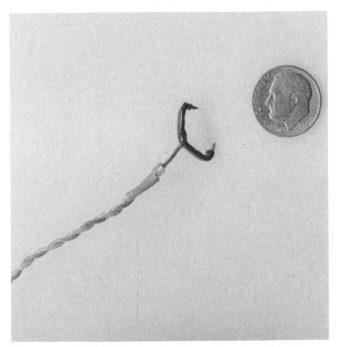

Figure 1.6. Vaginal fetal scalp electrode as described by Dr. Edward Hon.[16] This is a modification of a Michelle surgical skin clip. A specially made long forceps and a vaginal speculum are necessary for application.

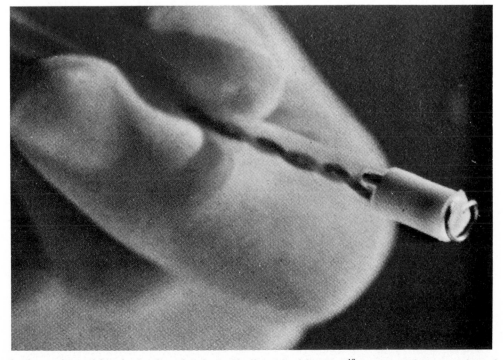

Figure 1.7. Spiral silver-silver chloride fetal scalp electrode described by Hon[17] in 1972. This is packaged within a plastic sheath which allows direct application without the aid of a speculum.

period of heightened government intervention into cost, risks, and benefits of medical care are further impetus to questioning electronic fetal monitoring.

Gastric freezing enjoyed a similarly rapid acceptance and boom in the sales of freezing machines. Their demise came rapidly when controlled studies failed to demonstrate benefit. Might this be the fate of fetal monitoring? Large, well-controlled studies are needed to resolve the issue.

Nevertheless, electronic fetal heart rate monitoring has become the standard of practice for high risk patients during labor, and antepartum electronic fetal heart rate monitoring is clearly the best current means available to assess the fetus at high risk for uteroplacental insufficiency before labor. Further applications will depend on continuing evaluation and adjustment of current methodologies as well as the development of new technology. It is clear, however, that the end result of the development of electronic fetal heart rate monitoring has been to allow assessment of the human fetus for hypoxia.

REFERENCES

1. Kennedy E: Observations on Obstetric Auscultation. Hodges and Smith, Dublin, 1833
2. Routh, Verardini: quoted in: Hirst BC: An American System of Obstetrics. Lea Brothers Co., Philadelphia, 1888
3. Hillis DS: Attachment for the stethoscope. JAMA 68:910, 1917
4. DeLee JB: Ein nues stethoskop für die Geburtshilfe besonders geeignet. Zentralbl Gynaekol 46:1688, 1922
5. Killian: quoted by Goodlin R, in: History of Fetal Monitoring. Am J Obstet Gynecol 133:325, 1979
6. Von Winckel F: Lehrbuch der Geburtshilfe, Weisbaden, 1893, p 634
7. Benson RC, Shubeck F, Deutschberger J, et al: Fetal heart rate as a predictor of fetal distress: a report from the collaborative project. Obstet Gynecol 32:529, 1968
8. Hon EH: The electronic evaluation of the fetal heart rate. Am J Obstet Gynecol 75:1215, 1958
9. Cremer M: Munch Med Wochenschr 53:811, 1906
10. Southern EM: Fetal anoxia and its possible relation to changes in the prenatal fetal electrocardiogram. Am J Obstet Gynecol 73:233, 1957
11. Hon EH: The clinical value of fetal electrocardiography. Am J Obstet Gynecol 79:1012, 1960
12. Pardi G, Brambati B, Dubini S, et al: Analysis of the fetal electrocardiogram by the group averaging technique. Proc 2nd Europ Congr Perinatal Med, London, 1970
13. Hon EH: Observations on "pathologic" fetal bradycardia. Am J Obstet Gynecol 77:1084, 1959
14. Caldeyro-Barcia R, Mendez-Bauer C, Poseiro JJ, et al: Control of human fetal heart rate during labor. In: Cassels D (editor) The Heart and Circulation in the Newborn Infant. New York, Grune & Stratton, Inc, 1966
15. Hammacher K: In: Kaser O, Friedberg V, Oberk editors: Gynakologie v Gerburtshilfe BD II. Stuttgard, Georg Thieme Verlag, 1967
16. Hon EH: Instrumentation of fetal heart rate and electrocardiography II. A vaginal electrode. Am J Obstet Gynecol 86:772, 1963
17. Hon EH, Paul RH, Hon RW: Electronic evaluation of fetal heart rate XI. Description of a spiral electrode. Obstet Gynecol 40:362, 1972
18. Williams RL, Hawes WE: Cesarean section, fetal monitoring and perinatal mortality in California. Am J Public Health 69:864, 1979
19. Task Force on Predictors of Fetal Distress, NICHD Consensus Development Committee on Antenatal Diagnosis, NIH Publication no 79-1973, 1979
20. Haverkamp AD, Thompson HE, McFee JG, et al: The evaluation of continuous fetal heart rate monitoring in high risk pregnancy. Am J Obstet Gynecol 125:310, 1976
21. Renou P, Chang A, Anderson I, et al: Controlled trial of fetal intensive care. Am J Obstet Gynecol 126:470, 1976
22. Kelso IM, Parsons RJ, Lawrence GF, et al: An assessment of continuous fetal heart rate monitoring in labor: a randomized trial. Am J Obstet Gynecol 131:526, 1978
23. Haverkamp AD, Orleans M, Langendoerfer S, et al: A controlled trial of the differential effects of intrapartum fetal monitoring. Am J Obstet Gynecol 134:399, 1979

CHAPTER 2

The Physiologic Basis of Fetal Monitoring

Clinical fetal heart rate (FHR) monitoring is actually an ongoing observation of human fetal physiology. The question that is being asked of the fetal monitor by the clinician is: What is the adequacy of fetal oxygenation? Because the FHR pattern appears to assume certain characteristics under the influence of various hypoxic and nonhypoxic stresses, it becomes important for the clinician to have a basic understanding of the physiology of fetal respiratory exchange and the physiologic control of the FHR. In this chapter, an attempt will be made to outline the principle factors involved in fetal oxygenation and carbon dioxide transfer as well as the basis for our current understanding of FHR responses to changes in fetal respiratory status.

THE ANATOMY OF MATERNOFETAL EXCHANGE

The placenta is an organ that serves as the fetus' extracorporeal life-support system. The placenta serves as the fetal lung (respiration), kidney (excretion), gastrointestinal tract (nutrition), skin (heat exchange), and is also a barrier against certain substances dangerous to the fetus. In addition, it is an endocrine organ that produces steroid (estrogen, progesterone) and protein (human chorionic gonadotropin, human placental lactogen) hormones.

Very early in gestation, the blastocyst implants in the decidualized endometrium and the trophoblast cells invade the maternal circulation, creating a lake of maternal blood that bathes the trophoblast and developing embryo. As the gestation grows, a number of spiral arteries that supply blood to the endometrium are penetrated and provide the basic architecture as the placenta develops with villi forming cotyledons arranged around these spiral arteries. The fetal chorionic villi develop many convolutions and float in the maternal blood that is supplied from the previously invaded spiral arteries. This maternal blood occupies an area referred to as the intervillous space and it is between this space and the fetal capillary (contained within the chorionic villus) that maternofetal and fetomaternal exchange occurs. The

human placenta is thus referred to as a hemochorial type because the mother's blood comes into direct contact with the fetal chorionic villus.[1] Oxygen, carbon dioxide, nutrients, waste products, water, and heat are exchanged at this level and must cross two layers of fetal trophoblast, the fetal connective tissue within the villus, and the fetal capillary wall (Fig. 2.1).

The uterine blood flow is supplied principally from the uterine arteries, but anastomoses occur between these vessels, other branches of the hypogastric arteries, and ovarian arteries. Significantly, the spiral arteries must traverse the full thickness of the myometrium in order to reach the intervillous space. Anything that affects maternal cardiac output will of course affect the flow through the spiral arteries. Additionally, as the uterus contracts, the intramyometrial pressure may exceed the intraarterial pressure, causing occlusion of these vessels and resulting

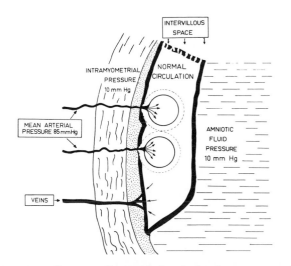

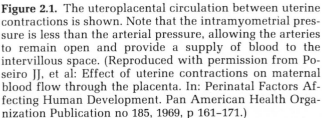

Figure 2.1. The uteroplacental circulation between uterine contractions is shown. Note that the intramyometrial pressure is less than the arterial pressure, allowing the arteries to remain open and provide a supply of blood to the intervillous space. (Reproduced with permission from Poseiro JJ, et al: Effect of uterine contractions on maternal blood flow through the placenta. In: Perinatal Factors Affecting Human Development. Pan American Health Organization Publication no 185, 1969, p 161–171.)

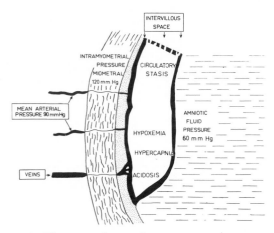

Figure 2.2. The uteroplacental circulation during a uterine contraction is shown. Note that the intramyometrial pressure exceeds the arterial pressure, causing circulatory stasis in the intervillous space. (Reproduced with permission from Poseiro JJ, et al: Effect of uterine contractions on maternal blood flow through the placenta. In: Perinatal Factors Affecting Human Development. Pan American Health Organization, Publication no 185, 1969, p 161–171.)

in cessation of blood flow to the intervillous space (Fig. 2.2).[2]

Most authorities agree that about 85% of the total uterine blood flow goes to supply the placental (intervillous) circulation and about 15% supplies the extra placental uterine musculature.[3] The intervillous space blood supplies the vascular support to the placenta itself and if the blood flow to any area is sufficiently compromised, an infarction of the placenta may occur.[4, 5]

For clinical purposes, the intervillous space circulation is probably maximal when the mother is at rest, in the lateral position. While estrogen administration to the pregnant ewe will increase uterine blood flow, it is not certain that this results in increased intervillous space flow.[6] Therefore, although we know of nothing that will increase effective uterine blood flow above that found in the resting lateral position, there are many things that will decrease uterine blood flow and these factors deserve some attention at this time.

FACTORS THAT DECREASE UTERINE BLOOD FLOW

Position

Changes in the mother's position may decrease blood flow to the uterus by at least two mechanisms. The supine position is characterized by an exaggeration of the lumbar lordotic curve resulting in uterine compression of the vena cava and/or the aortoiliac vessels. With vena caval occlusion, the return of blood to the heart is decreased and this may result in a fall in maternal cardiac output, maternal hypotension, and decreased uterine blood flow.[7, 8] Compression of the aorta against the spine or iliac vessels as

they cross the pelvic brim may result in decreases in uterine blood flow without maternal hypotension (Fig. 2.3).[2]

Exercise

Maternal exercise may serve to divert blood away from the uterus and to supply somatic muscle groups, resulting in decreased uterine blood flow. In the patient with normal uteroplacental function, this exercise diversion probably does not exceed the uteroplacental reserve. However, in a patient with decreased uteroplacental respiratory reserve, maximal maternal rest may be important.[9]

Uterine Contractions

The spiral arteries that traverse the myometrium are subject to collapse as the uterus contracts and the intramyometrial pressure exceeds the spiral arterial pressure. During normal pregnancy, the uterus has certain inherent contractility (Braxton-Hicks contractions) and as labor begins the contractions increase in intensity. If the uteroplacental reserve is normal, the Braxton-Hicks contractions and labor contractions do not appear to significantly compromise the total intervillous space blood flow. However, a normal fetoplacental unit may have its uteroplacental reserve exceeded if uterine activity is excessive as with spontaneous or oxytocin-induced uterine hypertonus and/or tetanic contractions.[10, 11] Patients with abruptio placenta may have hypertonus and polysystole, resulting in decreased intervillous space perfusion producing fetal hypoxia.

Surface Area

Anything that will decrease the effective surface area of the placenta will clearly increase the potential

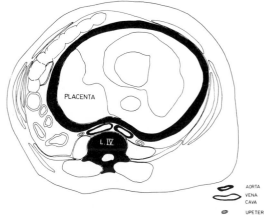

Figure 2.3. A cross-section of a pregnant uterus lying on the maternal vertebral column with the interposed great vessels which are subject to occlusion when the mother is supine. (Reproduced with permission from Poseiro JJ, et al: Effect of uterine contractions on maternal blood flow through the placenta. In: Perinatal Factors Affecting Human Development. Pan American Health Organization Publication no 185, 1969, p 161–171.)

for fetal hypoxia. Abruptio placenta is a classic example of reduced placental surface area available for exchange. Patients with multiple placental infarcts, as may be seen in hypertensive disorders and prolonged pregnancy, are also subject to having the fetus suffer from uteroplacental insufficiency.[4, 5]

Anesthesia

The administration of conduction anesthetics carries the potential for reduced intervillous space blood flow secondary to maternal hypotension, resulting from the sympathetic blockade that may occur to a greater or lesser degree in all such patients. The pharmacologic correction of such hypotension with alpha adrenergic agents may not restore uterine blood flow because the alpha adrenergic agents will increase uterine circulatory resistance along with the other somatic components of total peripheral resistance that are responsible for the rise in blood pressure. For this reason it is recommended that an agent such as ephedrine (a mixed alpha and beta adrenergic

stimulator) be used to restore maternal blood pressure after hypotension induced by the sympathectomy of conduction anesthesia.[12] Usually, however, the uterine blood flow is easily restored in such situations by correcting positional factors and volume expanding the mother, thus obviating the need for any pressor agents.

Hypertension

Maternal hypertensive syndromes may result in decreased intervillous space blood flow as a result of either acute vasospastic or chronic atheromatous changes in the uterine arterial blood supply. If one lowers blood pressure in the hypertensive patient either intentionally with antihypertensive agents or unintentionally as a result of administering a conduction anesthetic, one runs the risk of diverting blood away from the intervillous space if the caliber of the uterine arterial circulation remains diminished as other vascular beds are dilated.

Diffusion Distance

The thickness of the placental membrane between the intervillous space and the fetal capillary may also decrease the transfer of oxygen. An example of a clinical entity demonstrating this phenomenon can probably be found in erythroblastosis with placental edema. Perhaps this is also a factor in certain conditions of fetal dysmaturity where there is an increase in fibrin deposition between the intervillous space and the fetal capillary. Villous hemorrhage and edema in diabetics may also play a role in increasing the thickness of the placental membrane.

THE FETAL CIRCULATION

The anatomy and physiology of the fetal circulation is very complex. For the purposes of this chapter we will focus on the umbilical circulation and factors that affect placental exchange (Fig. 2.4).

The umbilical vessels are contained within the umbilical cord and are protected with an abundance of a substance called Wharton's jelly. There are two umbilical arteries that arise from the terminal ends of the hypogastric arteries and a single umbilical vein that returns blood to the fetus from the placenta channeling it partly through the liver and partly to the inferior vena cava via the ductus venosus. This well-oxygenated blood enters the right atrium and follows a course directing it mainly to the cephalic circulation, while blood returning from the upper body via the superior vena cava is channeled principally through the ductus arteriosus to the lower body and the placenta. About 30% of the fetal cardiac output goes to the placenta which comprises a low resistance vascular bed. The oxygen content of the umbilical venous blood closely approximates that of the uterine venous drainage which suggests that the

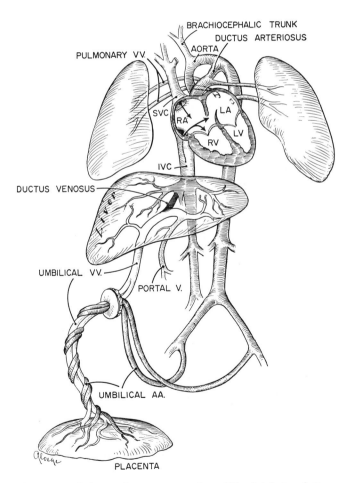

Figure 2.4. Schematic representation of the fetal circulation in the lamb. Note that the well-oxygenated blood returning from the placenta via the inferior vena cava (IVC) crosses into the left atrium while the superior vena cava (SVC) blood tends to run into the right ventricle. (Reproduced with permission from Assali NS: Fetal and neonatal circulation. In: Biology of Gestation II. Academic Press, New York, 1968, p. 254.)

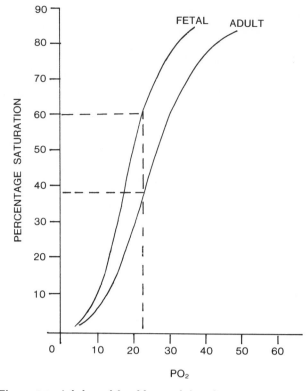

Figure 2.5. Adult and fetal hemoglobin dissociation curves.

pattern of umbilical and uterine flows follows functionally a concurrent relationship although the flow relationships are clearly much more complex and authorities in the field are not in total agreement concerning this fact.[13]

One must ask how the fetus can exist at a maximum pO_2 below that of the uterine vein (about 35 mm Hg) while the adult would be unable to survive under similar circumstances. The fetus has a number of unique characteristics that allow it to do well with such a low pO_2.

First, the fetal hemoglobin concentration is higher than the adult, allowing for a much greater oxygen-carrying capacity. Second, the fetal cardiac output far exceeds that of the adult on a volume per unit body weight basis. Third, the fetal hemoglobin dissociation curve favors a higher saturation at a given pO_2 (see Fig. 2.5). So, although the fetal pO_2 is lower, the fetus is able to compensate by having an increased oxygen content, due to the high hemoglobin concentration and the characteristic of the fetal hemoglobin dissociation curve. The more rapid circulation then increases the amount of oxygen that can be delivered to the fetal tissue per unit time.[14]

Oxygen crosses the placenta by simple diffusion. If the relative flows on the two sides of the placenta are held constant, the differential pO_2 between the intervillous space and the fetal capillary determines the rate of maternofetal oxygen transfer. Thus, administration of high concentrations of oxygen to the mother may raise her pO_2 several hundred millimeters of mercury and the maternofetal oxygen gradient

may be markedly increased by this maneuver.[15] Moreover, if the fetal pO_2 is increased by only a few millimeters of mercury, the fetal blood oxygen content may increase significantly because in either the physiologic or hypoxic range the fetal hemoglobin saturation curve is quite steep (see Fig. 2.5).[16]

Clinically, however, even though maternal hyperoxia may be of some help, most causes of fetal hypoxia are related to restriction of umbilical or intervillous space blood flow. Under conditions of diminished flow on either side of the placenta, changing the pO_2 gradient will not be of as much help as restoring the blood flow. It is still reasonable to administer oxygen to the mother[16] in such situations, but one must remember that restoration of flow is usually more important.

Control of FHR

The FHR, under physiologic conditions, represents the final product of intrinsic and extrinsic rate determining or modifying factors. Technically, the FHR represents the reciprocal of the interval between two successive beats, or more simply stated, the interval between beats is inversely related to the instantaneous rate. Most data on FHR utilize an electrical marker (specifically the peak of the fetal electrocardiograph (EKG) R wave) to signify the time of the beat. Unless otherwise stated, we will refer to the rate calculated from intervals between fetal EKG R waves. FHR changes constitute the basis for electronic fetal monitoring and for this reason one must look carefully at the factors that determine or modify the rate.

Schifferli and Caldeyro-Barcia[17] pointed to the fact that the baseline heart rate decreases with gestational age. At 15 weeks' gestation, the average baseline rate is about 160 beats per minute BPM (Fig. 2.6). It should be noted that although premature fetuses may have a slightly increased rate over that found at term, within the limits of fetal viability (from 28 weeks to term), the average baseline FHR difference is only about 10 BPM. One must, therefore, be careful not to attribute a baseline tachycardia to prematurity when it may well be a sign of fetal compromise. Surely any baseline FHR above 160 BPM must be explained on some basis other than fetal prematurity.

Schifferli further noted that if one administers atropine to a fetus, the resulting increase in heart rate is of greater magnitude as one approaches term, and the postatropine heart rate is usually in the range of 160. Because atropine is a parasympathetic blocking agent, it would appear that the gradual decrease in FHR that occurs with increasing gestational age can be explained as an increase in parasympathetic tone (see Fig. 2.6).

Renou et al.[18] have shown that if one administers atropine directly to a human fetus during labor, one observes three phenomena. First, there is a modest

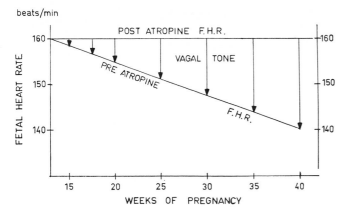

Figure 2.6. The preatropine FHR shows that the average FHR decreases as gestational age increases. The postatropine FHR shows that the FHR after atropine administration rises to approximately 160 BPM, regardless of gestational age, indicating increasing vagal tone as gestational age increases. (Reproduced with permission from Schifferli P, Caldeyro-Barcia R: Effects of atropine and beta adrenergic drugs on the heart rate of the human fetus. In: Boreus L (editor) Fetal Pharmacology. Raven Press, New York, 1973, p 264.)

increase in the baseline FHR, presumably due to blocking of the tonic parasympathetic effect described by Schifferli. Second, he noted a loss of the variability of the FHR, suggesting that a continuous balance between the parasympathetic slowing effect and the sympathetic accelerating effect may have been disturbed. Third, he noted that a majority of patients demonstrated the appearance of FHR accelerations during uterine contraction. This suggests that prior to release of parasympathetic tone by atropine, the accelerating forces were present but suppressed. Renou and coworkers then added a beta adrenergic blocking agent (propranolol) to these atropinized fetuses and noted abolition of the accelerations and a decrease in the baseline FHR (Fig. 2.7). It would thus appear that the acceleratory forces unmasked by atropine blockade were of beta sympathomimetic origin. With this information, it is then possible to think of the the baseline FHR to be a product of the modulated influences of the parasympathetic and sympathetic nervous systems. Furthermore, the baseline FHR variability probably represents an instantaneous product of these two forces that are constantly working in a push-pull relationship and the presence of good FHR variability probably requires the integrity of these two modulating forces.

Under normal circumstances, at term, the rate determined by the atrial pacemaker and modulated by parasympathetic and sympathetic factors usually ranges between 120 and 160 BPM. In a fetus with heart block, the rate is usually in the range of about 60 BPM which represents the intrinsic ventricular or nodal rate.

Parasympathetic impulses originate in the brain stem and are carried over the vagus nerve to the heart. Sympathetic impulses also originate in the brain stem and are carried via the cervical sympathetic fibers to the fetal heart. Sympathetic influences on the fetal heart may also come from humeral stimulation of the cardiac beta receptors via release of epinephrine from the adrenal medulla. In clinical practice, such conditions as fetal anencephaly, marked hydrocephaly, and anoxic brain damage may all be associated with an absence of FHR variability and a very "blunted" FHR response to stress. In the adult with cerebral death who is considered a brain stem preparation, the heart rate, when recorded instantaneously, has no variability. These clinical examples support the notion that heart rate variability is largely under central nervous system (CNS) influence. These examples further suggest that higher centers in the brain also play a role. While these mechanisms of CNS control of FHR cannot be completely understood with current available data, clinically it is important to recognize that the FHR pattern does depend on certain CNS controls and that factors influencing the CNS such as drugs, anatomic brain damage, or cerebral hypoxia may also affect the FHR pattern.

The Effect of Uterine Contractions on the FHR

FHR monitoring consists of a series of observed changes in instantaneous heart rate with and without uterine contractions. Uterine contractions subject the fetus to an intermittent hyperbaric state. They also cause intermittent decreases in intervillous space blood flow, they may influence cerebral blood flow under certain circumstances, and depending on the location of the umbilical cord, they may cause intermittent umbilical cord occlusion. These situations may all influence the FHR by giving rise to contraction-related or "periodic" FHR changes. The physiologic bases for these periodic changes are discussed below.

Early Deceleration. Pressure on the fetal head has been shown to cause slowing of the heart rate. It is believed that this is due to local changes in cerebral blood flow,[19] resulting in stimulation of the vagal centers. While the fetal head undoubtedly undergoes compression of a greater or lesser degree in all vaginal deliveries, the typical gradual onset, gradual offset FHR deceleration described as characteristic of fetal head compression is rather uncommon. Certainly during the second stage of labor, when pronounced variable FHR decelerations are commonly seen, it is not possible to say for sure that these decelerations may not be partially or entirely due to compression of the fetal head as it passes through the birth canal. Hon studied neonates, using different sized doughnut pessaries, and found that placing the circular pessary over the fetal vertex, when the center was 4 to 6 cm in diameter, usually resulted in point pressure from the edge of the pessary over the anterior fontanelle

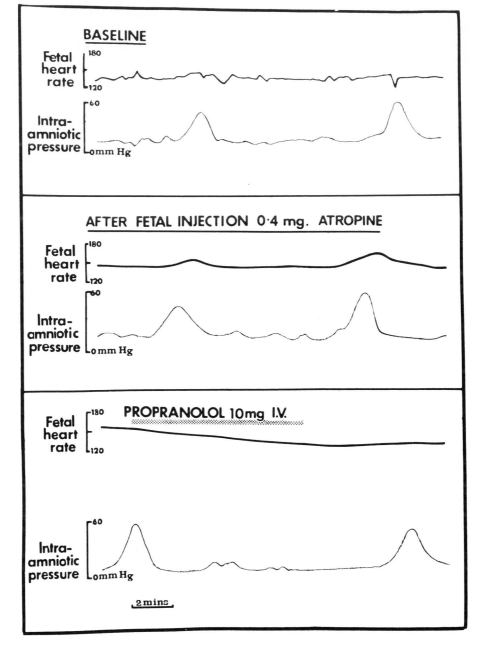

Figure 2.7. The **upper panel** shows a normal FHR-uterine contraction tracing. The **middle panel** shows that after atropine administration to a human fetus the FHR rises, the FHR variability decreases and accelerations appear with contractions. The **lower panel** shows that after maternal propranolol administration the FHR decreased and the FHR accelerations disappeared. (Reproduced with permission from Renou P, et al: Am J Obstet Gynecol 949:953, 1969.)

and that this was associated with an FHR deceleration.[20] This seemed to fit clinically with the fact that the FHR deceleration pattern that reflected the uterine pressure curve as a mirror image is usually found when patients are between 4 and 6 cm of cervical dilatation. The symmetrical deceleration pattern resulting from fetal head compression is called early deceleration and will be described in more detail in Chapter 6. Further studies have shown that early deceleration may be abolished or markedly altered by the administration of atropine,[21] thus confirming the theory that this is a vagal reflex. Although all authorities do not agree, there is good evidence that

this deceleration pattern does not carry asphyxic implications (see Fig. 2.8).[22]

Variable Deceleration. The umbilical cord is easily compressed as the fetus moves in relationship to the rest of the uterine contents. Uterine contractions are the usual cause of intermittent umbilical cord occlusion, especially if the cord is around the fetus' neck or fixed in another location, resulting in its impingement during contractions. The protective nature of amniotic fluid is suggested by the fact that it is quite unusual to see evidence of umbilical cord occlusion when there are adequate amounts of amniotic fluid present.

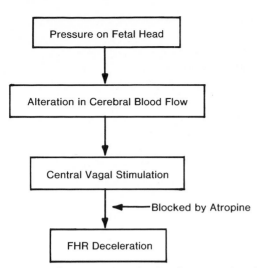

Figure 2.8. Mechanism of early deceleration (head compression).

Our understanding of the mechanism of FHR changes in association with umbilical cord occlusion began with the work of Barcroft.[23] He studied exteriorized fetal goats and showed that there was an almost instantaneous rapid and profound fall in the FHR when the umbilical cords of these fetal goats were occluded. Since the response was so rapid he reasoned that it may be due to a neurologic reflex. He then repeated the experiment after interrupting the vagus nerves of these fetal goats and found that there was a delay in the onset of the FHR deceleration. This then suggested that indeed the initial rapid deceleration associated with cord occlusion in the animal with intact vagi did appear to be caused by a vagal reflex, but the fact that a delayed deceleration was observed even with interruption of the vagal nerves suggested a second mechanism for the delayed portion of the deceleration (Fig. 2.9).

If one examines the hemodynamic effects of umbilical cord occlusion, some clues concerning the mechanism for the early component of the FHR deceleration emerge. When the umbilical arteries are suddenly occluded, there is a sudden increase in total fetal peripheral resistance resulting from a cutoff of the low resistance fetal placental circulation. This sudden increase in peripheral resistance in the fetal circulation causes sudden fetal hypertension.[24, 25] Stimulation of fetal baroreceptors occurs instantly, sending reflexes up the afferent limb of the neural reflex. The baroreceptor impulses affect the central vagal nuclei and result in a parasympathetic outflow that produces a sudden slowing effect on the fetal atrial pacemaker. Fetal EKG changes during cord occlusion show a gradual shortening of the P-R interval and with profound cord occlusion the P wave disappears, resulting in a ventricular rate of about 60 BPM.[26] With release of the cord occlusion, the atrial pacemaker returns with a gradual lengthening of the P-R interval back to predeceleration values. Hon et

al. have shown that atropine administered to the human will greatly alter, if not abolish, this profound deceleration associated with umbilical cord occlusion.[21] This tends to support Barcroft's hypothesis about the vagal reflex nature of at least one component of the FHR deceleration associated with umbilical cord compression.

This FHR deceleration problem may bear no consistent relationship to the contraction, presumably because the location of the umbilical cord may vary from one contraction to another. The pattern of cord occlusion has therefore been referred to as variable deceleration. Further description of the pattern will appear in a Chapter 6.

More recently, some work by Siasi et al.,[27] based on observations in neonates, suggested that the afferent limb of this reflex bradycardia, due to umbilical cord compression, may result from changes in arterial pO_2. Siasi noted that neonates on continuous heart rate monitors had heart rate changes similar to variable deceleration after apneic episodes. Since the deceleration seemed to follow the apnea, it appeared that one might explain this phenomenon by a fall in the neonatal arterial pO_2 (paO_2), causing a chemoreceptor initiation of the afferent limb to the vagal reflex. Next, he looked at neonates on respirators and noted that the delay in the onset of deceleration after

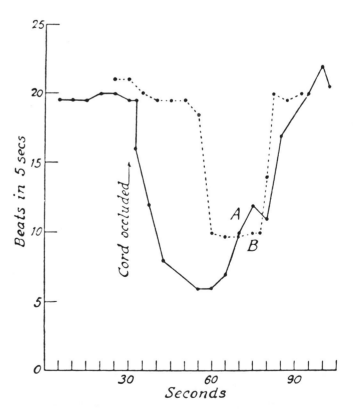

Figure 2.9. The **solid line** represents the FHR after total umbilical cord occlusion in the intact exteriorized fetal goat. The **broken line** represents the FHR after total umbilical cord occlusion in the vagectomized exteriorized fetal goat. (Reproduced with permission from Sir Barcroft J: Researches on Prenatal Life. Blackwell, Oxford, 1956.)

cessation of respiratory assistance was related to the level of the paO_2 before the cessation of breathing. The onset of the deceleration indeed appeared to occur at a critical paO_2. This observation would support Barcroft's theory and suggest that the delayed deceleration was possibly due to hypoxia.

Siasi expanded these studies by returning to exteriorized fetal sheep. By connecting the fetal umbilical circulation to a membrane oxygenator, he was able to show that the onset of variable deceleration after umbilical cord occlusion could be delayed by first raising the paO_2 of the fetus via the membrane oxygenator. Because these goats were anesthetized, however, one cannot say that the baroreceptor afferent limb does not play a role in variable deceleration. However, these experiments clearly point to the presence of a hypoxemic stimulus as at least having a role in variable deceleration. Certainly the paO_2 falls rapidly with total umbilical cord occlusion, but, fortunately, the paO_2 also rises rapidly with release of the occluded cord, accounting for the apparent clinical benignity of variable deceleration patterns in their mild to moderate forms.

Along with the sudden rise in pressure and the sudden fall in paO_2, there is an acute rise in the pCO_2 during umbilical cord occlusion.[22] This may result in varying degrees of respiratory acidosis and it is not clear what role this plays in the physiologic mechanism involved in the development of variable deceleration. It is not until cord occlusion is prolonged that a significant oxygen debt develops, resulting in fetal hypoxemia of a more than transient nature as evidenced by the development of metabolic acidosis reflecting significant anaerobic metabolism. When variable deceleration is severe, the late component of Barcroft comes into play. It is believed that this component is due to myocardial depression and represents significant hypoxemia and fetal metabolic acidosis (See discussion of Late Deceleration).

Recently it has been suggested that lesser degrees of umbilical cord compression may result in only occlusion of the low resistance venous return from the placenta. James et al.[28] and Lee et al.[29] have stated that this venous occlusion may result in a decreased return to the fetal heart, decreased fetal cardiac output, and a compensatory FHR acceleration (see Figs. 2.10 and 2.11). Clinical evidence to support this concept comes from the observation that periodic FHR acceleration associated with uterine contractions often leads to variable deceleration as labor progresses. Indeed, usually there are accelerations before and after variable decelerations.

In summary, the variable deceleration reflex appears to have both baroreceptor (hypertensive) and chemoreceptor (hypoxia) afferent limbs with the efferent limb being vagal. With severe hypoxemia and fetal metabolic acidosis, there may be a delayed deceleration component due to hypoxic fetal myo-

cardial depression. With mild forms of umbilical cord compression, only the vein may be occluded, resulting in FHR acceleration (Fig. 2.10).

Late Deceleration. Earlier in this chapter it was pointed out that intervillous space blood flow may be diminished by a number of causes. When intervillous space blood flow is decreased to a point that the fetus becomes hypoxemic, uteroplacental insufficiency (UPI) is said to exist. Clinical UPI may manifest itself in the chronic form with intrauterine growth retardation and/or antepartum fetal death, or in the acute form, the onset of fetal distress during labor, asphyxia neonatorum, and in the extreme, intrapartum fetal death.

Before electronic FHR monitoring, there was little known by practitioners of the art of obstetrics about characteristic FHR patterns that are associated with UPI. Among the first to describe FHR changes associated with UPI were Hon[30] and Caldeyro-Barcia et al.[31] They pointed to a slowing of the FHR that was related to uterine contractions with a gradual onset, usually after the peak of the contraction and a delayed return to baseline, usually after the end of the contraction. This was referred to as late deceleration by Hon and a Type II dip by Caldeyro-Barcia. This late deceleration pattern is believed to have both a reflex component and a hypoxic component some-

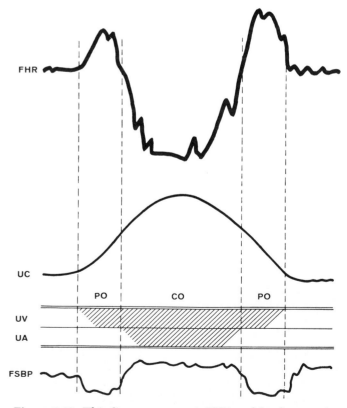

Figure 2.10. This figure represents FHR and fetal systemic blood pressure (FSBP) occurring during compression of the umbilical vein (UV) and the umbilical artery (UA). (Reproduced with permission from Lee C, et al: Obstet Gynecol 45:142, 1975.)

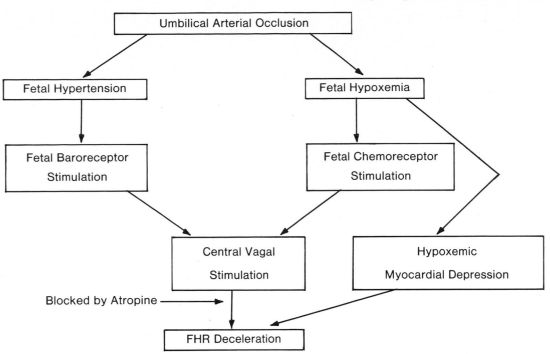

Figure 2.11. Mechanism of variable deceleration.

what similar to the mechanisms described in variable deceleration, but because of the nature and timing of the stimulus, the FHR pattern has different characteristics.

Recent work by Martin et al.[32] clarifies our understanding of the physiologic mechanisms involved in hypoxemic FHR changes. Martin devised a sheep model with an inflatable cuff that could be used to occlude the maternal sheep's common hypogastric artery and was able to measure blood pressure, heart rate, and blood gasses in this chronic fetal sheep preparation. Inflation of the implanted cuff around the common hypogastric artery resulted in cessation of blood flow through the uterine arteries. Intermittent compression could then simulate the changes in uterine blood flow that result from uterine contractions. The FHR changes noted with intermittent hypoxia in this model were a delayed FHR deceleration associated with transient fetal hypertension.

Treatment with phentolamine (alpha adrenergic blockade) resulted in a loss of the hypertensive response and a decrease in the late decelerations. Fetal atropine administration (parasympathetic blockade) resulted in periodic FHR accelerations in response to intermittent hypoxia. These accelerations were blocked by propranolol (beta adrenergic blockade). With combined blockade (alpha adrenergic, parasympathetic, and beta adrenergic) there was no change in FHR with intermittent hypoxia in the nonacidemic fetus. When the hypoxia was prolonged

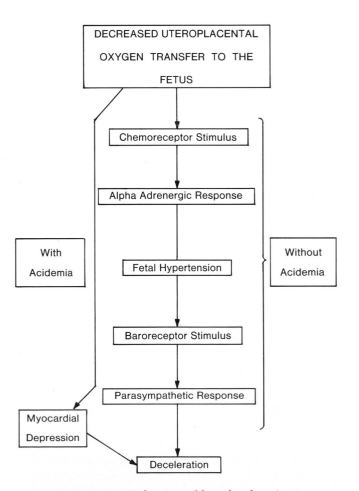

Figure 2.12. Mechanism of late deceleration.

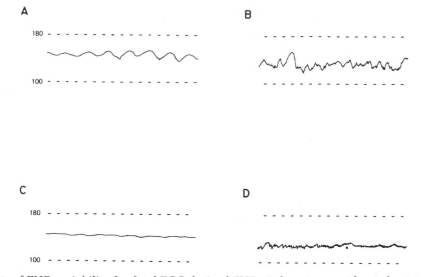

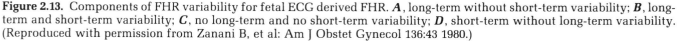

Figure 2.13. Components of FHR variability for fetal ECG derived FHR. *A*, long-term without short-term variability; *B*, long-term and short-term variability; *C*, no long-term and no short-term variability; *D*, short-term without long-term variability. (Reproduced with permission from Zanani B, et al: Am J Obstet Gynecol 136:43 1980.)

enough to produce acidemia, the initial hypertensive response was lost and the FHR deceleration occurred even in the presence of triple blockade, indicating that with hypoxia and acidemia the FHR deceleration is presumably due to myocardial depression.

With the knowledge of this work by Martin and coworkers, it would appear that late deceleration is primarily a reflex change with nonacidemic hypoxia but when hypoxia is severe enough to result in acidemia, the mechanism of late deceleration appears to be nonreflex myocardial depression. Clinically, the use of fetal scalp blood sampling may be of value to determine whether late deceleration is occurring in association with acidemia (Fig. 2.12).

Variability of the FHR

The interval between successive heart beats in the intact fetus is characterized by its nonuniformity. This beat-to-beat variability is known as short-term variability. Average interval differences are usually in the magnitude of 20 to 30 msec or 2 to 3 BPM when converted to rate. When variability is diminished, the usual beat-to-beat interval differences average about 1 BPM or less.

The long-term fluctuations in FHR have a cyclicity of 3 to 5 BPM, and the amplitude is usually from 5 to 20 BPM. A long-term variability of less than 5 BPM is considered to be reduced (see Fig. 2.13).

Parasympathetic influences tend to have a short time constant resulting in more rapid decelerations than the longer time constant sympathetic influences that cause slower and more sustained accelerations. Recent work by Druzen et al.[33] has shown that the parasympathetic system is more responsible for short-term variability while the sympathetic effect appears to be strongest on long-term variability. Recent studies by Modanlou et al.[34] suggested that short-term variability appeared to be reduced early in the course of neonatal hypoxemia with loss of long-term variability being a later change. Interestingly, with neonatal recovery, long-term variability reappeared first and the return of short-term variability was delayed.[34]

According to our understanding of the control of FHR, these changes in variability are probably related to changes in CNS status. Generally, the intact fetus has good short- and long-term variability. Drugs that depress the CNS or interfere with autonomic reflexes will tend to decrease FHR variability. There also appears to be a gradual increase in FHR variability as gestational age progresses. However, in the viable fetus who is more than 28 weeks' gestation, one should not attribute loss of variability to prematurity alone as most fetuses in the 28 to 32 weeks range will have reasonably good FHR variability but perhaps slightly less than the term fetus.

The major significance of FHR variability is that it may be affected by hypoxemia. Recent work by Druzen et al.[33] has shown that the earliest effect of fetal hypoxemia on FHR variability appears to be an *increase* in both long- and short-term variability. These investigators showed that mild hypoxia resulted in adrenergic discharge and fetal hypertension, causing stimulation of the fetal baroreceptors and a reflex vagal discharge. Thus a general increase in autonomic tone during early fetal hypoxia results in an increase in both short- and long-term variability. It has been known for a long time that prolonged and severe fetal hypoxia with acidemia will reduce FHR variability, presumably due to the CNS effects of hypoxia and acidosis.

A very curious pattern known as a sinusoidal FHR pattern is exceedingly rare. It is characterized by a very uniform "sinusoidal" long-term variability pattern and an absence of short-term variability. It has been seen with chronic fetal anemia associated with erythroblastosis.[35] It has also been reported with acute intrapartem fetal asphyxia,[36] after alphaprodine administration,[37] and in one case, of fetal-maternal hemorrhage.[38] The physiologic basis for this pattern is not clear but a recent report by Elliott et al.[39] showed that the pattern observed in the fetus with erythroblastosis was also seen in the neonate and did not respond to adequate neonatal oxygenation but disappeared after neonatal blood transfusion. They suggested that tissue hypoxia may have been relieved by raising the hemoglobin concentration.

In summary, the FHR is believed to be under the direct control of the fetal autonomic nervous system. We are beginning to understand the reflex mechanisms involved with hypoxic changes in FHR patterns and variability. With early hypoxia, whether caused by cord compression or uteroplacental insufficiency, the FHR patterns are primarily of neural reflex origin, whereas with severe hypoxia and fetal acidosis, the periodic FHR changes are probably primarily due to myocardial depression. The correlation between physiologic studies and clinical observations remains incomplete but clearly as we learn more about physiologic mechanisms involved in the control of the FHR, the clinical observations become more and more meaningful.

REFERENCES

1. Ramsey EM, Martin CB Jr, Donner MW: Fetal and maternal placental circulation. Am J Obstet Gynecol 98:419, 1967
2. Poseiro JJ, Mendez-Bauer C, Pose SV, et al: Effect of Uterine Contractions on Maternal Blood Flow Through the Placenta. Pan American World Health Organization, Scientific Publications no 185, Washington, D.C., 1969, p 161–171
3. Greiss FC Jr: Concepts of uterine blood flow. In: Wynn RM (editor) Obstet Gynecol Annual, New York, Appleton-Century-Crofts, 1973, vol. 2, p 55–83
4. Wallenburg HS, Stolte LAM, Janassens J: The pathogenesis of placental infarction I.; a morphologic study in the human placenta. Am J Obstet Gynecol 116:835, 1973
5. Wallenburg HS, Hutchinson DL, Schuler HM, et al: The pathogenesis of placental infarction II: an experimental study in the rhesus monkey placenta. Am J Obstet Gynecol 116:841, 1973
6. Greiss F, Marston E: The uterine vascular bed: effect of estrogens during ovine pregnancy. Am J Obstet Gynecol 93:720, 1965
7. Howard BK, Goodson JM, Mengert WF: Supine hypotensive syndrome in late pregnancy. Obstet Gynecol 1:371, 1953
8. Kerr NG: The mechanical effects of the gravid uterus in late pregnancy. J Obstet Gynecol Br Commonw 72:513, 1965
9. Emmanouilides G, Hobel C, Yashiro K, et al: Fetal response to maternal exercise in the sheep. Am J Obstet Gynecol 112:130, 1972
10. Lee MH, Hill JD, Ochsner AJ, et al: Maternal and placental myometrial blood flow of the rhesus monkey during uterine contractions. Am J Obstet Gynecol 110:68, 1971
11. Greiss FC Jr: Pressure flow relationship in the gravid uterine vascular bed. Am J Obstet Gynecol 96:41, 1966
12. Greiss FC Jr, Crandell DL: Therapy for hypotension induced by spinal anesthesia during pregnancy. JAMA 191:793, 1965
13. Dawes GS: Foetal and neonatal physiology. In: The Foetal Circulation. Year Book Medical Publishers, Chicago, 1968, p 91–105
14. Dawes GS: Foetal and neonatal physiology. In: Foetal Blood Gas Tensions and pH. Year Book Medical Publishers, Chicago, 1968, p 106–116
15. Longo LD: Placental transfer mechanisms. An overview. In: Wynn RM (editor) Obstetrics Gynecology Annual 1972. Appleton-Century-Crofts, New York, 1973
16. Khazin AF, Hon EH, Hehre FW: Effects of maternal hyperoxia on the foetus. Am J Obstet Gynecol 109:628, 1971
17. Schifferli P, Caldeyro-Barcia R: Effects of atropine and beta adrenergic drugs on the heart rate of the human fetus. In: Boreus L (editor) Fetal Pharmacology. Raven Press, New York, 1973, p 259–279
18. Renou P, Warwick N, Wood C: Autonomic control of fetal heart rate. Am J Obstet Gynecol 105:949, 1969
19. Paul WM, Quilligan EJ, MacLachlan T: Cardiovascular Phenomenon associated with fetal head compression. Am J Obstet Gynecol 90:824, 1964
20. Hon EH: Personal communication
21. Hon EH, Bradfield AH, Hess OW: The electronic evaluation of the fetal heart rate V. The vagal factor in fetal bradycardia. Am J Obstet Gynecol 82:291, 1961
22. Kubli FW, Hon EH: Observations on heart rate and pH in the human fetus during labor. Am J Obstet Gynecol 104:1190, 1969
23. Barcroft J: Researches on Prenatal Life. Blackwell Scientific Publications, Oxford, 1946
24. Lee ST, Hon EH: Fetal hemodynamic response to umbilical cord compression. Obstet Gynecol 22:554, 1963
25. Towell ME, Salvador HS: Compression of the umbilical cord. In: Crasignoni P, Pardi G (editors) An Experimental Model in the Fetal Goat, Fetal Evaluation During Pregnancy and Labor. Academic Press, New York, 1971, p 143–156
26. Yeh MN, Morishima HO, Niemann WE, et al: Myocardial conduction defects in association with compression of the umbilical cord. Experimental observations on fetal baboons. Am J Obstet Gynecol 121:951, 1975
27. Siassi B, et al: Effect of Arterial pO2 in the cardiovascular response to umbilical cord compression. Presented at the 20th Annual Meeting of the Society for Gynecological Investigation, Atlanta, Georgia, March 28–30, 1973
28. James LS, Yeh MN, Morishima HO, et al: Umbilical vein occlusion and transient acceleration of the fetal heart rate. Experimental observations in subhuman primates. Am J Obstet Gynecol 126:276, 1976
29. Lee CV, Di Loreto PC, O'Lane JM: A study of fetal heart rate acceleration patterns. Obstet Gynecol 45:142, 1975
30. Hon EH: Observations on "pathologic" fetal bradycardia. Am J Obstet Gynecol 77:1084, 1959
31. Caldeyro-Barcia R, Casacuberta C, Bustos R, et al: Correlation of intrapartum changes in fetal heart rate with fetal blood oxygen and acid base state. In: Adamsons K (editor) Diagnosis and Treatment of Fetal Disorders. New York, Springer-Verlag, 1968, p 205–225
32. Martin CB, De Haan J, Wilot BVD, et al: Mechanisms of late deceleration in the fetal heart rate. A study with autonomic blocking agents in fetal lambs. Eur J Obstet Gynecol Reprod Biol 9:361, 1979
33. Druzen M, Ikenoye T, Murata Y, et al: A possible mechanism for the increase in FHR variability following hypoxemia. Presented at the 26th Annual meeting of Society for Gynecological Investigation, San Diego, California, March 23, 1979
34. Modanlou H, Freeman RK, Braly P: A simple method of fetal and neonatal heart rate beat-to-beat variability quantitation (VQ) Am J Obstet Gynecol 127:861, 1977
35. Manseau P, Vaquier J, Chavinie J, et al: Le rythme cardiaque foetal sinusoidal aspect evocateur de souffrance foetale au cours de la grossesse. J Gynecol Obstet Biol Reprod 1:343, 1972

36. Gal D, Jacobson L, Ser H, et al: Sinusoidal pattern: an alarming sign of fetal distress. Am J Obstet Gynecol 132:903, 1978
37. Gray J, Cudmore D, Luther E, et al: Sinusoidal fetal heart rate pattern associated with alphaprodine administration. Obstet Gynecol 52:678, 1978
38. Modanlou H, Freeman RK, Ortiz O, et al: Sinusoidal fetal heart rate pattern and severe fetal anemia. Obstet Gynecol 49:537, 1977
39. Elliott JP, Modanlou HD, O'Keeffe DF, et al: The significance of fetal and neonatal sinusoidal heart rate pattern: further clinical observations in Rh incompatibility. Am J Obstet Gynecol (in press)

CHAPTER 3

Effects of Hypoxia and Asphyxia on the Fetus and Newborn

Since the intent of fetal monitoring is to identify the fetus suffering from hypoxia, one must first understand the effects of hypoxia and asphyxia (anoxia with concomitant biochemical changes) on the fetus and on its subsequent adaptation to extrauterine life. There is little argument that if profound hypoxia occurs for a sufficient length of time, death will result.

It has long been recognized that when fetal hypoxia occurs at sublethal levels, permanent damage to the fetus may result. However, the frequency with which this occurs in the intrapartum period and the ability of the clinician using fetal monitoring to prevent it is a subject of intense debate. References to perinatal brain damage can be found earlier, but the English orthopaedic surgeon, William John Little,[1] is credited with the first specific hypothesis suggesting adverse perinatal events were the main etiologic factors in infantile spastic palsies. He reviewed the histories of more than 200 cases of spasticity of congenital origin and presented his paper entitled *On the influence of abnormal parturition, difficult labours, premature birth and asphyxia neonatorum, on the mental and physical condition of the child, especially in relation to deformities* to the Obstetrical Society of London. He concluded that these 200 cases had one thing in common, i.e., some abnormal characteristic of parturition. The form of cerebral palsy (CP) described has often been called "Little's disease." Subsequently, other neurologic problems including mental retardation, epilepsy, and behavioral and learning disorders have been attributed to various intrapartum problems.

Animal data to corroborate the concept that perinatal asphyxia may cause profound sublethal neurologic damage can be found in the classic papers of William F. Windle. Windle had originally described the effect of asphyxia in guinea pigs.[2] Between 1954 and 1960, Windle[3] performed experimental asphyxiation of rhesus monkeys and evaluated the immediate, long-term, and neuropathologic effects. The monkeys were asphyxiated in one of two ways, both involving hysterotomy. Either the placenta and membranes were delivered with the fetus within the intact amniotic sac, or the fetal head was covered by a fluid-filled sac and the umbilical cord was completely occluded. The fetus was left anoxic for 5 to 20 min. Monkeys allowed to breathe in 6 min or less showed no neurologic deficits and no pathologic brain changes. Asphyxiation for more than 7 min produced at least transient motor and behavioral changes and relatively consistent brain pathology. There was necrosis of brain stem cells in the inferior colliculi and ventrolateral thalamic nuclei with secondary glial proliferative scarring. The most profound changes were found in monkeys left anoxic for 12 to 17 min. Resuscitation was invariably necessary. More severe brain stem lesions were created. Initially, the monkeys were hyporeactive and hypotonic. After 1 week, seizures developed in several. Ataxia and athetosis were often seen. As the monkeys matured, followed-up to 8 years, most deficits gradually improved leaving mainly hypoactivity and clumsiness. While this model indeed supported the hypothesis that perinatal asphyxia is associated with permanent neurologic damage, the pattern of damage did not seem to correspond with that seen in the human, i.e., mental retardation and spasticity. This was recognized by Ronald Myers who suggested that total asphyxia may not be the usual case in humans, and that prolonged partial asphyxia is more likely. Myers[4] was able to produce partial asphyxia in the rhesus monkey in a number of ways including uterine hyperstimulation with oxytocin, compression of the maternal abdominal aorta, maternal infusion of catecholamines, and allowing the pregnant monkey to inspire reduced oxygen concentrations. These were controlled by maintaining fetal PO_2 at 5 to 9 mm Hg. Myers et al.[5] later demonstrated that late deceleration of the fetal heart rate (FHR) was caused by this hypoxia. Fetuses were maintained in such partially asphyxic states for at least 1 hr, delivered, and resuscitated. The immediate effect on the newborn was flaccidity, which evolved after several hours into generalized hypertonus and decerebrate posturing at which time the newborns began to have periodic generalized seizures. Many fetuses developed ileus, cardiogenic shock, and died. A minority of fetuses survived. Extensive histopathologic examination of the brain led him to conclude that such prolonged partial hypoxia led to a vicious cycle of brain swelling causing decreased cerebral blood flow that further aggravated the brain swelling. Such diminished blood flow in extreme degrees led to total hemispheral cortical necrosis. In lesser degrees, cortical damage was seen in the middle third of the paracentral cerebral cortex and in the basal ganglia. Such lesions correspond closely with the intellectual deficits and spastic motor defects seen in asphyxiated humans and, therefore, this seems to be a much more reasonable model than that of Windle's total asphyxia.

ETIOLOGIC FACTORS IN CP

To establish what proportion anoxia contributes to damage and to distinguish between obstetric causes such as trauma and infection, many authors have reviewed obstetric histories of children with congenital neurologic damage. Early in his career, Sigmund Freud became interested in the etiology of cerebral palsy. In his 1893 monograph, *Die Infantile Cerebrallahmung*[6] he concluded that one-third of the cases were the result of traumatic birth, one-sixth consequent to prematurity, one-sixth of pre- or postnatal cause, and one-third unknown. Lilienfeld and Pasamanick[7] reviewed birth certificates of 561 congenitally spastic children and found a very high incidence of abruptio and placenta praevia. Eastman and DeLeon[8] reported on an analysis of 96 obstetrical records of infants who developed CP. Only 18 of these births were uncomplicated. Thirty-four babies were premature. Of the infants 30% had apnea of more than 30 sec at birth. There was a 3-fold increase in breech delivery among affected infants compared to controls; a doubling of third trimester hemorrhage, a 10-fold increase in shoulder dystocia, four times more

fetal distress by auscultation, and a 4-fold increase in anesthetic complications. Eastman's findings in a subsequent, more extensive review[9] of 753 cases are summarized in Table 3.1.

Finally, Steer and Bonney[10] in 1968 reviewed 317 patients with cerebral palsy and concluded 5% were a result of kernicterus, 8% were caused by congenital defects and neurologic infections, and 87% were cases "with possible obstetric causes".

FORMS OF CONGENITAL NEUROLOGIC DAMAGE

Hypoxia has been implicated in the etiology of several forms of neurologic damage.

CP

CP is probably the most specific problem secondary to perinatal hypoxic insults. CP will develop in about 5 infants per 1000 births with a prevalence of 1 to 2 per 1000 school-age children, which amounts to about 350,000 children in the United States today.[8, 11] CP is defined as "a persistent but not changing disorder of movement and posture, appearing in the early years of life and due to a non-progressive disorder of the brain."[9] It is estimated that about 50% of children with CP have mild intellectual retardation (IQ less than 70) and about one-fourth are severely affected (IQ less than 50).[12] CP is also described according to the distribution of extremities involved and the type of movement disorder. The classification according to distribution includes paraplegia, tetraplegia, and hemiplegia. Diplegia, a commonly used term, implies bilateral lower extremity involvement. Motor symptom classification describes the dominant movement disorder and includes spasticity, dyskinesia (athetosis), and ataxia. Spastic diplegia was the predominant form in prematurity but has declined steadily with improved neonatal care.[13] Ataxias are more likely in kernicterus. Perinatal infections such as cytomegalovirus and toxoplasmosis also can lead to spastic diplegias. Other nonperipartum conditions may lead to spastic diplegias including cretinism, mercury poisoning, and carbon monoxide poisoning.

Mental Retardation

Estimates of severe mental retardation are surprisingly uniform from country to country at about 3.5 per 1000 population.[14] Mild retardation is somewhat more variable, occurring in 23 to 31 per 1000, probably because of testing inaccuracy and the effect of environment in this group.[14] Mental retardation is a much less specific result of perinatal asphyxia than is CP. Perinatal causes probably are only responsible for about 10% of mental retardation alone.[15, 16] Chromosome abnormalities and various hereditary disorders account for 65%, infection about 5%, prenatal causes

Table 3.1.
Obstetric Background of 753 Cases of CP[9]

	CP (%)	Control (%)
Postnatally Acquired	8.5	
Premature (Less than 2500 g)	29.0	8.0
Twins	7.0	1.0
(Rate Twin A = Rate Twin B)		
Mid/High Forceps	8.0	5.0
Breech	9.0	3.5
Resuscitated at Birth	27.0	3.0
Hypoxia	11.0	4.0
Cord Prolapse	3.0	0.3
Abruptio Placenta	4.0	1.3
Toxemia	5.0	2.0
Prolonged Labor	2.4	1.6
Hemolytic Disease	6.0	0.3
Congenital Anomalies	5.0	1.3

such as toxins and maternal disease about 10%, and the rest are unknown.[17] Many studies, including the Collaborative Perinatal Project,[18] have looked prospectively at children determined to be asphyxic at birth, by several criteria including Apgar score, neonatal apnea, shock, or acidosis. The vast majority (generally greater than 90%) has normal IQ's and the mean IQ is usually only 5 to 10 points below average.[18]

Epilepsy

Although the potential for hypoxia to cause seizures in both newborns and adults is clear, there is not a strong relationship between perinatal events and epilepsy. This is true only if one looks at epilepsy in the absence of CP and mental retardation. The Collaborative Perinatal Project did not demonstrate an increase in epilepsy in low birth weight infants or in depressed infants.[19] However, epilepsy is more common in individuals with CP and mental retardation.

BEHAVIORAL AND LEARNING DISORDERS

Because most depressed neonates do not have demonstrable intellectual impairment, many have questioned whether indeed such infants do eventually reach their full intellectual potentials. The data would suggest the opposite, however, since many children born hypoxic who demonstrated intellectual impairment in infancy and preschool periods will be normal later on. Whether or not this actually implies dissipation of the effects of hypoxia with catch-up intellectual growth, or limitations of testing is open to question. Some of Windle's severely asphyxiated monkeys had structural brain defects despite apparent normal behavior. The subtleties of behavioral difficulties and learning disorders make the problem very difficult to analyze and data are not presently available.

OTHER CAUSES OF NEUROLOGIC DAMAGE

As has already been pointed out, hypoxia is certainly not the only cause of prenatal and perinatal neurologic damage. Other causes may be entirely separate or additive; or indeed as pointed out by Freud,[6] in babies apparently distressed and hypoxic at birth, the cause may have been precedent damage or anomaly unrelated to hypoxia.

Prematurity

The association of prematurity and perinatal neurologic insults and their sequelae have long been recognized. In Shakespeare's King Richard III, Richard, then Duke of Gloucester proclaimed:

"I that am curtail'd of this fair proportion
Cheated of feature by this dissembling nature
Deform'd, unfinish'd *sent before my time*
Into this breathing world, scarce half made up
And that so lamely and unfashionableThat dogs bark at me as I halt by them."

Little pointed this passage out in presenting his paper and documented a high association between spastic rigidity and prematurity.

Intrauterine Growth Retardation (IUGR)

IUGR may be caused by perinatal infections, teratogens, congenital anomalies, inadequate nutrition, or uteroplacental insufficiency. It is associated with a high incidence of birth asphyxia. Fitzhardinge and Steven[20] followed 96 full-term growth retarded infants (excluding anomalies and congenital infections) up to 8 years of age. CP only occurred in 1% of the infants and epilepsy occurred in 6%. However, "minimal cerebral dysfunction (learning difficulties, hyperactivity and poor coordination) were found in 25%". Of the infants 30% had speech problems and 40% had poor school performance. Because this group of fetuses/newborns does have a high incidence of perinatal asphyxia, it is difficult to know whether the antepartum or intrapartum insult or some combination is responsible for such neurologic damage.

Traumatic Birth

The relatively high incidences of mid and high forceps and of breech deliveries in retrospective studies[8, 9] of neurologically damaged babies suggest that birth trauma may have contributed to this damage. Further evidence in breech births is provided by reduced incidences of these problems with elective cesarean section. In this era of liberal cesarean section rates, such data regarding the contribution of trauma to neurological damage may now be considerably less significant.

Prolonged Labor

Friedman et al.,[21-23] in his series of studies concerning the effects of prolonged labor on adverse developmental outcome, has demonstrated that this may indeed also have contributed to sublethal CNS damage. However, he suggests this may not be as important as the means of delivery (e.g., mid forceps). Again, changing practices and liberalization of cesarean section will hopefully lessen this factor's impact.

Anesthesia and Analgesia

Drugs and anesthesia may contribute to such damage in one of two ways. Regional anesthesias may cause maternal hypotension resulting in fetal hypoxia from decreased uterine perfusion. Alternatively, depressants, whether anesthetic agents or narcotics, may cause neonatal apnea. In a setting where good neonatal resuscitation is available, however, this should contribute little to hypoxic damage.

Genetic Factors

Congenital anomalies are indeed associated with high incidences of CP, mental retardation, epilepsy, and developmental disabilities. Generally series evaluating mental retardation report higher incidences of associated congenital defects than do series on CP. In a series of 1410 autopsies from three hospitals for the mentally retarded Malamud[24] reports a 61% incidence of anomalies. Down's syndrome was the most frequent single cause. However, in most cases, associated somatic anomalies are apparent and central nervous system (CNS) anomalies are inferred and can be excluded from analysis of obstetric factors.

Congenital Infections

Indeed congenital infections can be associated with CNS damage with or without microcephaly or hydrocephaly. Rubella, cytomegalic virus, syphillis, toxoplasmosis, among others, are well-known causes. These, similar to anomalies, are more likely to contribute to mental retardation than CP, and to somatic growth retardation and probably account for about 10% of mentally retarded children in developed countries.[14]

Antenatal Insults

Finally the most controversial, and difficult to analyze, contributing factor to neurologic damage is the role that antenatal factors play. Certainly, as has been pointed out, when IUGR is associated, antenatal insult probably contributes. In addition, when one observes the high incidence of antepartum bleeding and toxemia in the histories of affected children, the question of the contribution of prepartum damage becomes apparent. These babies will often appear depressed at birth and have intrapartum fetal distress, but the damage may have occurred before the onset of labor.

Therefore, factors other than intrapartum hypoxia do seem very important in the pathogenesis of congenitally acquired neurologic damage. In assessing what contribution one may make by intrapartum assessment techniques, consideration must be given to such insults which may have occurred before the onset of labor.

OTHER FORMS OF HYPOXIC/ ASPHYXIC DAMAGE

Neurologic damage is not the only sublethal result of perinatal hypoxia. It is well known that the lungs, kidney, and gastrointestinal tract are also sensitive to ischemia and hypoxia and that newborn sequelae may result.

Respiratory Distress Syndrome

In the premature baby, the respiratory distress syndrome is the leading cause of neonatal death and serious morbidity. This is generally thought to be due to inadequate pulmonary surfactant as the primary etiologic factor. Pulmonary lecithin (the major component of surfactant) synthesis is significantly diminished by hypoxia and acidosis.[25] Even in babies with mature lecithin:sphingomyelin ratios, depressed and acidotic babies are more likely to have respiratory distress syndrome (RDS).[26] Hobel et al.[27] and Martin et al.[28] have pointed out that in premature newborns, acidotic babies and those with abnormal heart rate patterns suggesting hypoxia, had higher incidences of RDS and higher mortalities from RDS. Furthermore, Martin found ominous FHR patterns to be even more predictive of RDS than Apgar scores.

Renal Damage

The association between renal damage and asphyxiated newborns has been known since 1920. Anuria and renal failure similar to that in the adult may be seen. Animal data suggest such ischemic damage may be the result of decreased renal blood flow that occurs in the fetuses during the redistribution of blood flow seen during hypoxia.[29] Premature fetuses seem more susceptible to renal damage from ischemia.

Gastrointestinal Damage

Similarly, when the blood flow is redistributed during periods of fetal hypoxia, blood flow to the fetal gastrointestinal tract is particularly diminished. Alward et al.[30] have shown in animal fetuses that asphyxia could lead to decreased blood flow to the gastrointestinal tract resulting in dilation of segments of the large and small bowel and scattered mucosal necrosis. Towbin and Turner,[31] in looking at autopsies with other hypoxic damage, found intestinal injuries due to venous stasis and infarction with lesions ranging from focal mucosal necrosis to massive gross intestinal infarction. Necrotizing enterocolitis (NEC), seen most frequently in prematures, may at least in part be the result of such damage. Preliminary data suggests ominous FHR patterns are often seen in fetuses destined to develop NEC.[32]

EVIDENCE THAT ABNORMAL FHR PATTERNS CORRELATE WITH HYPOXIA/ASPHYXIA

Knowing that hypoxia and asphyxia in addition to other intrapartum events correlate with sublethal damage, one must demonstrate that abnormal FHR patterns correlate with hypoxia and acidosis if they are to be used to detect such problems. Furthermore, if one uses Apgar scores as a measurement of neonatal depression, one must demonstrate that such depression is also correlated with hypoxia and acidosis. The latter was well demonstrated by Modanlou et al.[33] As one can see in Figures 3.1 A to C, biochemical changes, especially pH and base deficit, are significantly correlated with depressed newborns.

While it is not within the realm of this Chapter to discuss the mechanisms responsible for the genesis of FHR patterns, it should be established that these changes are caused by fetal hypoxemia and acidemia and are correlated with fetal distress and neonatal depression. Barcroft[34] first demonstrated typical variable type deceleration caused by umbilical cord occlusion in the fetal goat (Fig. 3.2). Subsequently, Lee and Hon[35] were able to reproduce this in the human fetus. Myers et al.[5] were able to reproduce late decelerations in the rhesus monkey by causing uterine hypotension and demonstrated clearly that such decelerations were only seen with "marked impairment of fetal oxygenation".

Kubli et al.[36] correlated fetal scalp pH in the human with various FHR patterns as shown in Figure 3.3 demonstrating that the more severe the pattern, the more likely the fetus is to be acidemic. Paul et al.[37] further refined this work. Looking at late decelerations only, they found FHR variability to correlate even better than the severity of the late deceleration with both acidosis and depressed Apgar scores. Since then, many other studies have demonstrated a correlation with ominous FHR patterns and acidosis.

In terms of looking at outcome there are many studies correlating various monitor patterns with Apgar scores, showing generally that the more ominous the tracing, the more likely one is to have a depressed baby. Since there are really no studies where fetal monitor patterns are blinded and not acted upon, intervention may indeed have decreased the degree of correlation, because in most patterns a period of time is necessary from the development of intermittent hypoxia to the development of the metabolic acidosis. Bisonette[38] produced one of the most detailed analyses of FHR patterns and Apgar scores, as shown in Figure 3.4. However, this correlation is far from 100%. Schifrin and Dame[39] attempted to predict Apgar scores from FHR patterns obtained within 30 min of delivery without regard to clinical circumstances during labor. As can be seen in Figure 3.5, when a normal baby was predicted, they were nearly always right; when a depressed baby was predicted they were more often wrong; but when a baby was born depressed, it was nearly always predicted. Since there are indeed other causes of neonatal depression besides intrapartum hypoxia/asphyxia (Table 3.2) one would not expect to find 100% correlation between a predicted healthy baby and a normal Apgar score. The high degree of correlation does point out the sensitivity of FHR monitoring.

The only follow-up study available that relates EFM in any degree to long-term sequelae is that of Painter et al.[40] They followed 50 high risk infants who were monitored electronically in labor at frequent intervals up to 1 year of age. Twelve infants had normal FHR patterns, 16 moderate to severe variable decelerations, and 22 with severe variable or late decelerations. Twelve of the 19 infants in the moderate to severe variable group had abnormal exams at some point despite normal Apgar scores, and 1 infant was abnormal at 12 months of age with delay in gross and fine motor development. In the severe group, 6 of the 22 children had some neurologic abnormality at 1 year. All the patients with normal FHR patterns were normal at 1 year. Furthermore, FHR patterns were more predictive of abnormal examinations than were Apgar scores.

It can be concluded, therefore, that FHR patterns suggesting fetal hypoxia and/or acidosis do correlate with depression at birth and at least with the minimal data available also have correlation with adverse outcome in long-term (1 year) follow-up. One must be careful to point out that, first, not all abnormal patterns correlate with poor outcome, and what is not known is to what extent intervention ameliorates or prevents adverse outcome. Finally, it is obvious that EFM correlates best and is most valuable when the pattern is reassuring.

DIFFICULTY AND LIMITATIONS WITH EARLY ASSESSMENT

What makes all these data particularly hard to analyze is the problems inherent with generally available immediate newborn assessment techniques. The Apgar score, as originally developed, was intended to assess the newborn for effects of drugs and anesthesia and was limited to term babies. While it has proven to be a valuable and easily applicable index; it is far from the ultimate in newborn evaluation. Suggestions such as those of Painter that ominous electronic fetal monitoring (EFM) patterns correlate better with adverse outcome than do Apgar scores, leads one to question whether correlating monitor patterns with Apgar scores leads to a wrong impression, and that indeed normal Apgar score might be questioned in light of an abnormal monitor pattern.

Another problem in correlating such monitoring with newborn sequelae is the general tendency for abnormal exams early in life to normalize later. This may be real or a problem related to the limitations of neurologic testing.

And finally, data which were obtained in previous years may become relatively inapplicable as improvement in treatment techniques develop. This is particularly true in prematures where at one time follow-up in extremely small prematures revealed 60% were abnormal, the figure is now reversed and over 80% are normal.[41]

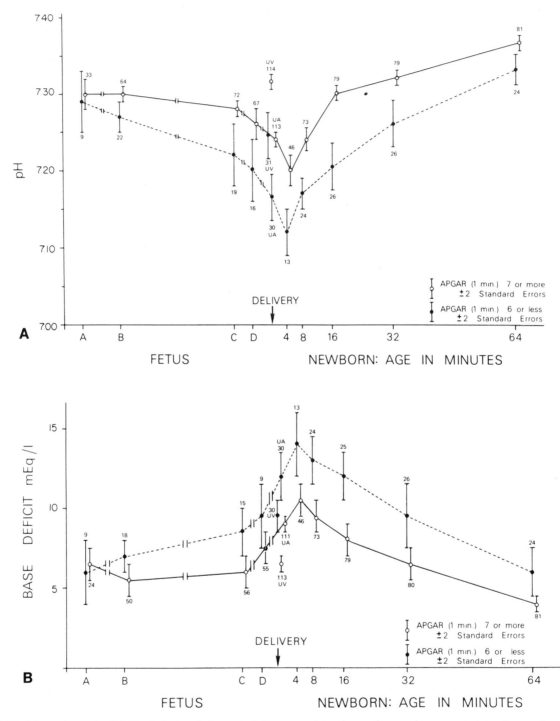

Figure 3.1A. Normal pH (***solid line***) during labor, at delivery and in the early newborn period is shown. In addition, the ***dotted line*** represents pH from fetuses and newborns delivered with 1 min Apgar of 6 or less. Point ***A*** is early labor, ***B*** is at 5 cm dilation, ***C*** is at complete dilation and D is just prior to delivery. (Reproduced with permission from Reference 33.)
Figure 3.1B. This is the normal course of base deficit in labor (***dark line***). As in Figure 1A, the ***dotted line*** represents base deficit from depressed babies. (Reproduced with permission from Reference 33.)

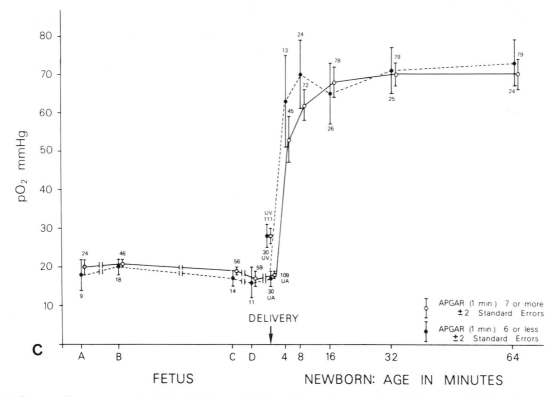

Figure 3.1C. The two **lines** represent pO₂'s in labor and after delivery in normal and depressed babies. As opposed to pH and base deficit, intrapartum pO₂ does not differ significantly in these two groups. However, in depressed babies there is a wider range in pO₂ values. (Reproduced with permission from Reference 33.)

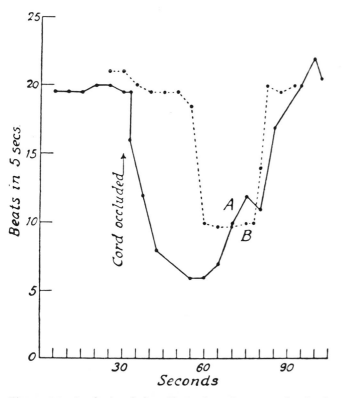

Figure 3.2. Analysis of the effect of asphyxia in the fetal goat produced by ligature at the umbilical cord. **Dark line** vagus nerves intact; **broken line** vagus nerves cut. (Reproduced with permission from Reference 34.)

Group	FHR pattern	Mean ± S.D.	Averaged samples* (No.)
I	Variable deceleration (CC)—mild	7.29 ± 0.046	42
	No deceleration	7.30 ± 0.042	71
	Early deceleration (HC)	7.30 ± 0.041	16
II	Variable deceleration (CC)—moderate	7.26 ± 0.044	35
III	Late deceleration (UPI)—mild	7.22 ± 0.060	27
	Late deceleration (UPI)—moderate	7.21 ± 0.054	7
IV	Variable deceleration (CC)—severe	7.15 ± 0.069	10
	Late deceleration (UPI)—severe	7.12 ± 0.066	10

*218 averaged pH samples from 618 single pH samples.

Figure 3.3. Correlation of FHR patterns and pH values. (Reproduced with permission from Reference 36.)

FHR pattern	Number	Per cent	Mean Apgar	Apgar 4–6 (moderate depression)		Apgar 0–3 (marked depression)	
				Number	Per cent	Number	Per cent
Normal	322	45·0	8·2	16	5·0	3	0·9
Uncomplicated baseline tachycardia	24	3·4	7·9	1	4·2	1	4·2
Uncomplicated baseline bradycardia	38	5·3	8·1	3	7·9	0	0
Uncomplicated loss of beat-to-beat variation	40	5·6	7·2	7	17·5	2	5·0
Complicated loss of beat-to-beat variation	11	1·5	6·7	2	18·2	2	18·2
Acceleration	52	7·3	8·4	1	1·9	0	0
Early deceleration	122	17·1	8·0	6	4·9	1	0·8
Late deceleration	20	2·8	5·4	7	35·0	5	25·0
Variable deceleration with normal baseline	71	9·9	7·7	9	12·7	2	2·8
Variable deceleration with abnormal baseline	14	2·0	5·9	0	0	7	50·0

Figure 3.4. Relationship between FHR pattern and 1 min Apgar score. (Reproduced with permission from Reference 38.)

Normal Apgar Predicted
  1 Min - 93% Correct
  5 Min - 99% Correct

Low Apgar Predicted
  1 Min - 43% Correct
  5 Min - 20% Correct

Low Apgar Baby Delivered
  1 Min - 54% Predicted
  5 Min - 83% Predicted*

Figure 3.5. Reliability of prediction of Apgar score from FHR tracings. *, 100% when corrected for congenital anomalies. (Reproduced with permission from Reference 39.)

Table 3.2.
Causes of Neonatal Depression Other than Intrapartum Hypoxia/Acidosis

Upper Airway Obstruction
Congenital Infection
Prematurity
Drugs/Anesthesia
Congenital Anomalies
Trauma/CNS Hemorrhage
Shock

As is true with most areas of scientific investigation; new information always generates new questions. In addition, many of the original questions are only partially answered.

The concept of the antenatal contribution to fetal neurologic damage is an important one. If intervention is to improve outcome, the damage must not have occurred before evaluation and intervention take place. This also points out the potential importance of antepartum fetal monitoring. Not only do the majority of fetal deaths occurs in the antepartum period, but the potential for eliminating antepartum damage also exists.

We are in need of information that establishes that intervention does indeed improve outcome and prevent damage. This is extremely difficult data to procure since the methodology must involve blinding fetal monitoring data and the incidence of such problems is sufficiently infrequent to necessitate studying large numbers of patients.

And finally, we must have long-term follow-up data in monitored patients to determine correlation of FHR with long-term outcome; to determine what early damage is truly reversible; to determine what types and frequencies there are of more subtle damage such as learning difficulties; and to answer many other questions.

Fetal monitoring and the prevention of asphyxic damage presents a perplexing complex of questions which are not only medical but socioeconomic and moral. Not only must we establish a potential for benefits, but we must decide to what extent we are willing to invest in such technology, with its associated costs and problems, in order to attack a problem where the frequency may be quite low once nonhypoxic/asphyxic factors are eliminated.

REFERENCES

1. Little WJ: On the influence of abnormal parturition, difficult labours, premature birth and asphyxia neonatorum, on the mental and physical condition of the child, especially in relation to deformities. Trans Obstet Soc London 3:293, 1862
2. Windle WF, Becker RF: Asphyxia neonatorum. An experimental study in the guinea pig. Am J Obstet Gynecol 45:183, 1943
3. Windle WF, Neuropathology of certain forms of mental retardation. Science 140:1186, 1963
4. Myers RE: Two patterns of perinatal brain damage and their conditions of occurrence. Am J Obstet Gynecol 112:246, 1972
5. Myers RE, Mueller-Huebach E, Adamsons K: Predictability of the state of fetal oxygenation from quantatative analysis of the components of late decelerations. Am J Obstet Gynecol 115:1083, 1973
6. Freud S: Die Infantile Cerebrallahmung. Vienna: A. Hoelder, 1897
7. Lilienfeld AM, Pasamanick B: The association of maternal and

fetal factors with the development of cerebral palsy and epilepsy. Am J Obstet Gynecol 70:93, 1955

8. Eastman NJ, DeLeon M: The etiology of cerebral palsy. Am J Obstet Gynecol 69:950, 1955

9. Eastman NJ, Kohl SG, Maisel JE, et al: The obstetrical background of 753 cases of cerebral palsy. Obstet Gynecol Survey 17:459, 1962

10. Steer CW, Bonney W: Obstetric factors in cerebral palsy. Am J Obstet Gynecol 83:526, 1962

11. Nelson KB, Ellenberg JH: Epidemiology of cerebral palsy. In: Schoenberg BS (editor) Advances in Neurology, vol 19. Raven Press, New York, 1979

12. Alberman E: Main causes of major mental handicap: prevalence and epidemiology. In: Ciba Foundation Symposium 59: Major Mental Handicap: Methods and Costs of Prevention. Elsevier-Excerpta Medica, Amsterdam, 1978

13. Hagberg G, Hagberg B, Olow I: The changing panorama of cerebral palsy in Sweden, 1954–1970. I. Analysis of the general changes. Acta Paedriat Scand 64:187, 1975

14. Stein Z, Susser M: Mental retardation. In: Last JM (editor) Preventive Medicine and Public Health. Appleton Century Croft, New York (in press)

15. McDonald AD: Severely retarded children in Quebec: prevalence, cause and care. Am J Ment Defic 78:205, 1973

16. Drillien CB: Studies in mental handicap II. Some obstetric factors of possible aetiological significance. Arch Dis Child 43:283, 1968

17. Warkany J: Mental retardation. In: Congenital Malformations. Year Book Medical Publishers, Inc., Chicago, 1971, p 262–267

18. Drage JS, Kennedy S, Berendes H, et al: The Apgar score as an index of infant morbidity. A report from the Collaborative Study of Cerebral Palsy. Dev Med Child Neurol 8:141, 1966

19. Ellenberg J, Nelson K: Birthweight and gestational age in children with cerebral palsy or seizure disorders. Am J Dis Child 133:1044, 1979

20. Fitzhardinge PM, Steven EM: The small for date infant: II Neurological and intellectual sequelae. Pediatrics 50:50, 1972

21. Friedman EA, Niswander KR, Sachtleben MR, et al: Dysfunctional labor X. Immediate results to infant. Obstet Gynecol 33:776, 1969

22. Friedman EA, Miswander KR, Sachtleben MR: Dysfunctional labor XI. Neurologic and developmental effects on surviving infants. Obstet Gynecol 33:785, 1969

23. Friedman EA, Sachtleben MR, Bresky PA: Dysfunctional labor XII. Long term effects on infant. Am J Obstet Gynecol 127:779, 1977

24. Malamud N: Neuropathology. In: Stevens HA and Heber R (editors) Mental Retardation. The University of Chicago Press, Chicago, 1964

25. Merritt TA, Farrell PM: Diminished pulmonary lecithin synthesis in acidosis: experimental findings as related to the respiratory distress syndrome. Pediatrics 57:32, 1976

26. Cruz, AC, Bohi WC, Birk SA et al: Respiratory distress syndrome with mature lecithin/sphingomyelin ratios: diabetes mellitus and low Apgar scores. Am J Obstet Gynecol 126:78, 1976

27. Hobel CJ, Hyvarinen M, Oh W: Abnormal fetal heart rate patterns and fetal acid-base balance in low birth weight infants in relation to respiratory distress syndrome. Obstet Gynecol 39:83, 1972

28. Martin CB, Siassi B, Hon EH: Fetal heart rate patterns and neonatal death in low birthweight infants. Obstet Gynecol 44:503, 1974

29. Cohn HJ, Sacks EJ, Heymann MA, et al: Cardiovascular responses to hypoxemia and acidemia in fetal lambs. Am J Obstet Gynecol 120:817, 1974

30. Alward CT, Hook JB, Helmrath TA, et al: Effects of asphyxia on cardiac output and organ blood flow in the newborn piglet. Pediat Res 12:824, 1978

31. Towbin A, Turner GL: Obstetric factors in fetal-neonatal visceral injury. Obstet Gynecol 52:113, 1978

32. Braly P, German J, Garite T: Fetal heart rate patterns in infants who develop necrotizing enterocolitis. Arch Surg (in press)

33. Modanlou H, Yeh SY, Hon EH, et al: Fetal and neonatal biochemistry and Apgar scores. Am J Obstet Gynecol 117:942, 1973

34. Barcroft J: Researches on Perinatal Life. Blackwell Scientific Publications Ltd, Oxford, 1946, p 124

35. Lee ST, Hon EH: Fetal hemodynamic response to umbilical cord compression. Obstet Gynecol 22:533, 1963

36. Kubli FH, Hon EH, Khazin AF, et al: Observations on fetal heart rate and pH in the human fetus during labor. Am J Obstet Gynecol 104:1190, 1969

37. Paul RH, Suidan AK, Yeh SY, et al: Clinical fetal monitoring VII. The evaluation and significance of intrapartum FHR variability. Am J Obstet Gynecol 123:206, 1975

38. Bisonette JM: Relationship between continuous fetal heart rate patterns and Apgar score in the newborn. Br J Obstet Gynecol 82:24, 1975

39. Schifrin BS, Dame L: Fetal heart rate patterns. Prediction of Apgar score. JAMA 219:1322, 1972

40. Painter MJ, Depp R, O'Donoghue: Fetal heart rate patterns and development in the first year of life. Am J Obstet Gynecol 132:271, 1978

41. Hack M, Faranoff AA, Merkatz IR: The low birthweight infant—evaluation of a changing outlook. N Engl J Med 301:1162, 1979

CHAPTER 4

Instrumentation, Artifact Detection, and Fetal Arrhythmias

INSTRUMENTATION

In order for the obstetrician or obstetrical nurse to fully interpret fetal monitor tracings, it is necessary that they have some understanding of the processes involved in acquisition and processing of fetal heart rate (FHR) and uterine activity data. Fetal monitors are designed to handle most situations but there are times when their output can be misleading unless one understands the limitations of the instrumentation he is using. Clearly, most errors we see in FHR interpretation are related to the quality of the data acquisition and presentation, and for this reason we believe an understanding of this Chapter is critical for the clinician who is using electronic fetal monitoring in the management of obstetrical patients.

Direct (Internal) Fetal Electrocardiographic (FECG) Derived FHR

FHR tracings derived from the FECG obtained from a fetal scalp electrode provide the FHR as defined by the interval between fetal R waves. In order for the clinician to understand the significance of FHR recordings, he must be acquainted with the way in which an electronic FHR monitor acquires its signal, processes the acquired signal, and then how it is displayed. It is also important to understand what the monitor can count and what it can't count.

The FECG signal provides the clinician with a measure of the electrical activity of the fetal heart. It does not necessarily represent mechanical activity.

The FECG signal obtained from the fetal scalp is obtained with a bipolar electrode that penetrates the skin of the fetal scalp for one pole and has a second conductor that resides in the secretions of the maternal vagina providing the other pole. It is believed that the potential difference (voltage) being measured is between these two points and the circuit is probably completed through the fetal umbilical cord, placenta, and the maternal circulation. Originally a modified skin clip was used for this electrode but now a convenient spiral electrode is used. This signal is then amplified and fed into an instantaneous beat-to-beat cardiotachometer (Fig. 4.1).

The raw FECG signal must first be amplified before it can be counted. This is done by an electronic amplifier with an automatic gain control circuit. The FECG signal is thus amplified to a predetermined voltage before electronic counting. One must bear in mind that all electronic signals will be equally amplified and the result will be to amplify noise as well as FECG signals. Once the FECG signal has been filtered and amplified, the interval between R wave peaks must be measured. In order to convert the interval between R waves to rate in beats per minute, the reciprocal of this interval must be computed. With

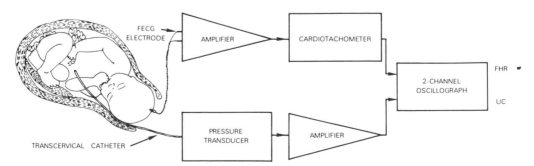

Figure 4.1. Schematic diagram of a direct fetal monitoring system. The FECG is obtained from a fetal scalp electrode and counted in a cardiotachometer. The actual uterine pressure is recorded directly from a transcervical intrauterine catheter.

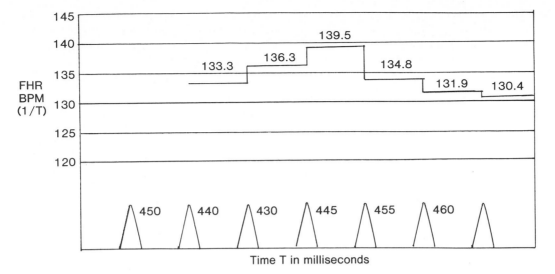

Figure 4.2 This represents a "blown up" FHR tracing demonstrating that a new rate is set with each FECG R wave constituting a series of square waves that indicate beat-to-beat changes.

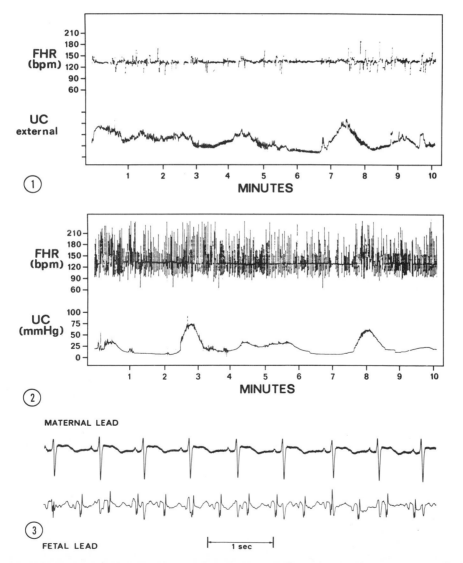

Figure 4.3. The ***upper tracing*** is FHR obtained with Doppler ultrasound showing a moderate amount of artifact. The ***middle tracing*** shows the same fetus monitored with an internal FECG electrode, resulting in a grossly irregular pattern caused by maternal ECG artifact. The ***lower tracing*** shows simultaneously-recorded maternal and fetal scalp electrocardiograms. Note the large maternal ECG artifact on the fetal ECG tracing which explains the grossly irregular FHR in the ***middle tracing***. (Reproduced with permission from Reference 1.)

internal FHR monitors, a new rate is set each time an R wave is detected. As each new wave arrives, the rate is recalculated from the reciprocal of the previous R-R interval and the FHR recording is reset. The result of this instantaneous calculation of the rate with each new R wave is a series of square waves being plotted (Fig. 4.2). The minute rate differences between beats are referred to as beat-to-beat or short-term variability, and can only be appreciated when the FHR is computed with an instantaneous beat-to-beat cardiotachometer as described above. Long-term changes in heart rate with a cyclicity of 3 to 5 per minute are referred to as long term variability and still longer term changes such as those occurring in response to uterine contractions or fetal movement are referred to as periodic changes. Long-term variability and periodic changes can be detected with Doppler systems but short-term variability can only be appreciated with direct FECG systems.

Most FECG counting systems cannot count from R-R intervals less than 250 msec which corresponds to a rate of 240 beats per minute (BPM). If the FHR exceeds 240 BPM, even a direct FECG system will not count every beat and may halve such rates. This only occurs with fetal tachyarrhythmias, such as paroxysmal, atrial tachycardia, or with intermittent premature atrial or ventricular contractions, where the premature beat may have an interval of less than 250 msec and therefore go undetected. This will be further discussed in the section on fetal arrhythmias.

The FECG wave form has identifiable P waves, QRS complexes, and T waves, providing the signal-to-noise ratio is adequate. The peak of the R wave is the most easily counted portion of the FECG. Its amplitude usually varies from 50 to 100 μv, the peak of the R wave is very sharp and its frequency allows it to be easily separated from other electrical impulses coming from the fetal scalp. Occasionally, the relative amplitude of maternal ECG complexes derived from the fetal scalp may increase above their usual level of about one-fifth the fetal R wave amplitude and counting off the maternal R wave can occur.[1] Since the maternal R wave bears no defined relationship to the fetal R wave, the recording resulting from maternal ECG will appear to have random rate changes that are very abrupt as one would see with other electronic noise or fetal arrhythmias (see Fig. 4.3). If the fetal ECG wave form is unusual with a notched R wave, or high peaked P wave, the resulting FHR tracing may also reflect this artifact with a "noisy tracing".

Older FHR monitors had a polarity switch that allowed the monitor operator to reverse the electrical polarity of the signal in case the FECG was inverted and artifact occurred because the monitor was counting off the Q and S waves. Newer monitors make this adjustment automatically (see Fig. 4.4).

In the rare event that the fetus is dead, and there is no FECG signal, the amplifier will continue to increase its gain until something reaches the desired amplitude for counting. In about 50% of such cases, the maternal R wave will be amplified sufficiently to be counted, with the result being the maternal heart rate being recorded from the dead fetus's scalp (see Fig. 4.5).[2, 3]

Doppler Ultrasound

When it is not feasible to record the FHR from the fetal scalp ECG signal, the most common method currently used is Doppler ultrasound (see Fig. 4.6). The Doppler method allows recording of the FHR from the maternal abdominal wall but the signal is not nearly as precise as the fetal scalp ECG (Fig. 4.7) and in order to produce a heart rate tracing, it is necessary to interpose a great deal of electronic logic which at times may actually cause the monitor output to be misleading. In this section there will first be a description of how Doppler ultrasound works, followed by a look at clinical interpretation problems introduced by the Doppler monitoring system.

The principles involved in Doppler FHR monitoring include the following.

1. Ultrasonic signals will penetrate human tissues,

2. When the ultrasonic beam encounters an interface with increased density to the transmission of the signal, a portion of the signal will be reflected at a 90 degree angle to that surface and a portion will be transmitted to the next interface.

3. The reflected signal will undergo a frequency

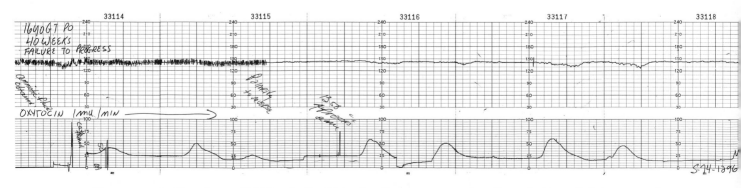

Figure 4.4. Artifact due to FECG polarity. Note the disappearance when the polarity switch is reversed.

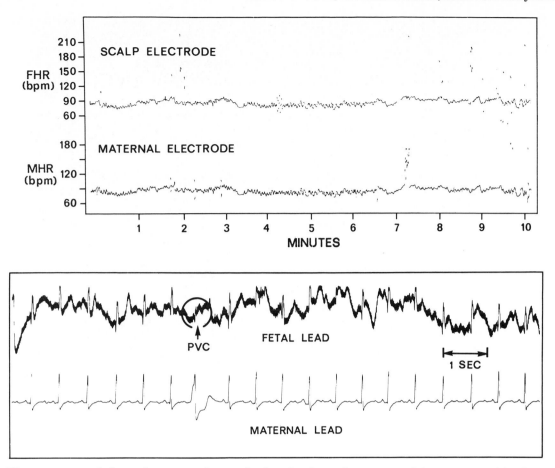

Figure 4.5. The *upper panel* shows heart rate from a fetal scalp electrode (FHR) and from maternal leads (MHR) with a dead fetus. Note the two rates are identical in detail. The *lower panel* shows the fetal scalp lead and the maternal lead ECG tracing indicating that the dead fetus is transmitting the maternal ECG to the fetal lead. (Reproduced with permission from Reference 1.)

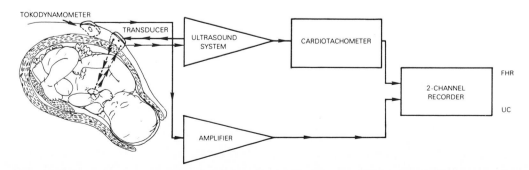

Figure 4.6. Schematic diagram of an indirect fetal monitoring system. The fetal ultrasonogram is obtained from an abdominal wall transducer, conditioned, and then counted by a cardiotachometer. The semiquantitative uterine activity is measured by an external tocodynamometer.

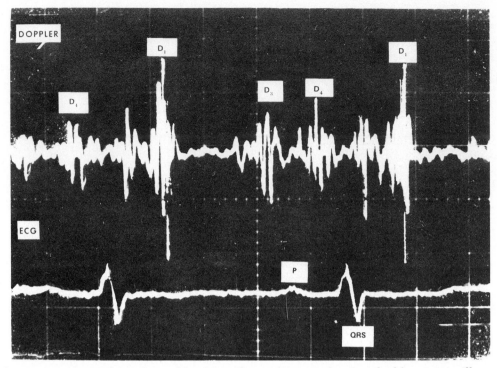

Figure 4.7. Simultaneous tracing of the FECG and fetal Doppler cardiogram photographed from an oscilloscope. (Reproduced with permission from Lauersen, N, et al: Am J Obstet Gynecol 125:1125, 1976.)

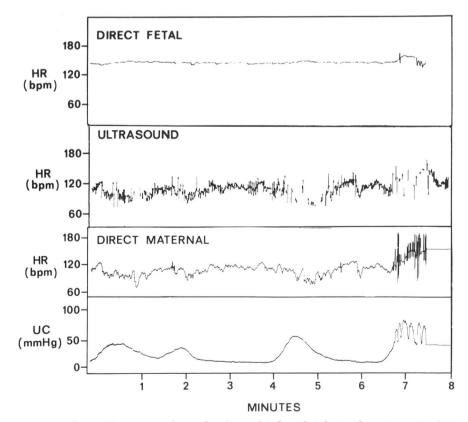

Figure 4.8. Simultaneous recording of heart rate from the direct fetal scalp electrode (***upper tracing***), abdominal Doppler (***middle tracing***), and direct maternal (***lower tracing***). Note that the abdominal Doppler signal is recording the maternal heart rate from a maternal vessel in the abdomen. (Reproduced with permission from Klapholz, H, et al: Obstet Gynecol 44: 373, 1974.)

change (Doppler shift) if the reflecting interface is moving. The frequency will increase if the reflecting interface is moving toward the signal source and will decrease if the reflecting interface is moving away from the signal source.

Utilizing these principles, the Doppler transducer contains a transmitter or signal source and a receiver. The signal is continuously being transmitted and the reflected signals are continuously being received. As long as the reflecting interfaces are not in motion, the reflected signal has the same frequency as the transmitted signal. However, if the reflecting interface is the surface of a moving organ such as the fetal heart, there will be a frequency change (Doppler shift) in the reflected signal and the electronics of the fetal monitor will sense this frequency change and convert it to an electronic signal. This electronic signal can then be used as a marker of the fetal heart beat as well as the source for development of an audible signal that provides the sound that we hear clinically when listening with a Doppler device. It is important for the clinician to understand that one is not listening to the fetal heart when using the Doppler method but one is actually hearing a sound that symbolizes frequency changes in the reflected ultrasonic signal and, therefore, actually represents movement.

Because Doppler ultrasound detects movement of a reflecting interface, one must be aware of the fact that maternal heart rate can also be counted off the abdominal Doppler signal if the transducer is inadvertently directed at a moving maternal vessel (Fig. 4.8). For this reason, the physician or nurse placing the Doppler should always check the maternal pulse to be sure it is not the source of the recorded heart rate.

As the fetal heart beats, there is a to-and-fro action with each beat as the heart goes through a contracting systole, followed by a dilating diastole. Hence there are two major components to the cardiac cycle that give rise to two separate frequency change complexes in the reflected Doppler signal (see Fig. 4.7).

The fact that there are two components to each cardiac cycle makes the electronic counting of the FHR difficult. If the same counting logic used for FHR computation from the direct fetal ECG signal were used, the heart rate would be doubled because of the two signals arising from each cardiac cycle. In order to avoid this problem, the electronic logic inserts a "refractory window" following the first component of the complex Doppler signal in order to avoid counting the second component as a separate beat. This works well most of the time, but if the FHR slows and the interval between the two components of the reflected signal becomes very long, the counting circuit in the monitor may begin "seeing" the second component outside the refractory period and the result will be an erroneous doubling of the FHR. This may happen at rates under about 90 BPM. Conversely, when rates get very high, the following cardiac cycle may be obscured in the refractory window and the counting circuit may only be able to see every other heart beat with the result being an erroneous halving of the FHR (Figs. 4.9 and 4.10).

The most common artifact that is introduced by Doppler ultrasound systems is the apparent increased FHR variability (Fig. 4.11). This occurs because the complexity and variability of the Doppler signal is so great that a sensing device cannot count at the same point in each cardiac cycle. The beat-to-beat variability of the FHR calculated from the fetal ECG usually averages about 3 to 5 BPM, but the Doppler signal has an inherent variability much greater than that.

There have been many attempts made to avoid this artifactual "jitter" characteristic of Doppler-derived FHR tracings. If one averages heart rate over a sufficiently long time, the jitter can be eliminated completely, but one then also loses short-term changes in heart rate that may be of clinical significance. If there is too much logic, the tracing can be very misleading (see Fig. 4.12). Most Doppler systems today employ a running average of, say, 3 beats with electronic updating with each new beat reflecting the average of the immediately preceding three valid intervals. There may also be different weight assigned to the more recent interval in the averaging process. While the rate is updated with each successive beat, the variability displayed still represents an average figure and, therefore, should never be considered to reflect

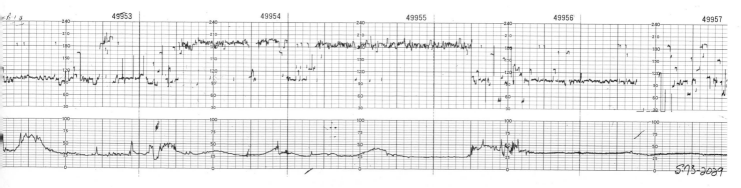

Figure 4.9. Tracing from a Doppler system showing halving of the FHR at rates over 180 BPM.

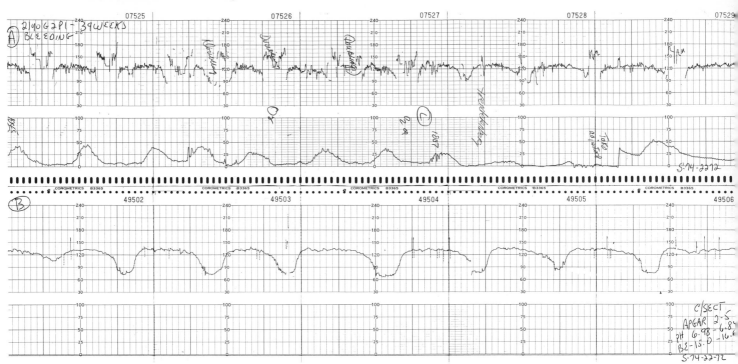

Figure 4.10. The *upper tracing* is taken from a Doppler signal source. At first glance it appears to be a poor quality, erratic tracing, but if one looks closer one can see that there are late decelerations, but the FHR doubles whenever it goes below 90 BPM, putting the trough of the late decelerations above the baseline. The *lower tracing* shows a continuation of the *upper tracing* after the fetal scalp electrode signal source was begun, showing the deep decelerations that were previously unrecognized because of the artifactual doubling of the FHR by the Doppler logic system.

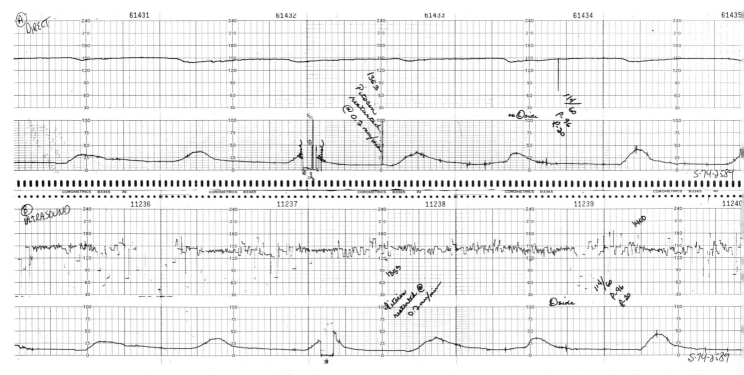

Figure 4.11. Simultaneous recordings with Doppler (*lower tracing*) and direct FECG (*upper tracing*) signal sources. Note the apparent increased variability and obscuring of periodic changes on the Doppler tracing.

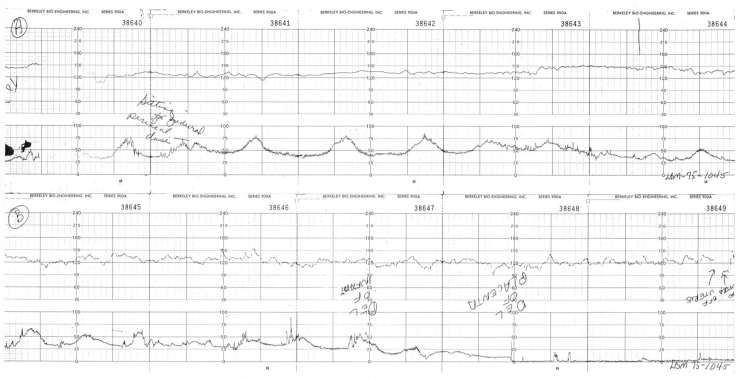

Figure 4.12. This tracing shows a Doppler record from a monitor with an excessive amount of electronic logic. Note that in the ***lower panel*** the baby delivers and then the placenta delivers and an apparent FHR can still be seen on the tracing.

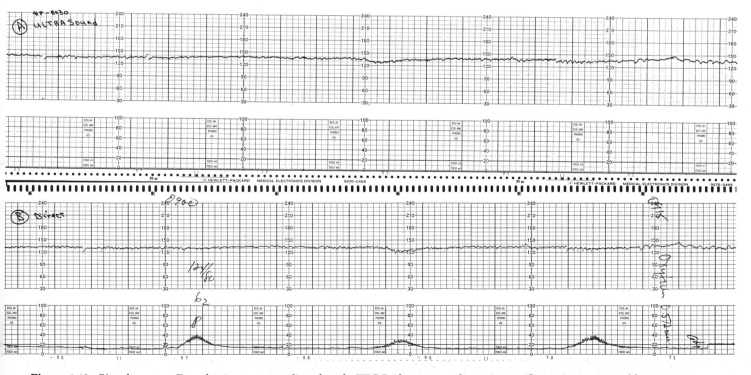

Figure 4.13. Simultaneous Doppler (***upper panel***) and scalp FECG (***lower panel***) tracings utilizing an improved logic system that has a small amount of averaging over 2 to 3 beats. The usual Doppler artifact is decreased and the two tracings are quite comparable.

true beat-to-beat variability which can only be measured from the fetal ECG signal. With the improved logic offered on currently available Doppler systems, the FHR recording more closely resembles the true FECG-derived pattern (Fig. 4.13) than the older systems which contained too much artifact. In general, the Doppler system will still reflect more apparent FHR variability than is actually present which means that unless excessive averaging is used, the Doppler tracing that shows reduced FHR variability is probably valid, whereas increased or "normal" variability seen on a Doppler tracing may or may not be valid.

Abdominal FECG-derived FHR Tracings

Abdominal FECG signals were first recorded by Cremer in 1916.[4] The original application of this method was for the diagnosis of fetal life. Larks and Dasgupta[5] and Hon and Hess[6] later showed that the presentation of the fetus could be predicted by the polarity of the fetal QRS complex in relation to the maternal signal obtained from the maternal abdomen. With a breech presentation, the FECG complex would be similar in polarity to that of the mother whereas with a cephalic presentation, the R wave would be opposite that of the maternal polarity. In addition, abdominal FECG tracings could also be used to diagnose twins, in some instances, by comparing the fetal complexes determining two separate rate patterns among the fetal complexes.

From the maternal abdomen, the FECG complex is much smaller than the maternal ECG (Fig. 4.14). Often, if the electrical noise level is high, one may not be able to see a FECG signal.

The FECG signal may be seen early in pregnancy but is often lost between about 28 and 30 weeks. At term and beyond, the signal is usually quite strong. In order to maximize the chance of recording an FECG from the maternal abdomen, it is necessary to minimize the electrical resistance of the mother's abdominal wall skin and to place the electrodes in the optimal position for maximal signal amplitude. Unfortunately, the electromyographic muscle noise produced by the muscles of the maternal abdominal wall will completely obscure the FECG obtained from the maternal abdomen.

Because the mother is at rest during antepartum testing, this usually does not cause a problem before labor. However, after labor starts, if the mother is actively moving her abdominal muscles, the interference makes the technique virtually impossible. During antepartum testing, however, when a good signal is obtained, this method appears to give the best recordings of any method available and once the electrode placement is completed, there is very little need to make readjustments, even with some fetal movement (Fig. 4.15).

In order to count the FHR from the abdominal FECG complex, the electronic logic used must allow for the coincidence that occurs between the fetal and maternal ECG complexes every few beats. In order to avoid counting the maternal rate plus the fetal rate, a peripheral maternal ECG source is obtained from another maternal lead. The counting circuit can then determine when not to count the maternal ECG signal. It also makes it possible, through electronic logic, to detect a fetal maternal coincidence, using the premise that the expected fetal R-R interval is known, based on the preceding R-R intervals. When coincidence occurs, the electronic logic will then insert one R-R interval equal to the last true fetal R-R interval and go on counting, utilizing the interval to calculate rate during maternal FECG coincidence. Strictly speaking, this introduces false data, making the interval preceding and following the coincidence to be derived based on the expected fetal R wave, rather than the real one that was obscured by the maternal ECG complex. In reality, this compensation for lost fetal R waves (during fetal-maternal ECG coincidences) does not significantly alter the appearance of the FHR trace when compared with a simultaneously derived direct fetal scalp ECG FHR pattern (Fig. 4.15). However, if one were to quantitate short-term variability electronically by measuring fetal R-R interval differences, there would be considerable error introduced with a tendency to decrease the apparent FHR short-term variability proportionately to the number of derived R-R intervals used.

Another problem that may occur with abdominal FECG heart rate monitoring may arise if the maternal and fetal rates are similar or one is half or double the other. As one can imagine, with similar rates the amount of coincidence would be very high when the beats were synchronous and with rates that were multiples, the uniform coincidence patterns could also make it impossible to measure true R-R intervals.

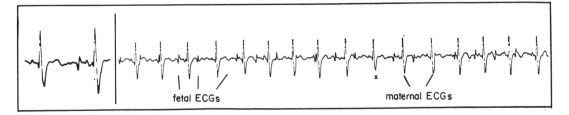

fetal ECGs   maternal ECGs

Figure 4.14. An abdominal tracing showing the large maternal ECG complexes and the clear but much smaller fetal complexes. (Reproduced with permission from Hon E, Lee S: Am J Obstet Gynecol 87:804, 1963.)

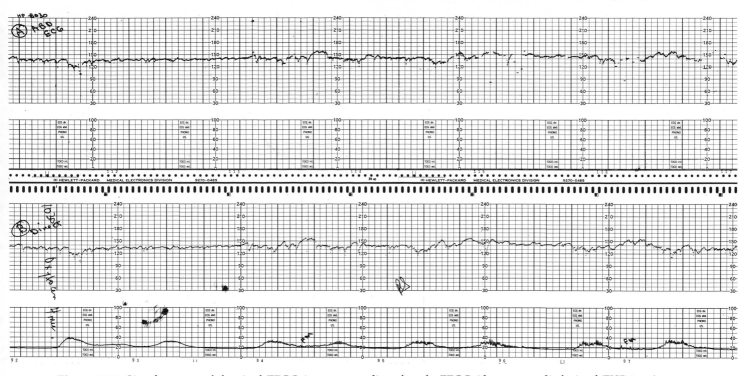

Figure 4.15. Simultaneous abdominal FECG (*upper panel*) and scalp FECG (*lower panel*) derived FHR tracings.

In the commercially available monitors we have tested, the electronic logic will only allow one derived fetal R-R interval to be inserted without at least one intervening true R-R interval. The result is that when rates are similar or harmonically related, the tracing may be rejected as synchrony occurs but will not be plotted based on consecutive derived fetal R-R intervals.

Phonocardiographically-derived FHR

As the fetal heart beats, the closure of the valves produces sound that may be detected by listening with a suitable stethoscope through the mother's abdominal wall. This mechanical energy may be sensed by a microphone and amplified, producing an electrical signal that may then be reconverted to sound or the signal may be used to produce an oscillographic tracing of the heart sounds known as a phonocardiogram. The amplified electrical signal can also be used as a counting source for an FHR monitor. Phonocardiography was indeed the first method used to record FHR electronically from the mother's abdominal wall.

There are two major components to the signal. With ventricular systole, the atrioventricular valves close, producing the first heart sound and with the onset of diastole, the aortic and pulmonary valves close, producing the second heart sound. The phonocardiographic signal is clearer than the Doppler signal, resulting in less artifactual "jitter". For this reason, phonocardiography has been extensively used for antepartum FHR monitoring.

The main drawback to phonocardiographically-derived FHR systems is that they are extremely sensitive to ambient noise such as maternal bowel sounds, voices in the room, certain air conditioning systems, and especially noise produced by any motion of the microphone or of the bed clothing against the microphone. In addition, any fetal kicking or motion produces a very loud noise that will "saturate" the automatic gain system on the monitor's amplifier, resulting in complete loss of recording for several seconds while awaiting the amplifier to "open up" again. For this reason, a manual gain control offers a great advantage when using abdominal fetal phonocardiography for recording heart rate. Also, because of the high sensitivity to ambient noise, the technique is unsatisfactory for monitoring during the active phase of labor (Fig. 4.16). The current role of phonocardiographic FHR recording is quite limited but should be considered if abdominal FECG and Doppler do not give satisfactory recordings during antepartum testing. Certainly, with careful technique, this method will give quite satisfactory recordings but would have to be considered today below abdominal FECG and Doppler as a preferred method of antepartum FHR monitoring.

Scaling Factors

The appearance of the FHR and uterine contraction (UC) recording is dependent on the vertical and horizontal scale. In the United States, the standard factors are 30 BPM/cm on the vertical scale and 3 cm/min on the horizontal scale. In Europe, standard

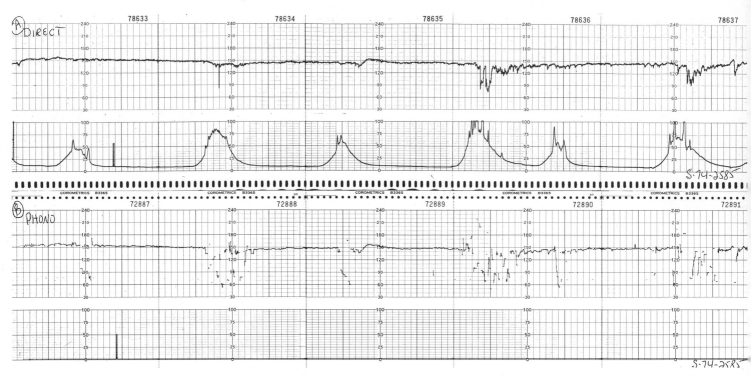

Figure 4.16. Simultaneous phonocardiographic (*upper tracing*) and scalp FECG (*lower panel*) derived FHR tracings. Note the signal loss during contractions with the phono recording.

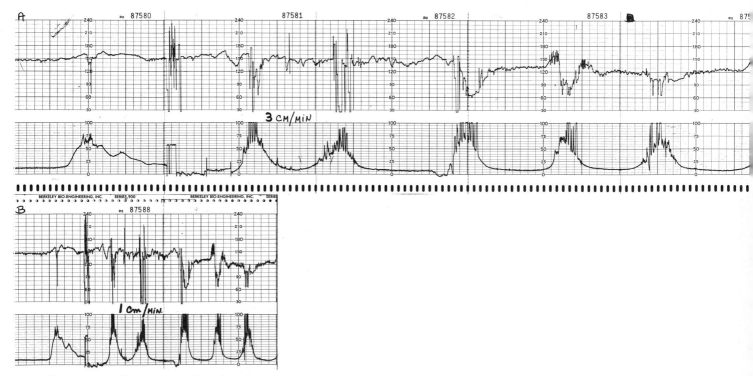

Figure 4.17. The *upper* and *shorter lower tracings* are taken from a tape recorded FHR-UC pattern which was played back to a monitor running at 3 cm/min (*upper tracing*) and 1 cm/min (*lower tracing*).

factors are 20 BPM/cm vertical and 1 or 2 cm/min horizontal. The European scaling factors accentuate apparent FHR variability and tend to make periodic changes appear more abrupt than with the American scaling factors.

In the United States, most monitors have a choice of 1 or 3 cm/min paper speed. It is our opinion that 1 cm/min tracings are very hard to read and the small savings on paper are not justified. Figure 4.17 shows how a 1 cm paper speed can significantly change the appearance of a tracing.

Artifact Detection

All fetal monitors contain a system designed to reject artifact. The basis for these systems is electronic logic that rejects data when a variation that is greater than expected occurs between successive heart beats. The logic circuit first samples each interval, compares it with the previous interval and if it varies from that previous interval by more than, say, 25%, it is not accepted and the monitor will go into a "hold" mode which instructs the recorder to keep the rate set at the same rate that corresponded to the previously accepted interval between beats. If the succeeding beat also varies by more than the accepted amount, it also will be rejected, and after an arbitrary number of beats or an arbitrary time interval, the monitor will go from the "hold" mode to a

nonrecord mode which is accomplished by either lifting the pen off the chart or by turning the heat off on the recorder pen. The pen-lift or heat-off mode will remain in operation until the monitor receives an arbitrary number of beats whose interval differences are less than the accepted level of variation. When electronic "credence" is again established, the recorder will again begin recording, either by lowering the pen back onto the paper or by turning the heat back on.

This artifact rejection system is always in operation when using external modes such as Doppler, phonocardiography or abdominal fetal electrocardiography. It can be defeated when on internal direct-fetal ECG mode. The reason for this choice is that artifact is so common with external techniques that to not use the logic would make it virtually impossible to read the tracing under most circumstances. However, when using the direct fetal ECG mode, artifact is relatively rare in most circumstances so the logic system will only result in missing true fetal heart rate changes that exceed the arbitrarily-defined limits for the logic system. Specifically, this occurs with fetal arrhythmias where the intervals between beats may actually change by large amounts but not be artifact.

This logic system for internal FECG monitoring is controlled by a switch on the back of some fetal monitors. Other monitors have the logic always in

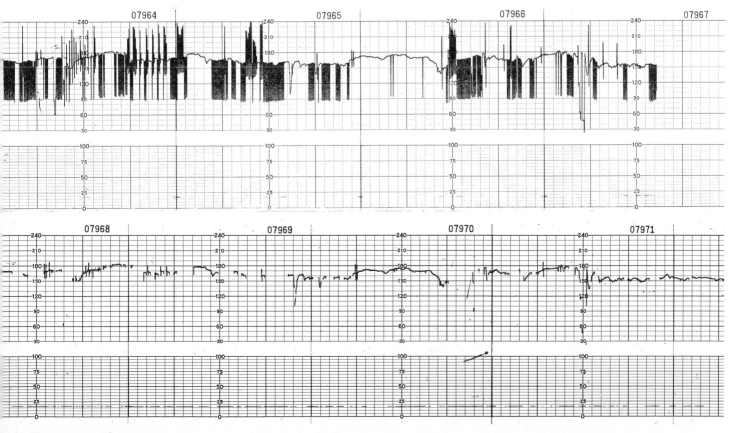

Figure 4.18. The *upper* tracing is a recording of a fetal arrhythmia with the pen lift out. The *lower tracing* is the same recording run with the pen lift in.

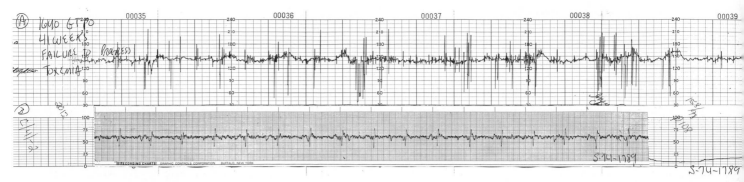

Figure 4.19. The FHR upper tracing shows many vertical deflections caused by a poor signal-to-noise ratio as can be seen on the lower simultaneous FECG tracing demonstrating a biphasic QRS and much extraneous electrical noise which explains the "dirty" FHR tracing above.

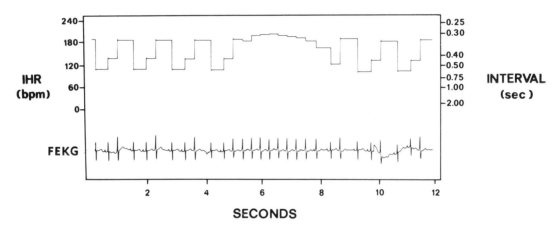

Figure 4.20. A tracing with the horizontal scale expanded by increasing the chart speed to 150 cm/min shows the FECG (below) and instantaneous heart rate (IHR) above during supraventricular extra systoles and an episode of fetal supraventricular tachycardia. (Reproduced with permission from Klapholz H, et al: Obstet Gynecol 43:718, 1973.)

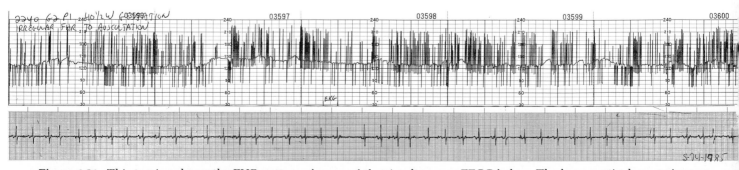

Figure 4.21. This tracing shows the FHR pattern above and the simultaneous FECG below. The large vertical excursions on the FHR scale are caused by the fetal arrhythmia which is shown on the FECG tracing to be due to premature multifocal atrial contractions. Note the biphasic P waves.

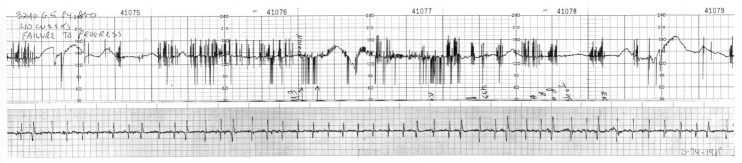

Figure 4.22. This tracing shows the FHR patterns above and the simultaneous FECG below. The large vertical excursions on the FHR scale are caused by the fetal arrhythmia which is shown on the FECG tracing to be due to premature ventricular contractions. Note the changing configuration of the fetal QRS complexes with each premature beat.

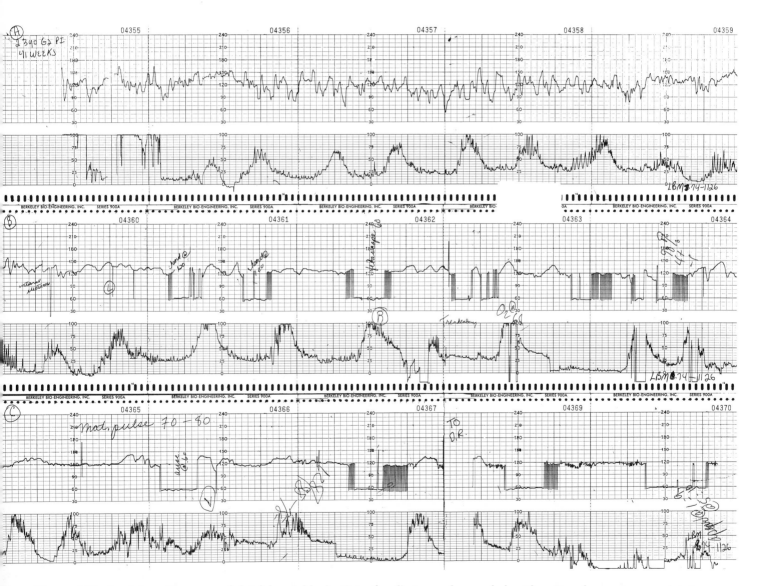

Figure 4.23. An interesting case of fetal heart block. Note the **first panel** recorded with a Doppler system containing excessive logic shows an erratic pattern. The **middle** and **lower panels** are from a direct fetal scalp ECG. There are intermittent abrupt drops to 60 BPM from the 120 BPM baseline. Where it says 'heard at 120 BPM, the nurse was using a Doppler listening device and counting the atrial rate. With the third episode of 60 BPM FHR, the nurse listened with a fetoscope (phono) and the rate of 60 agreed with the FECG rate of 60 indicating the ventricular rate. Thus, a diagnosis of an intermittent 2-to-1 heart block was made.

operation, regardless of mode being used, and others have it always in operation when using external modes, and not in operation when using internal modes. On those monitors with a switch, it is recommended to have the monitor in the no-logic mode when using the internal monitor in order to detect arrhythmias (Fig. 4.18) and only using the logic on internal recording when there is true artifact such as with a poor signal-to-noise ratio (Fig. 4.19) or where there is a large maternal R wave that is intermittently being counted. This can usually be determined by looking at the signal on the scope if one is provided, or to write out the FECG signal on those monitors with this option.

Fetal Arrhythmias

Fetal arrhythmias occur fairly commonly but will not be appreciated if the previously mentioned logic system is operational when recording with direct fetal ECG. Arrhythmias will never be recordable when using external techniques, because on all clinical monitors the external systems have logic in operation at all times in order to make the recording readable.

Figure 4.20 shows an expanded view of the recording of a fetal arrhythmia when the premature beat causes a sudden rise in the rate and the following pause causes a sudden drop in the rate, resulting in the characteristic vertical lines associated with the instantaneous FHR recording of fetal arrhythmias. Since electrical noise or maternal ECG artifact can cause the same FHR tracing appearance, it is important to examine the raw FECG tracing on the scope in order to differentiate between arrhythmia and artifact.

There are a number of fetal arrhythmias that have been reported.[7-10] The following is a list: (1) premature atrial contractions (Fig. 4.21); (2) premature ventricular contractions (Fig. 4.22); (3) paroxysmal atrial tachycardia; (4) heart block (Fig. 4.23); (5) vagal cardial arrest (Fig. 4.24). The clinical significance of these arrhythmias should be appreciated. Premature atrial contractions and premature ventricular contractions probably have very little clinical significance, except for a possible slight increase in fetal cardiac anomalies. They are not to be considered a sign of fetal hypoxia and do not carry any significance as far as intervention. Sometimes a terminal FHR pattern will show some premature ventricular contractions (PVC's) or premature atrial contractions (PAC's),[11] but the significance of the pattern does not come from these findings but rather from the periodic and baseline FHR characteristics.

Paroxysmal fetal atrial tachycardia (PAT) is often diagnosed prior to labor and is usually diagnosed because of a rate in excess of 250 beats per minute. Management of patients with fetal PAT may be difficult. There are documented cases of fetal hydrops developing in such fetuses because of heart failure.[12, 13] This may lead to fetal death in some instances. Therefore, if a patient has a mature fetus with this diagnosis, it would be wise to effect delivery, probably by cesarean section, because the fetal cardiac reserve is compromised and one cannot monitor the fetus during labor when fetal PAT is present. The neonate usually responds very well to digitalis, but we have not been successful in digitalizing the fetus via the mother. If the fetus is not mature, we have followed such patients with serial sonograms to look for the development of hydrops as evidenced by the development of fetal ascites or thickening of the

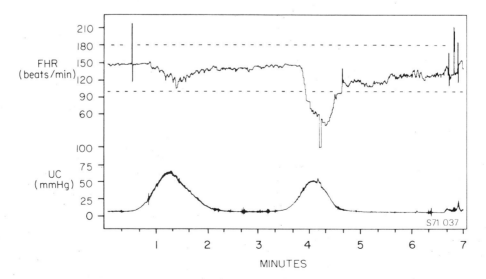

Figure 4.24. An example of a FHR/UC tracing containing an episode of transient fetal cardiac arrest. At the 4-min mark, during the course of severe variable deceleration, there was a transient fall of FHR to the zero level. Concomitant examination of FECG tracing proved the episode of transient fetal cardiac arrest. (Reproduced with permission from Yeh S, et al: Obstet Gynecol. 50:571, 1977.)

placenta. Once hydrops is detectable, it would probably be best to deliver even a premature fetus, although we have not yet had to do this.

Congenital heart block is associated with a very high incidence of fetal anomalies and has been reported to have an increased incidence in mothers with disseminated lupus erythematosis.[14] Heart block may either be intermittent or fixed. It is suspected when a fetal bradycardia is noted, usually at a prenatal visit. The rate is usually in the 60 to 80 BPM range. When a heart block is present, it is possible to make the diagnosis positively by a simple technique. If the rate is found to be, say, 60 with the DeLee stethescope, one can assume that that is the ventricular rate since the phono signal being heard reflects the closure of heart valves which are controlled by the ventricular action. If the rate heard with a Doppler instrument is twice the rate of the ventricular rate, one can assume that the Doppler instrument is counting the atrial rate since it counts movement, and with the heart block the atrial rate will usually be at least twice the ventricular rate (Fig. 4.23).[15] Confirmation can be made with real time ultrasound[16] and it may also be possible to confirm a congenital heart malformation with the real time instrument, depending on the experience of the ultrasonographer. When congenital heart block is diagnosed, the fetus should be delivered in a center where cardiac surgery is performed, in order to offer the neonate the possibility of a pacemaker at the time of birth as this may be lifesaving. Sometimes congenital heart block disappears at the time of birth, and sometimes, even though it did not reverse at birth, a pacemaker may not be necessary. Certainly, in all cases of heart block a careful evaluation of the neonate for congenital cardiac anomalies should be made. Vagal cardiac arrest may occur during variable deceleration.[17] It is characterized by several seconds of cardiac asystole. If one looks at the fetal ECG changes that occur during variable deceleration, one will notice that the amplitude of the fetal P wave diminishes and when the fetal rate reaches about 60 BPM the P wave disappears. The nodal rhythm is then about 60 BPM and represents sinus arrest in the fetus. Almost always, as the heart rate returns at the end of a variable deceleration, the P wave returns and a sinus rhythm is restored. Occasionally the nodal rhythm will cease when the heart rate is at 60, resulting in a complete cardiac standstill. This would appear to be a serious problem. However, with a limited experience with such cases, no serious sequalae have occurred as a result of these episodes which only last a few seconds. Therefore this cannot be considered an indication for intervention at this

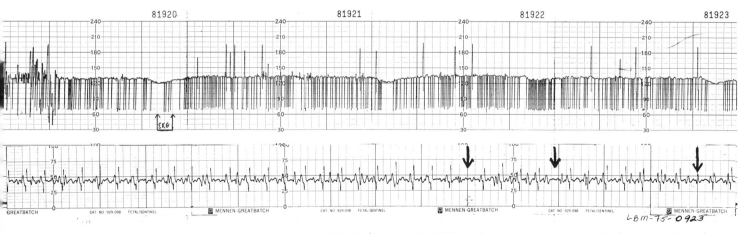

Figure 4.25. This tracing shows a series of downward deflections of the FHR in the upper tracing and the lower tracing of the simultaneous FECG shows absent QRS complexes or dropped beats.

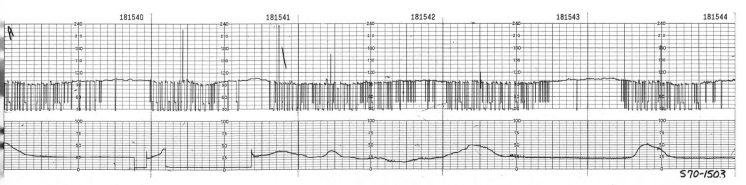

Figure 4.26. This tracing also shows a series of downward reflections. In this instance, the heart rate is maternal from a dead fetus' scalp electrode. The downward deflections represent a weak maternal signal with intermittent noncounted beats. (Reproduced from Paul R, Freeman R: Selected Records of Intrapartum Fetal Monitoring. USC Pub. 1971.)

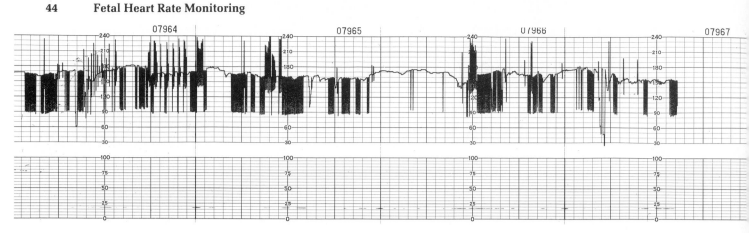

Figure 4.27. This tracing is an example of premature ventricular contractions of multifocal origin. At times the deflections are all downward because the premature beat occurred at less than 250 msec from the previous beat and the monitor cannot detect such a short interval and only the compensatory pause is recorded. When an upward deflection precedes the downward deflections, it is because the interval is greater than 250 msec.

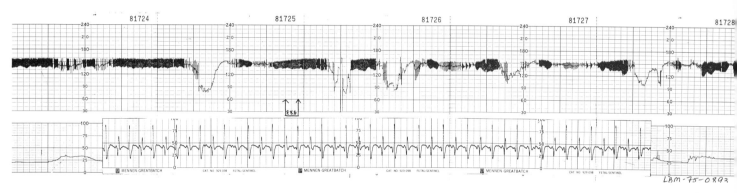

Figure 4.28. This tracing shows an FHR tracing above with rapid excursions above and below the baseline, representing unifocal premature ventricular contractions in a bigeminal rhythm as shown on the simultaneous FECG in the *lower tracing*.

time. Some have advocated giving atropine to the mother to prevent such problems, but I am not aware of the results of such a venture, and since these brief arrests do not appear to have serious sequelae, I am not sure what is to be accomplished.

Occasionally one will see a tracing with all downward deflections. This may be due to dropped beats (Fig. 4.25). A very low amplitude signal (Fig. 4.26) or premature beats where the interval is too short to be counted (less than 250 msec), resulting in only the compensatory pause being shown (Fig. 4.27).

Rarely PVC's will occur every other beat, creating a bigeminal rhythm as noted in Fig. 4.28.

An understanding of fetal monitor instrumentation is key to interpreting artifacts and arrhythmias. As one becomes more aware of such things, the chance of being technologically misled will decrease.

APPLICATION OF MONITORING DEVICES

Uterine Contraction Monitors

Clinically, uterine contractions can be monitored by two techniques; external tocodynamometry or by intrauterine pressure measurement. Both methods have advantages and disadvantages and each is most applicable to certain clinical situations. This section will deal with the methodology involved in the clinical application of these techniques.

Intrauterine Pressure Monitoring. The pregnant uterus is a closed fluid-filled space and hydrostatic pressure within the uterus is equal at all points. Therefore, an open-ended catheter filled with fluid and inserted into the amniotic sac will carry a pressure equal throughout to the pressure of the amniotic fluid at its open intrauterine end minus the algebraic pressure in cm of water that represents the difference in level between the intra and extrauterine ends of the catheter. This assumes an open system without catheter occlusion by solid matter or by kinking or entrapment between the uterus and fetus.

The pressure within the uterine cavity is proportional to the tension in the uterine wall and inversely proportional to the diameter of the uterus at any given tension. Thus the larger the uterus, the lower the intrauterine pressure for any given tension in the uterine wall. This is borne out by the clinical observation that pressure in the nonpregnant uterus may exceed 200 mm Hg during menstruation while intrauterine pressure with twins may never exceed 25 or 30 mm Hg, even in active labor with good progress.

The usual pressures observed in the pregnant uterus during active labor at term are in the range of 50 to 100 mm Hg at the peak of contractions with a baseline tone of 5 to 15 mm Hg. Premature labors often have much higher pressures because of the smaller uterine size.

A pressure transducer is used to quantitate the pressures from the extrauterine end of the intrauterine catheter. The transducer has a pressure input and an electrical output with voltage proportional to this pressure. The output of the transducer is the actual signal used by the recorder after appropriate amplification. There are several different types of pressure transducers available, including some very small ones that are inserted into the uterus themselves. However, the commonly used transducers consist of a closed chamber with a removable (and sometimes disposable) plastic dome which has two connections. One is for the uterine catheter and the other is used for flushing or calibration. Within this closed chamber there is a diaphragm at its base. As the pressure in the closed chamber changes, the diaphragm is distorted to a greater or lesser degree and the voltage output of the transducer is proportional to the amount of pressure which distorts this diaphragm. For this reason, the transducer is often referred to as a strain gauge.

The intrauterine catheter may either be inserted

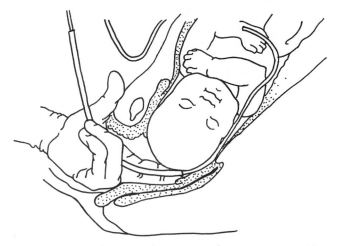

Figure 4.30. Technique of uterine catheter insertion. Note that the introducer is only inserted about 1 centimeter inside the cervix.

transabdominally or transcervically. Transabdominal insertion allows direct measurement of pressure without rupturing the membranes at the cervical os. Because of the small catheter size necessitated by this approach, however, pressure recording is more susceptible to interference because of catheter plugging and kinking. The discomfort and increased risk of transabdominal insertion render this technique of no current clinical use.

Transcervical insertion involves inserting the catheter through an introducer tube into the uterine cavity. Before inserting the catheter into the introducer, a 10 ml syringe filled with sterile bacteriostatic water (not saline) should be attached to the extrauterine end of the catheter with a needle adapter which will eventually attach to the strain gauge pressure transducer. Saline is not used because it will corrode the transducer. The patency of the catheter should be tested and the air cleared from the system by flushing the catheter with the sterile water before insertion (Fig. 4.29).

Transcervical insertion of the uterine pressure catheter is accomplished by first placing it into a sterile introducer tube that is inserted just inside the uterine cervix and next to the presenting part (Fig. 4.30). This allows for the sterile introduction of the more flexible polyethylene catheter into the uterus without vaginal contamination. It is especially important not to insert the introducer more than 1 cm inside the cervix as it is quite rigid and uterine perforation can occur with the introducer. The more flexible intrauterine catheter is usually advanced into the uterus quite easily but on occasion resistance will be met. In this situation, one should move the introducer 90 degrees in its orientation to the cervix and try again. Usually one begins posterior to the presenting part, but the catheter can be inserted anywhere in the 360 degree circumference of the cervix. When the catheter advances easily, it should be in-

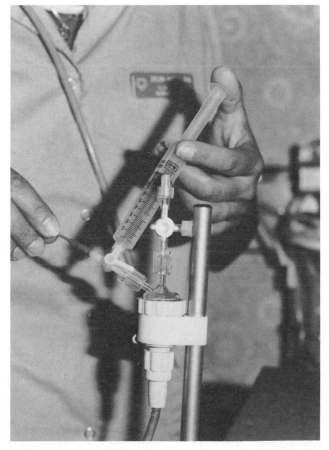

Figure 4.29. Uterine pressure strain gauge transducer.

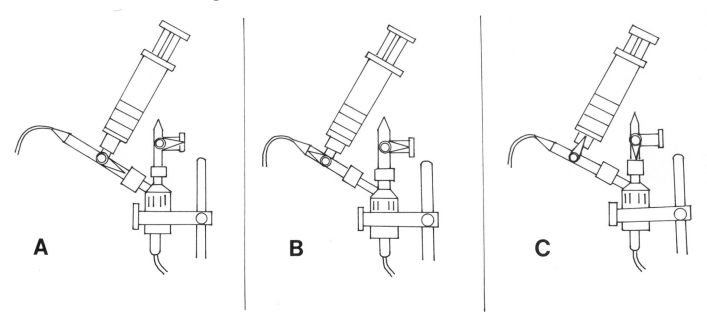

Figure 4.31. A, The pressure transducer is open to air, allowing the zero setting and calibration to be computed.. With the system closed between the syringe and the pressure transducer, the catheter to the patient is flushed to remove any air or debris. B, With the system closed to the catheter and open to air, the dome of the pressure transducer is back flushed to clear any air from this part of the system. C, The system is then closed to air and opened to the patient's catheter and recording of uterine pressure can begin.

serted about 18 inches to the point of the mark on the catheter which should be just visible at the introitus.

Once the catheter is in place, the syringe should be removed from the catheter and the catheter attached to one of the two ports of the chamber on the strain gauge pressure transducer using a 3-way stopcock. A 10-ml syringe filled with sterile water is then attached to the other port on the 3-way stopcock. A 2-way stopcock or pressure "pop-off" valve is then attached to the other port of the strain gauge dome to allow for back flushing and opening the system to air (Fig. 4.31).

Calibration is accomplished by following these steps.

1. Flush the catheter to the patient to be sure the system is patent.

2. Back flush the system through the strain gauge by first opening the other port to air, then closing the 3-way stopcock to the patient and running 2 to 3 ml of sterile water back through the transducer from the syringe. Be sure all air is released.

3. The diaphragm of the strain gauge pressure transducer is placed at a level approximately equal to a point level with the patient's xiphoid process with her in the supine position. This is estimated to be approximately the level of the tip of the intrauterine end of the catheter.

4. With the system still open to air, the new setting on the monitor should be adjusted to read zero.

5. With the system open to air, the calibration button (usually 50 mm Hg) on the monitor should be pressed to show that the fetal monitor is responding appropriately.

6. The system is again back flushed slowly and while the water is running out of the other port of the transducer, the stopcock is closed. This will make sure no air is trapped. The 3-way stopcock to which the syringe is attached should now be opened to the patient and closed to the syringe. At this point, the pressure channel should record approximately 5 to 15 mm Hg pressure which is considered normal uterine tone. If there is a contraction in progress, of course the pressure may be higher. If you have the patient cough at this point, you should see a sharp 10 to 20 mm deflection on the monitor recorder, indicating probable patency. The system should now be recording (Fig. 4.32).

If the tracing does not show symmetrical smooth pressure changes with contractions, there may be a plugged or kinked catheter (Fig. 4.33). One should first flush the intrauterine catheter, and if that does not work, one should try to pull the catheter out 2 to 3 cm in case there is a kink. Occasionally one will have to replace the catheter if one cannot get a good recording with simple manipulation. Sometimes the baseline uterine pressure may appear quite high with the patient in the supine position but on repositioning to the lateral position, the pressure will usually return to a more normal level. This is partially due to the height of the catheter tip in the uterus, and partly due to actual changes in tone. If the pressure remains high in the lateral position, and it is not due to true hypertonus, it may also be due to a plugged or kinked catheter.

The previously described system for calibration does not guarantee that the pressure transducer is

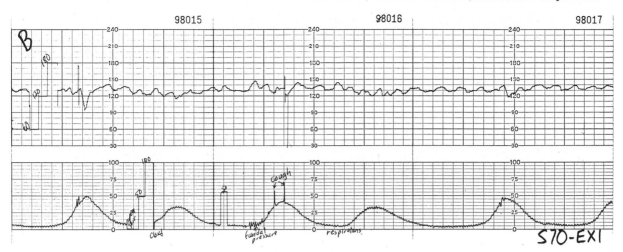

Figure 4.32. This tracing shows the calibration of the FHR at 60, 120, and 180 on the **upper tracing** and calibration of the uterine pressure channel below. Note that after the first uterine contractions the system is opened to air, zeroed, calibrated at 50 and 100 mm Hg, and then closed. After calibration the patient is asked to cough and sharp spikes are seen. (Reproduced with permission from Paul R, Freeman R: Selected Records of Intrapartum Fetal Monitoring. USC Pub. 1971.)

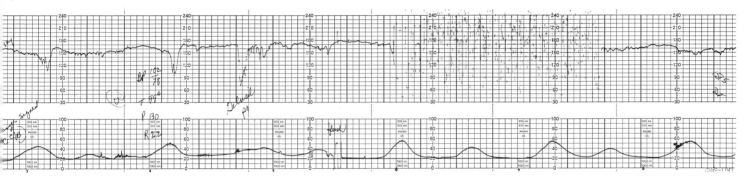

Figure 4.33. This tracing shows a uterine pressure tracing from a plugged catheter corrected by flushing.

working properly or is calibrated. If one suspects that the pressure transducer is not recording accurately, one can adapt a sphygmomanometer to the transducer and put in a given pressure and see what actually records on the monitor. Since strain gauge pressure transducers have been implicated in transmission of infection, one should be careful to follow the manufacturer's recommendation for cleaning and sterilizing.

The External Tocodynamometer. If membranes are not yet ruptured, the external tocodynamometer allows the patient's uterine activity to be monitored in a nonquantitative way which is usually satisfactory in patients who are progressing well and are not requiring oxytocin augmentation. Occasionally, FHR deceleration may be observed in a very obese patient when contractions cannot be recorded with an external tocotransducer and intrauterine pressure monitoring may clarify this situation.

External tocotransducers come in many different sizes and shapes. They are attached by an elastic belt around the patient's abdomen and when the uterus contracts the change in shape and hardness of the

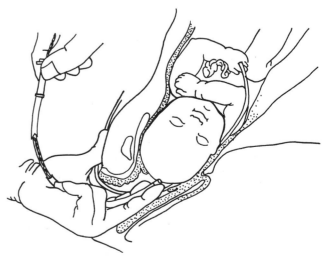

Figure 4.34. Technique for application of the spiral electrode.

uterus depresses a plunger which moves a slight distance and causes a change in the voltage of a small electrical current which is passing through. These voltage changes are proportional to the uterine activity and are represented qualitatively by the fetal

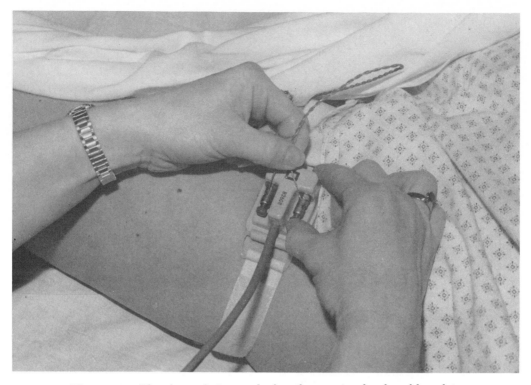

Figure 4.35. The electrode is attached to the previously-placed leg plate.

monitor as contractions. Since one does not ever know the true pressures by this method, it usually works well to arbitrarily set the uterine activity channel at about 25 mm Hg between contractions by adjusting the pen position. Positioning of the external tocotransducer is most important because if it is not over the proper part of the uterus, it may not detect uterine activity at all. One should palpate to find where contractions are the most easily felt and place the transducer there with careful attention to adjustment of the elastic belt to an appropriate tension (Fig. 4.36). Often where the uterus is quite small as with premature or growth retarded fetuses, the external tocotransducer may be very poor at picking up uterine activity. One must not be afraid to palpate and pay attention to the patient's complaints of contractions in such situations. This is also especially true with obesity (Fig. 4.37).

The external tocotransducer can give fairly reliable estimates of the frequency and duration of contractions. The baseline tone and actual contraction amplitude, of course, cannot be measured at all with the external tocotransducer. When routinely monitoring patients, the external tocotransducer will be adequate in over 90% of patients and it doesn't carry any apparent risk of infection as may theoretically be the case with the intrauterine pressure catheter.

The Spiral Fetal Scalp Electrode

The most commonly used fetal scalp electrode consists of a spiral or "corkscrew" placed inside two concentric tubes with the wires trailing through the center tube. The whole assembly is placed through the vagina and cervix against the presenting part which should be clearly identified by the person placing the electrode. The inner tube is then rotated clockwise one full turn and this causes the electrode to turn in a similar manner with the sharp tip penetrating the fetal presenting part and continuing as a corkscrew for one turn to achieve retention qualities (Fig. 4.34). The wires are then attached to the leg plate which is usually placed on the mother's thigh with electrode paste to provide a common ground and help prevent electrical noise (Fig. 4.35). The leg plate is attached to the fetal monitor at the appropriate place.

If the signal is not clear, one should check to be sure the electrode is well attached, that the leg plate is appropriately grounded, and if available on that particular monitor, the leg plate circuit should be checked by plugging it into the check point on the monitor and running a test signal through it.

Precautions that should be taken when inserting an internal electrode include the following.

1. Use of sterile technique.

2. Do not attempt placement if you aren't sure of the exact site of placement.

3. Do not place over facial structure or fontanelle.

4. Avoid the genitalia in breech presentation.

5. Never try to reinsert an electrode by manually twisting because sometimes the spiral is stretched out and the depth of insertion may exceed the safe depth set on nonstretched electrodes.

When removing the electrode, simply twist the

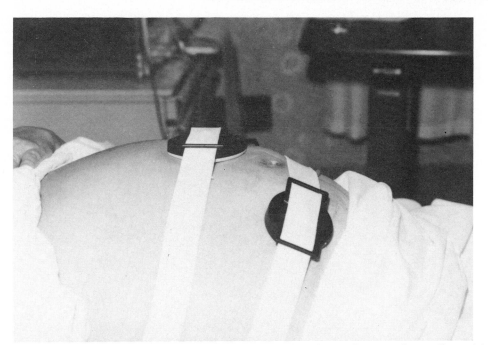

Figure 4.36. Patient with external tocodynomometer (*upper*) and Doppler transducer (*lower*) in place.

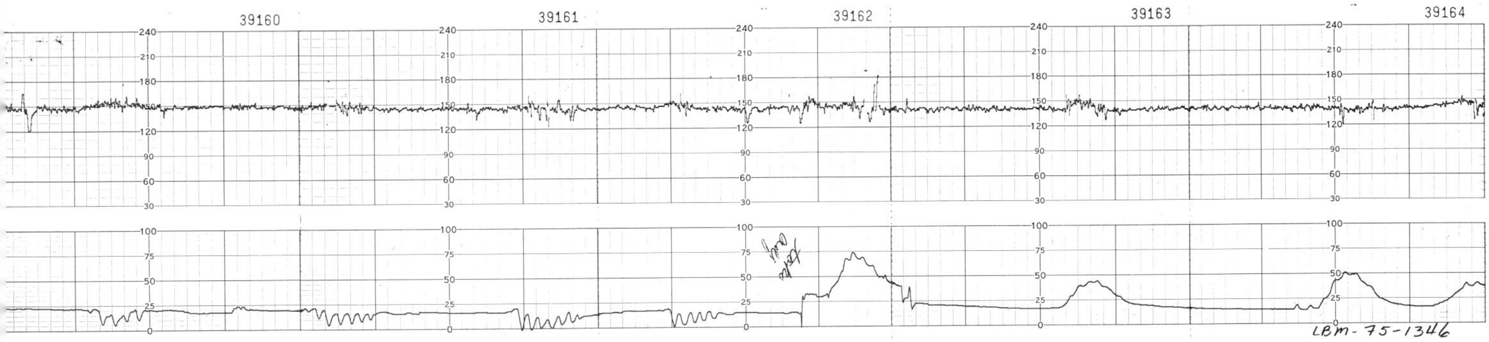

Figure 4.37. This tracing shows that contractions are evident only as irregular areas on the pressure tracing until the toco was adjusted and repositioned after which subsequent contraction recording is satisfactory.

wires counter clockwise. This can be done just before delivery or after delivery on the neonate. At cesarean section, the electrode should be removed just before delivery, and not left attached, and brought up through the wound. It's a good idea to cleanse the area of application on the baby's scalp after birth.

The Doppler Transducer

The Doppler transducer is usually secured to the patient with an elastic adjustable retaining strap that encircles the maternal abdomen. Selection of the optimum location for the transducer should include the following steps.

1. First place the retaining strap under the patient in supine position.

2. Place an adequate amount of ultrasonic coupling gel over the transducer face and apply to the maternal abdomen.

3. Begin searching for the strongest signal by lis-

tening with the monitor audio turned on. In cephalic presentation, this is usually found to be below the umbilicus in a term pregnancy, but with a breech it may be higher on the maternal abdomen.

4. When the optimal area is located, secure the transducer to the retaining strap and adjust for final placement at the location where the signal is clearest and the monitor is able to count well.

Because the Doppler transducer has a transmitter of ultrasonic signals as well as a receiver of the reflected signal, the exact angle of the transducer is very important. By the laws of physics, the beam is reflected from a moving interface where the angle of incidence equals the angle of reflection. Therefore the beam will only return to the transducer when it is arranged perpendicular to the moving interface. One can use this principle by tilting the transducer (Fig. 4.38) to get the optimal signal then moving it to a point where the tangential placement would allow reception of the reflected beam without transducer

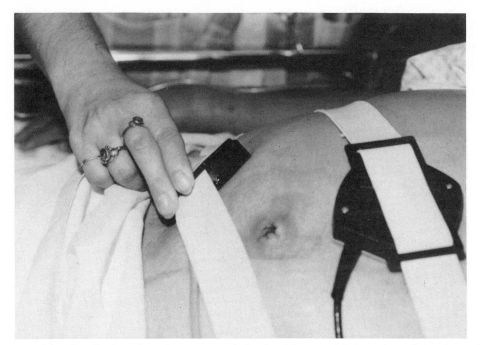

Figure 4.38. When searching for the best location to record the fetal heart with Doppler, often tilting the transducer will give a clue as to the direction to move for better recording.

tilt. Once the transducer placement is optimal, one must constantly recheck because if the fetus moves, or the mother changes position, the signal may be lost and the transducer may have to be repositioned.

The Phono Transducer

The phono transducer is applied similarly to the Doppler transducer but one should not use the coupling gel. The phono is much less directional than the Doppler but it is much more subject to extraneous noise. Ideally the patient should be monitored in a quiet area where extrinsic sounds will not interfere. One must be very careful not to let the patient's clothing or bed clothing touch the phono transducer because the rustling sound interferes with the recording. Today there are few if any situations where the phono offers significant advantage over the abdominal ECG and Doppler combination. Because of its great sensitivity to interference from outside sounds, the technique is not practical for patients in active labor and should be reserved for antepartum monitoring.

If one is using a phonosystem with manual gain control, one should adjust the gain so it is just adequate for counting because if the amplitude is increased above that point, the possibility for extrinsic sound interference becomes greater.

The Abdominal FECG Technique

The abdominal FECG technique requires three electrodes on the maternal abdomen or two on the maternal abdomen and a third on a maternal extrem-

ity. Two of the maternal abdominal electrodes pick up maternal and FECG signals and the maternal extremity electrode picks up the maternal ECG separately. This is then used in the logic circuits to determine when maternal-fetal ECG coincidence occurs, requiring compensation to be used.

The greatest problem with signal acquisition when using abdominal-fetal ECG signal sources is the signal-to-noise ratio. Since the abdominal FECG is of such low amplitude, the electrical resistance of the maternal abdominal skin may obscure the fetal signal in the ambient electrical noise. Therefore, it is very important to decrease maternal abdominal electrical skin resistance as much as possible. Many techniques have been advocated, including abrading the skin, degreasing the skin and rubbing in conductive electrode paste. We have found that abrading the skin is not as important as cleaning it carefully with alcohol to remove all grease and then rubbing in the paste. The excess paste should be removed before applying the electrode in order to promote adhesion of the electrode to the skin. The signal will usually improve with time as the electrode paste works its way into the skin. Before placing the abdominal electrodes, the leg electrode is secured by a strap around the mother's leg.

Usually the sites for the maternal abdominal electrodes will be suprapubic and infraumbilical in the midline (Fig. 4.39). However, one usually begins with suction electrodes that are movable until the optimal signal is found. Usually the suprapubic electrode is left stationery and the infraumbilical electrode is moved from side to side. The signal will usually be

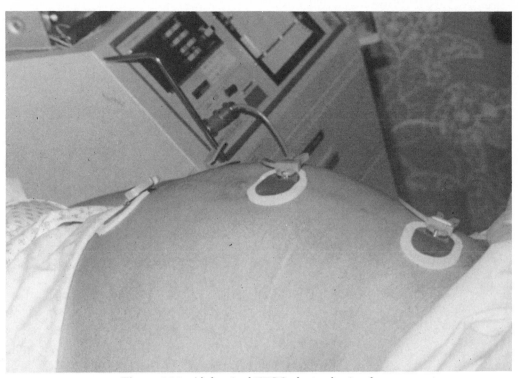

Figure 4.39. Abdominal FECG electrodes in place.

best if the infraumbilical electrode is moved to the side away from the fetal small parts.

Once the signal is found, the paste-on electrodes are put in place and monitoring is begun. Often slight tilt of the mother's position may improve a signal that is not optimal but one must use trial and error here.

POSSIBLE FUTURE APPROACHES TO FETAL MONITORING

Continuous Fetal Scalp pH Monitoring

In Chapter 7 on fetal acid base monitoring, the standard method described was intermittent fetal scalp blood sampling. As was pointed out, this method has several limitations that make its clinical applicability difficult. A summary of these problems follows. (1) Noncontinuous data; (2) difficult procedure; (3) scalp data may not reflect that from the central circulation; (4) risks of bleeding and infection; (5) influenced by maternal acid base status; (6) influenced by CO_2 retention.

The concept of continuous fetal pH assessment would only eliminate the first problem. However, this is probably the most serious limitation to the applicability of fetal pH monitoring. If one could have continuous data, it would be possible to make a very careful minute-to-minute assessment of fetal pH in patients with nonreassuring FHR patterns and also eliminate another related problem with pH monitoring which is the loss of time between sampling,

pH determination, repeat sampling for verification and clinical decision for intervention. Since there is a good theoretical advantage to the clinical use of continuous pH monitoring, we will include a discussion of the current state of the art of this approach, even though it is not yet clinically available at the time of this writing.[18, 19]

The principle involved in continuous fetal scalp pH monitoring is that a pH electrode imbedded into the fetal scalp tissue will reflect the acid base status of that fetus and allow the clinician to make an assessment of the degree of anaerobic glycolysis and lactic acid production that is occurring.

First it should be noted that this method is not measuring fetal blood pH per se, but it is measuring the pH of the subcutaneous tissue of the fetal scalp. Some say that the tissue pH may more accurately reflect the overall state of fetal oxygenation because the blood pH may only reflect the state of the circulation but not that of the perfused tissues. In addition, local pH in the fetal scalp may be influenced by both generalized peripheral vasoconstriction with poor tissue perfusion or local changes in tissue perfusion. When the fetus is becoming hypoxic, we know that initially there is an increase in alpha adrenergic activity with fetal hypertension. If this is true, the local tissues may develop acidosis more rapidly than the central circulation because of this phenomenon. Conversely, there may be a lag in recovery of local tissue pH levels as hypoxia is corrected for the same reason.

There is also the problem of local tissue injury at

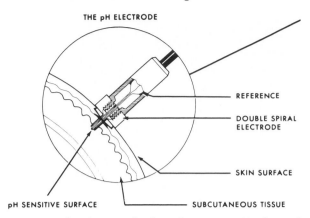

Figure 4.40. Continuous fetal scalp tissue pH electrode. (Reproduced with permission of Lauersen N, et al: Am J Obstet Gynecol 133:45, 1979.)

the site of the electrode, producing an acidotic reaction that may merely reflect this reaction to the technique. Since the standard for fetal pH monitoring is based on studies of fetal capillary blood pH from intermittent sampling, it seems that information relating the continuous scalp tissue pH to the fetal scalp capillary blood pH would be helpful as we learn to interpret the numbers produced.

At the time of this writing, there are numerous clinical trials involving a comparison of fetal scalp capillary pH, continuous fetal tissue pH and continuous FHR monitoring. Several studies have shown reasonably good correlation between continuous fetal tissue pH and continuous FHR monitoring. Several studies have also shown reasonably good correlation between continuous tissue pH and capillary blood pH, both in neonates and fetuses.[20–22] Unfortunately, most of the studies have few, if any, acidotic fetuses and it is this situation where the potential for error is the greatest, and of course it is where the correlation is the most important. Technically the method involves the application of a retaining device with a spiral electrode retention system. An incision is made into the fetal scalp through the retention ring, and the pH electrode is inserted through the ring and fixed in place with the electrode tip in the incised fetal scalp tissue (Fig. 4.40). Apparently, there is considerable skill involved in this maneuver as the success improves as any given investigator gains more experience.[23] Of concern is the fact that the glass electrode tip has broken off in the scalp on numerous occasions.[24] The FDA panel on monitoring devices has not yet released this device for general use because of issues involving safety and efficacy.

CONTINUOUS TRANSCUTANEOUS FETAL SCALP PO₂ MONITORING

Since the development of the transcutaneous pO_2 electrode by Huch et al.,[25] the monitoring of continuous transcutaneous pO_2 in neonates has enjoyed

generally good success. It has become obvious that intermittent pO_2 sampling from arterial or capillary sources in the neonate may often be quite misleading, and the fluctuation from minute-to-minute is so great that to be able to look at the continuous arterial pO_2 would be of much greater value. Studies correlating arterial pO_2 with transcutaneous pO_2 have shown close agreement, but in certain situations where there is a discrepancy between the circulatory pattern in the skin and in the central circulation, the potential exists for wide variations between the arterial and transcutaneous pO_2 values. One may ask, however, if low pO_2 values measured transcutaneously during peripheral vasoconstriction are misleading or if transcutaneous pO_2 values may actually give a better measurement of overall condition of the fetal organism because of this discrepancy during shock-like states.

Technically, the system is rather difficult to use in the fetus because the size of the electrode requires the cervix to be 4 to 5 cm dilated, the scalp hair must be shaved, and the device must be bonded to the fetal scalp with a glue-like substance. The electrode has a small heater surrounding it because the temperature of the skin is critical for an accurate measurement. The skin is heated to about 40 degrees centigrade. The temperature is controlled by a servo-control mechanism to very close tolerances. Interestingly, one can monitor the current being used to maintain the skin temperature and use this as a measure of the local circulation by the principle of heat dissipation.

There have only been limited studies of this technique but the results are very interesting in that it appears that the pO_2 system responds more rapidly to changes in the overall oxygen status of the fetus than does pH.[26] Clearly, since it is fetal oxygenation that we are most concerned with, this method offers the theoretical advantage over other monitoring methods of being the most specific. At the time of this writing, however, there is a great deal of work that must be done to gain enough experience with the method to learn its advantages, limitations, and risks. Application of the electrode will also probably have to be greatly simplified before it will have clinical value outside of research settings.

Fetal Breathing Movements

The development of diagnostic ultrasound gave rise to studies by Dawes and Boddy[27–29] involving fetal breathing movements. Originally they used only single dimensional, A-scan technique that was very difficult, but more recently the use of real time ultrasound has allowed the clinician to study fetal breathing movements much more easily.[30]

There have been a large number of studies reported where fetal breathing movements were characterized and correlated with various fetal states. Most investigators agree that fetal breathing movements are usually found a high percentage of the time in well fetuses. As a fetus deteriorates, the percent of time that fetal breathing can be seen decreases, and before fetal death fetal breathing movements are absent for varying periods of time. In acute distress and agonally, the fetus may make gasping movements that are clearly different from "normal" fetal breathing movements.

The actual clinical application of this technique has yet to gain wide use. Manning and Platt[31] have suggested that fetal breathing studies may help to distinguish between true and false positive contraction stress tests. However, FHR reactivity measurement appears to give similar information and is much easier to obtain.

At the time of this writing, fetal breathing measurements would have to be considered still experimental in nature. Larger clinical studies are necessary before the use of this technique can be fully evaluated.

As technology improves, there will undoubtedly be more sophisticated methods that will become available to the clinician interested in fetal assessment. The major task is to properly evaluate each new technology, test it clinically, and if it appears to be useful, to educate the clinician in its proper use and limitations.

FETAL SYSTOLIC TIME INTERVAL MONITORING

The electro-mechanical interval of the cardiac cycle is that time which elapses between initiation of the electrical impulse (ECG) and the beginning of mechanical activity. This period is also known as the isometric phase of the cardiac cycle because there is no motion during this interval. This interval may be influenced by a number of factors, including fetal condition. There has been very limited clinical work done with this approach which involves detecting the fetal ECG and the time of valve movement usually by ultrasonic techniques.[32-34] At the present time, instrumentation is not available that will continuously compute the electro-mechanical interval of the fetal heart but the possibility exists.

Murata et al.[35, 36] have shown very good correlation between the electro-mechanical interval and pH in animal fetuses, and for this reason the method should have great promise clinically when the instrumentation is developed to allow for continuous automated measurement.

Thus we can see that fetal monitoring technology is getting more and more sophisticated and complex. Certainly, we will be able to learn more about our intrauterine patient with future methods, but the main problem at present is to keep the clinician's knowledge of available equipment updated so that it may be used to maximal advantage for the patient.

REFERENCES

1. Klapholz H, Schifrin BS, Myrick R, et al: Role of maternal artifact in fetal heart rate pattern interpretation. Obstet Gynecol 44:373, 1974
2. Schneiderman C, Waxman B, Goodman C: Maternal fetal electrocardiogram conduction with intrapartum death. Am J Obstet Gynecol 113:1130, 1972
3. Lackritz R, Schiff I, Gibson M, et al: Decelerations on fetal electrocardiography with fetal demise. Obstet Gynecol 51:367, 1978
4. Cremer M: Munch Med Wochenschr 53:811, 1906
5. Larks SD, Dasgupta K: Fetal electrocardiography with special reference to early pregnancy. Am Heart J 56:701, 1958
6. Hon EH, Hess OW: The clinical value of fetal electrocardiography. Am J Obstet Gynecol 79:1012, 1960
7. Hon EH, Huang HS: The electronic evaluation of fetal heart rate. VII Premature and missed beats. Obstet Gynecol 20:81, 1962
8. Shenker, Lewis: Fetal cardiac arrhythmias. Obstet Gynecol Surv 34:561, 1979
9. Sugarman RG, Rawlinson KF, Schifrin BS: Fetal arrhythmia. Obstet Gynecol 52:301, 1978
10. Komaromy B, Gaal J, Lampe L: Fetal arrhythmia during pregnancy and labor. Br J Obstet Gynecol 84:492, 1977
11. Cetrulo C, Schifrin BS: Fetal heart rate patterns preceding death in utero. Obstet Gynecol 48:521, 1976
12. Heovall G: Congenital paroxysmal tachycardia; a report of three cases. Acta Paediat Scand 62:550, 1973
13. Klein A, Holzman I, Austin E: Fetal tachycardia prior to the development of hydrops—attempted pharmacologic cardioversion: case report. Am J Obstet Gynecol 134:347, 1979
14. Berube S, Lister G, Towes W, et al: Congenital heart block and maternal systemic lupus erythematosis. Am J Obstet Gynecol 130:595, 1978
15. Armstrong D, Murata Y, Martin C, et al: Antepartum selection of congenital complete heart block; a case report. Am J Obstet Gynecol 126:291, 1976
16. Platt L, Manning F, Craigan G, et al: Antenatal detection of fetal A-V dissociation utilizing real time B-mode ultrasound. Obstet Gynecol 53:595, 1979
17. Hon EH: Perinatal Factors Affecting Human Development. Pan American World Health Organization, Scientific Publications no 185, Washington, D.C., 1969, p 161
18. Stamm O, Latscha U, Janecek P, et al: Development of a special electrode for continuous subcutaneous pH measurement in the infant scalp. Am J Obstet Gynecol 124:193, 1976
19. Lumley J, Potter M, Nerman W, et al: The unreliability of a single estimation of fetal scalp blood pH. J Lab Clin Med 77: 535, 1971
20. Young B, Katz M, Klein S: The relationship of fetal heart rate patterns and tissue pH in the human fetus. Am J Obstet Gynecol 134:685, 1979
21. Sturbois G, Uzan S, Rotten D, et al: Continuous subcutaneous pH measurement in human fetuses. Am J Obstet Gynecol 128: 901, 1977
22. Young B, Noumoff J, Klein S, et al: Continuous tissue pH monitoring in the human fetus in labor. Obstet Gynecol 52:533, 1978
23. Lauerson JN, Miller FO, Paul R: Continuous intrapartum monitoring of fetal scalp pH. Am J Obstet Gynecol 133:411, 1979
24. Summary of Minutes of Fetal Monitoring Devices Subcommittee of the Obstetrical-Gynecological Device Classification Panel, F.D.A., Silver Spring, Maryland, March 8, 1977
25. Huch A, Huch R, Schneider H, et al: Continuous transcutaneous monitoring of fetal oxygen tension during labor. Br J Obstet Gynecol (Suppl) 84:1, 1977
26. Baxi LV, Petrie R, James LS: Human fetal oxygenation following paracervical block. Am J Obstet Gynecol 135:1109, 1979
27. Boddy K, Robinson JS: External method for detection of fetal

breathing in utero. Lancet 2:1231, 1971

28. Boddy K, Dawes GS: Fetal breathing. Br Med Bull 31:3, 1975

29. Dawes G, Fox H, Leduc B, et al: Respiratory movements and parodoxical sleep in the foetal lamb. J Physiol 210:478, 1970

30. Platt L, Manning F, Lemay M, et al: Human fetal breathing: relationship to fetal condition. Am J Obstet Gynecol 132:514, 1978

31. Manning F, Platt L: Fetal breathing movements and the abnormal contraction stress test. Am J Obstet Gynecol 133:590, 1979

32. Murata Y, Martin C: Systolic time intervals of the fetal cardiac cycle. Obstet Gynecol 44:224, 1974

33. Wolfson R, Zador I, Pillay S, et al: Antenatal investigation of human fetal systolic time intervals. Am J Obstet Gynecol 129: 203, 1977

34. Murata Y, Martin C, Ikenoue T, et al: Antepartum evaluation of the pre-ejection period of the fetal cardiac cycle. Am J Obstet Gynecol 132:278, 1978

35. Murata Y, Martin C, Ikenoue T, et al: Cardiac systolic intervals in fetal monkeys: pre-ejection period. Am J Obstet Gynecol. 132:285, 1978

36. Murata Y, Miyake K, Quilligan E: Pre-ejection of cardiac cycles in fetal lamb. Am J Obstet Gynecol 133:509, 1979

CHAPTER 5

Uterine Contraction Monitoring

It is interesting that in discussions on the benefits of fetal monitoring, uterine contraction monitoring is most often ignored. It is true that the development of fetal heart rate monitoring was aimed at detecting fetal distress and that contraction patterns were included so that the various decelerative patterns could be timed in relation to contractions. It became apparent, however, with the often routine use of monitors in labor, that one principle benefit of such routine monitoring was the data it provided relative to uterine activity.

Uterine activity may be assumed to be adequate if progress in labor, as defined by progressive cervical dilation and descent, is adequate. However, there arise the two other extremes. Failure to progress in labor may or may not be due to inadequate uterine contractions. On the other end, excessive uterine activity may be present, as in abruptio placentae, and cause inadequate placental perfusion, thus giving rise to fetal hypoxia. When it is necessary to induce or augment labor, one must be especially aware of uterine activity to reach an optimum of adequate stimulation without excessive activity, which could lead to fetal distress or even uterine rupture. Any of the above conditions require close monitoring of uterine contractions.

Manual palpation has been the traditional method of monitoring such contractions. This method can be used to measure contraction frequency and duration, but it can measure intensity only relatively. It is time consuming, requires constant attendance, and provides no permanent record. This process becomes so tedious that realistically what occurs in most cases, at best, is intermittent manual palpation for short intervals. Fortunately, the fetal monitor has provided us with a tool which can significantly improve our ability to monitor uterine contractions.

PHYSIOLOGY OF UTERINE CONTRACTIONS

Uterine contractions have as a primary function the expulsion of the intrauterine contents. Prior to the onset of active labor, however, there is also uterine activity for which the function may be preparation of the cervix for labor. Although it may serve this latter function, the uterus is a smooth-muscle organ under progressive stretch, and contractions may be a physiologic response to this stretch, perhaps dampened by the organism's physiologic mechanisms which normally inhibit the premature onset of labor. These preparatory contractions have been described by Caldeyro-Barcia and Poseiro[1] to occur in two types. The first are small, weak contractions of short duration, localized to isolated small areas of the uterus, occurring about once a minute. These begin in early pregnancy and seem to disappear near term. They may be related to or the same as localized periodic thickening of the uterine wall described by new ultrasound techniques.[2, 3] The other type of contractions are the better known Braxton-Hicks' contractions, which have a higher magnitude of strength (10 to 20 mm Hg), are more generalized, and have a frequency which increases from 1 contraction/hr at 30 weeks to every 5 to 10 min at term.[1] The transition into the regular rhythmical contractions of labor may be insidious or abrupt.

Contractions must be defined by their characteristics of frequency, duration, strength (amplitude), uniformity, and shape. During normal labor, the strength of contractions varies from an average of 30 mm Hg in early labor to 50 mm Hg in late first stage and 20 to 30 mm Hg more during second stage.[4] It must be realized that the uterus is not a flaccid sac but has the characteristic of baseline tone. At and near term, this baseline tone is generally 8 to 12 mm Hg, and values in excess of 15 to 20 mm Hg are defined as hypertonus (or, redundantly, baseline hypertonus).[4] The smaller nonpregnant uterus will generate very large uterine pressures, since according to the law of Laplace, at a given amount of work, the amount of intracavitary pressure is inversely proportional to the radius of the cavity. This is true for the uterus only to a point, however. With excessively large volumes, as in polyhydramnios, tonus may begin to rise because of excessive stretching of the muscle fibers.[5]

Once actual labor begins, contractions become more frequent, more coordinated, and stronger. The propagation of uterine contractions is the result of pacemaker-like activity originating usually from the area of the uterotubal junction, more often on the right. For the contraction to fulfill its purpose most efficiently, i.e., expulsion of the fetus via cervical dilation and fetal descent, the contraction must start in the fundus and progressively propagate towards the cervix. Reynolds et al.[6] described this as "fundal dominance," which, simply stated, says that because of the lesser curvature at the fundus and the greater muscle mass, the strength of contractions is greatest at the fundus and least at the cervix. Caldeyro-Barcia and Poseiro[1] further refined this description. They described a triple descending gradient of wave propagation, intensity, and duration, such that the origin of the contraction is in the fundus and the direction of the contractile wave is toward the cervix and that not only is the contraction more intense in the fundus

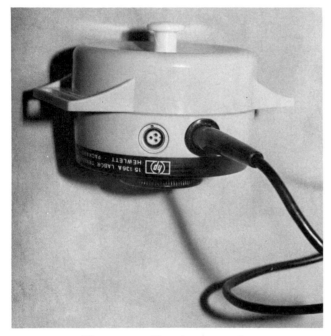

Figure 5.1. Tocodynamometer.

but also the duration of the contraction is progressively shorter from the fundus to midcorpus to cervix.

MONITORING OF UTERINE ACTIVITY

External Techniques

Contractions are most conveniently monitored externally with a tocodynamometer. Mechanical devices for monitoring contractions externally were introduced as early as 1861. Murphy[7] described a ring tocodynamometer, and subsequently, Reynolds et al.[8] used three such instruments on various portions of the uterus to describe normal contraction physiology. The tocodynamometer is essentially a weight with a centrally placed pressure-sensitive button, secured to the abdominal wall with a strap (Fig. 5.1). The "toco" is positioned near the fundus and adjusted to a position which records contractions best. A sensitivity adjustment, usually present on the "toco" is adjusted to place the resting pressure at 15 to 20 mm Hg to obtain the best tracing. It must always be remembered that the contraction strength is only relatively accurate and that it varies greatly with maternal position, relative obesity, and the tightness of the belt. These factors also affect the sensitivity of the recording, so that the apparent duration of the contraction will vary; the more sensitive the "toco," the longer the apparent contraction duration (Fig. 5.2). The frequency is, therefore, most accurately recorded externally; the duration, less accurately; and the intensity, least accurately.

The external technique has the advantages of being noninvasive, thus being applicable to patients with intact membranes. This allows application to the antepartum patient, the patient in premature labor, or the patient during the early intrapartum period. There are, however, disadvantages. Patient mobility is limited. The best tracings are obtained in the supine position, thus causing nurses and physicians to encourage laboring in this less desirable position. Gen-

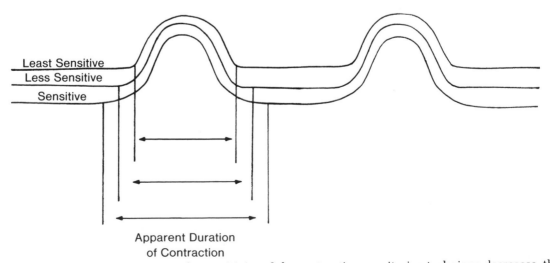

Least Sensitive
Less Sensitive
Sensitive

Apparent Duration
of Contraction

Figure 5.2. This drawing illustrates that as the sensitivity of the contraction monitoring technique decreases, the apparent duration of the contraction shortens.

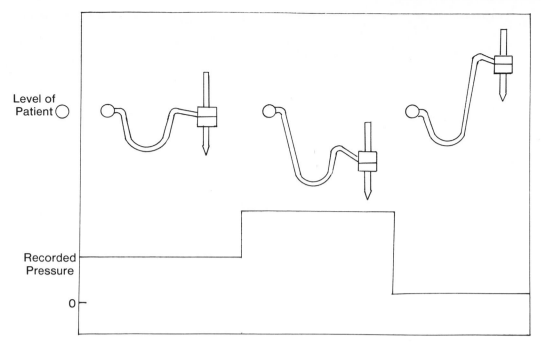

Level of
Patient ◯

Recorded
Pressure

0

Figure 5.3. Illustration of the effect of the relative height of the pressure transducer to that of the patient on the recorded pressure. If the transducer is below the patient, the recording is artifactually elevated, and if the transducer is above the patient, the pressure recording will be low.

erally, external monitors are more uncomfortable for the patient. Some obese patients give poor to nonexistent tracings. The limitations with regard to intensity and duration have been discussed. At times, when fetal heart rate patterns consistent with fetal distress occur and position is changed, loss of a previously good contraction tracing results, thus making decelerations difficult to time.

Internal Monitoring

According to the law of Pascal, if a closed spheroid is fluid filled, pressure is equal at all points. This describes the uterus quite well, and therefore, the pregnant uterus is ideal for contraction pressure monitoring. As early as 1872, Schatz[9] used a hydrostatic bag in the lower uterine segment after membranes had ruptured, for pressure recording. Bourne and Burn,[10] in 1927, used the hydrostatic bag extraovularly (between the membranes and the lower uterine segment). Alvarez and Caldeyro-Barcia[4] described a transabdominal technique for inserting open fluid-filled catheters in the amniotic cavity for recording contractions. Other techniques described include electrohysterography and intramyometrial pressure recording. In 1952, Williams and Stallworthy[9] suggested the use of a Drew-Smythe metal cannula (originally designed for high amniotomy) as a guide to introduce a polyethylene tubing transcervically into the amniotic cavity. This then was the forerunner for the technique now commonly used for internal contraction monitoring.

Currently, sterile disposable kits are available with flexible plastic catheters and guides for internal contraction monitoring. The details of insertion, instru-

mentation, and calibration are described in Chapter 4. This method can be used to describe and record accurately the frequency, duration, strength, and tonus of the uterus and its contractions. It is less confining and uncomfortable for the patient and is unaffected by position except as contraction pressures actually change with position change. The pressure recording is only accurate if the level of the catheter tip is at the level of the transducer. Raising the tip above the level of the transducer will raise the pressure artifactually, and if the transducer is above the catheter tip, the reading will be inaccurately low (Fig. 5.3).

One must wait for membrane rupture or perform amniotomy to use commonly available internal techniques. On the use of this technique, the literature is somewhat controversial, but certainly there is some suggestion that internal monitoring is associated with an increased risk of infection. Uterine perforation has been described but is usually caused by insertion of the less flexible insertion guide. For avoidance of this complication, the guide should never be inserted more than 1 cm beyond the fingertips. Finally, for the patient there is discomfort associated with introduction of the catheter. The alternative to electronic contraction monitoring is manual palpation or the patient's sensation. Caldeyro-Barcia and Poseiro[1] have said the contractions are palpable to the examiner at a minimum pressure of 10 mm Hg and that the patient senses the pain of contractions at a minimum of 15 mm Hg. As with external monitoring, palpation and patient sensation will be reliable with regard to frequency but will be less so for duration and intensity (Fig. 5.4).

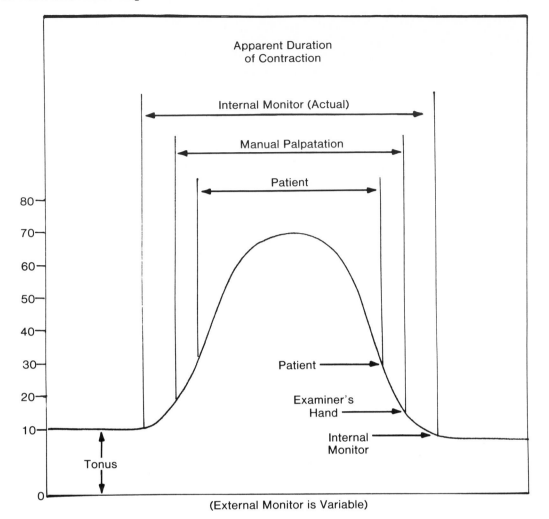

Figure 5.4. Relative sensitivity of various methods available to detect uterine contractions.

Quantitation of Uterine Activity

For many reasons, it may be important actually to quantitate the amount of uterine activity per unit time. The most practical reason would be to determine whether uterine contractions are sufficient in evaluating poor progress in labor. Because failure to progress in a clinically adequate pelvis is an indication for oxytocin if contractions are deemed inadequate and because one is going to try to achieve adequate forces, one must define adequacy. In 1957, Caldeyro-Barcia et al.[5] defined the "Montevideo unit." This unit is defined as the product of the average amplitude (in mm Hg) multiplied by the number of contractions in 10 minutes. Shifrin[11] has defined adequate uterine activity in labor to be greater than 200 Montevideo units. This has been the most extensively used quantitation measure by investigators. It does have the limitation of not including duration of contractions in its calculation. El-Sahwi et al.[12] defined the "Alexandria unit" to overcome this problem, which unit is the average amplitude (in mm Hg) multiplied by the average duration (in minutes) multiplied by the average number of contractions in 10 minutes. Both of these methods

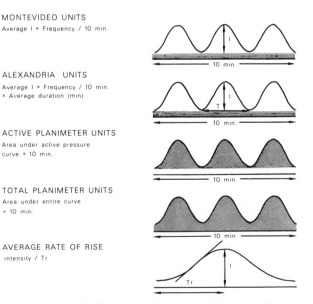

Figure 5.5. Available methods for quantitation of uterine activity. (Reprinted with permission from Reference 13.)

are very time consuming. Miller et al.[13] have described a computerized method of quantitating uterine activity by integrating the entire area under the curve (Fig. 5.5).

Besides inadequate uterine activity, problems may occur with abnormal rhythmicity or excessive uterine activity. These may occur spontaneously, as a result of abnormal pregnancy as in hydramnios, abruptions, or preeclampsia, or with excess oxytocin stimulation. The terminology, which is not universally agreed upon, is described in Fig. 5.6.

There are two characteristics of these nonsynchronous abnormal contraction patterns. The first is their effect on the progress in labor. This will depend on cause. Some may be noted with protracted active phases of labor or secondary arrest of labor.[14] In these cases, the patterns may be a result rather than a cause of abnormal labor. Other causes may include injudicious oxytocin administration, polyhydramnios, and abruption in which case the effect of these contraction patterns on labor may be to shorten it,

although, generally, this is unpredictable. The other consideration is the effect that these contraction patterns may have on intervillous blood flow, fetal oxygenation, and fetal heart rate. Intramyometrial pressure usually is about 2 to 3 times that of intraamniotic pressure. Mean maternal arterial pressure is about 85 to 90 mm Hg in labor. Therefore, the duration of contractions of intraamniotic pressure exceeding 30 to 40 mm Hg (corresponding to myometrial pressures in excess of mean arterial pressure) determines how long the maternal spiral arteries are compressed and, therefore, how long freshly oxygenated blood will not be getting to the intervillous space. Another important aspect is how much relaxation time is available for recovery. The effects that these contraction patterns may have on the fetus are perhaps most immediately reflected in heart rate and may be manifest by increased variability, delayed (late) decelerations, or prolonged decelerations (Fig. 5.7). Shenker[15] has suggested that the most frequent cause of late decelerations is excessive uterine activity. If these excessive contractions and their resultant fetal hypoxia are prolonged, fetal acidemia may result, manifesting in decreased variability and fetal tachycardia.

OTHER FACTORS AFFECTING UTERINE CONTRACTIONS

To understand and correct abnormal contraction patterns and heart rate reactions to them, one must be aware of the common factors, both intrinsic and extrinsic, which affect uterine contractility. The factors may manifest by decreasing or increasing contraction strength and/or frequency. Intrinsic factors include pathologic state and maternal position. The most common diseases that alter uterine contractions include polyhydramnios, preeclampsia, and abruption. Abruption usually causes the greatest degree of hyperactivity (Fig. 5.8). Polysystole, tachysystole, hypertonus, or any form of hyperactivity may be seen. In abruptio placentae, it may be the uterine hyperactivity, the loss of placental surface area, or both, which results in the fetal distress which is often seen. In preeclampsia and eclampsia, Alvarez et al.[16] have

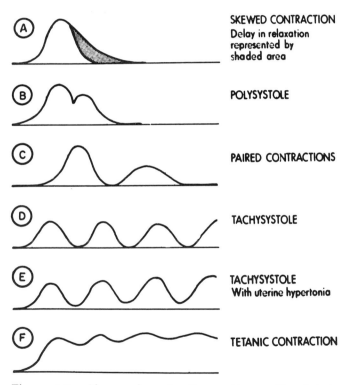

Figure 5.6. Abnormal contraction patterns. (Reprinted with permission from Reference 14.)

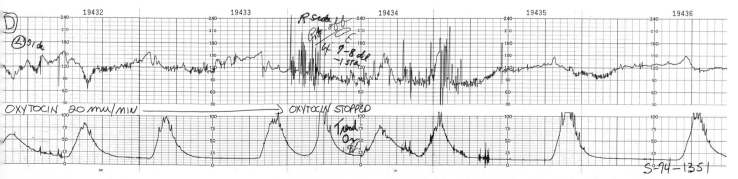

Figure 5.7. Note the prolonged deceleration of the fetal heart rate associated with oxytocin hyperstimulation. As commonly occurs, a period of late decelerations and some decrease in fetal heart rate variability is seen following the prolonged deceleration.

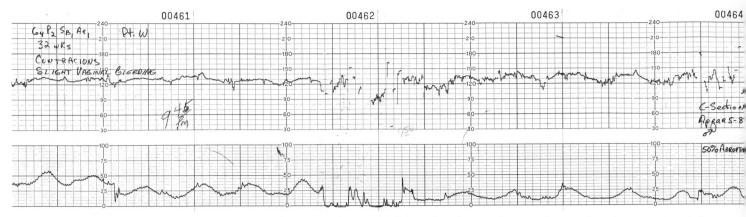

Figure 5.8.   This is an example of uterine hyperactivity in the form of tachysystole, seen in a patient in premature labor with vaginal bleeding. In this case, it is very difficult to interpret the occurrence of late decelerations. Both fetal heart rate and contractions are being monitored externally. The cause of uterine hyperactivity and late decelerations was a 50% abruptio placentae.

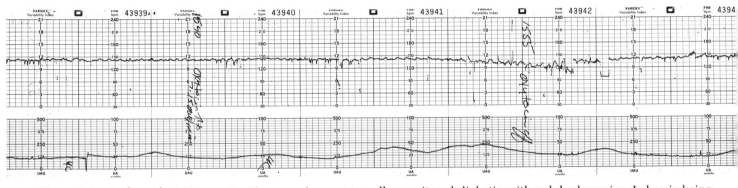

Figure 5.9.   Prolonged uterine contraction seen in an externally monitored diabetic with polyhydramnios. Labor is being augmented with oxytocin, and such prolonged contractions in response to oxytocin are commonly seen with polyhydramnios.

pointed out that uterine tonus is unaffected but that frequency and intensity of contractions are often increased. Polyhydramnios has a variable effect on tonus; until the uterus is severely stretched, baseline tone is often low to low normal, but as the condition worsens, a hypertonus may develop. Uterine contractions often are quite prolonged with hydramnios (Fig. 5.9).

Position has a relatively consistent effect on uterine activity. It is clear that uteroplacental perfusion is poorer in the supine position than in either lateral position. Caldeyro-Barcia et al.[17] have shown that generally, when the patient is turned from her back to her side, contractions become stronger and less frequent (Fig. 5.10). Finally, maternal pushing efforts during labor are commonly seen on contraction tracings and can add 20 mm Hg or more to the recorded intensity of contractions. They are usually seen as rapid, brief elevations of intrauterine pressure superimposed on the uterine contraction (Fig. 5.11).

Many extrinsic factors may affect uterine contractions. There has always been conjecture and debate as to whether oxytocin reproduces a physiologic con-

traction pattern. Much of this debate stems from the fact that many clinicians use dose rates far in excess of physiologic values. Caldeyro-Barcia et al.[18, 19] and Poseiro and Noriega-Guerra[20] have shown that oxytocin both accelerates and coordinates uterine contractions and that at physiologic doses of 1 to 8 m-units/min, this occurs without elevation of tonus. These studies have shown no difference between contractions, with or without oxytocin, with data from intraamniotic pressure, intramyometrial pressure, and electrohysterography. Alvarez and Cibils[21] have shown that both types of contractions have equivalent efficiency in producing cervical dilation. When doses of oxytocin exceed physiologic requirements, however, all forms of hyperactivity as well as hypertonus can be seen. Many other drugs affect uterine activity. The more common ones are listed in Table 1.

SUMMARY

The study of fetal monitoring is incomplete without detailed knowledge of uterine activity and its effects

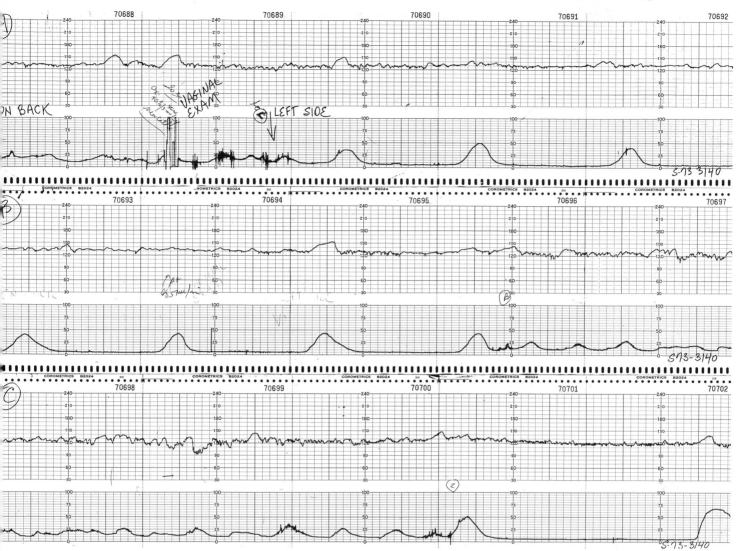

Figure 5.10. On *panel A*, frequent uterine contractions are occurring. When the patient is turned to her left side, the contractions become less frequent and increase in strength. The patient has turned and is lying on her back in *panel B*, and the contractions have become frequent and smaller. Finally, again on her left side in *panel C*, the contractions are spaced out as before in *panel A*.

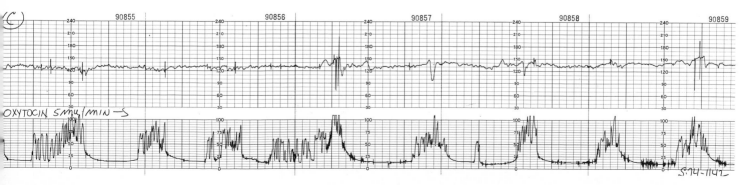

Figure 5.11. Small spikes (intermittent short elevations of pressure) seen on top of uterine contractions represent maternal pushing.

Table 5.1.
Drugs Affecting Uterine Contractions

Stimulating Drugs
  Acetylcholine
  Ergonovine
  Estrogen
  Meperidine (Demerol)
  Norepinephrine
  Oxytocin
  Propranalol
  Prostaglandins
  Quinine
  Sparteine Sulfate
  Vasopressin
Inhibiting Drugs
  Beta Sympathomimetics
    Ritodrine, Orciprenaline, Isoxsuprine, Salbutamol, Fenoterol,
    Epinephrine, etc.
  Diazoxide
  Ethanol
  Halothane
  Magnesium Sulfate
  Progesterone
  Prostaglandin Inhibitors

on fetal oxygenation and heart rate. Most periodic changes in the fetal heart rate occur at or after the time of the uterine contraction. The intent of this chapter has been to describe the details of contraction monitoring and the physiologic mechanisms of labor so that the student might better be able to integrate this knowledge and understand the physiologic and pathophysiologic basis of fetal monitoring.

References

1. Caldeyro-Barcia R, Poseiro JJ: Physiology of the uterine contraction. Clin Obstet Gynecol 3:386, 1960
2. Sample WF: The unsoftened portion of the uterus. Radiology 126:227, 1978
3. Buttery B, Davison G: The dynamic uterus revealed by time lapse echography. J Clin Ultrasound 6:19, 1978
4. Alvarez H, Caldeyro-Barcia R: Contractility of the human uterus recorded by new methods. Surg Gynecol Obstet 91:1, 1950
5. Caldeyro-Barcia R, Pose SV, Alvarez H: Uterine contractility in polyhydramnios and the effects of the withdrawal of the excess of amniotic fluid. Am J Obstet Gynecol 73:1238, 1957
6. Reynolds SRM, Hellman LM, Bruns P: Patterns of uterine contractility in women during pregnancy. Obstet Gynecol Surv 3:629, 1948
7. Murphy D: Uterine Contractility. New York, Lippincott, 1947
8. Reynolds SRM, Heard OO, Bruns P: Recording uterine contraction patterns in pregnant women; applications of strain gauge in multi-channel tokodynamometer. Science 106:427, 1947
9. Williams EA, Stallworthy JA: A simple method of internal tocography. Lancet 330, 1952
10. Bourne AW, Burn JH: Dosage and action of pituitary extract in labour with note on action of adrenalin. J Obstet Gynecol Br Emp 34:249, 1927
11. Schifrin BS: The case against pelvimetry. Contemp Obstet Gynecol 4:77, 1974
12. El-Sahwi S, Gaafar A, Toppozada HK: A new unit for evaluation of uterine activity. Am J Obstet Gynecol 98:900, 1967
13. Miller FC, Yeh SY, Schifrin BS, et al: Quantitation of uterine activity in 100 primiparous patients. Am J Obstet Gynecol 124:398, 1976
14. Stookey RA, Sokol RJ, Rosen MJ: Abnormal contraction patterns in patients monitored during labor. Obstet Gynecol 42:359, 1973
15. Shenker L: Clinical experience with fetal heart rate monitoring of 1000 patients in labor, Am J Obstet Gynecol 115:1111, 1973
16. Alvarez H, Pose SV, Caldeyro-Barcia R: La contractilidad uterina en la toxemia gravidica. Proc First Peruv Cong Obstet Gynecol 2:281, 1959
17. Caldeyro-Barcia R, Noriega-Guerra L, Cibils LA, et al: Effects of position change on the intensity and frequency of uterine contractions during labor. Am J Obstet Gynecol 80:284, 1960
18. Caldeyro-Barcia R, Sica-Blanco Y, Poseiro JJ, et al: A quantitative study of the action of synthetic oxytocin on the pregnant human uterus. J Pharmacol Exp Ther 121:18, 1957
19. Caldeyro-Barcia R, Poseiro JJ: Oxytocin and contractility of the human pregnant uterus. Ann NY Acad Sci 75:813, 1959
20. Poseiro JJ, Noriega-Guerra L: Dose response relationships in uterine effect of oxytocin infusion. In: Oxytocin. London, Pergamon Press, 1960
21. Alvarez H, Cibils LA: Cervical dilation and uterine work in labor induced with oxytocin. In: Oxytocin. London, Pergamon Press, 1960

CHAPTER 6

Basic Pattern Recognition

INTRODUCTION

The evaluation of the fetus in labor by electronic heart rate monitoring is a complex process. In determining if the pattern is reassuring or nonreassuring and what must be done, many factors must be evaluated. The fetal heart rate is evaluated for baseline rate, variability, accelerations, decelerations, and the progression of each. Contraction frequency and strength must be considered. The parity of the patient, her rate of progress in labor, and an estimate of the anticipated time of delivery, as well as maternal and obstetrical complications, all go into this rather complex equation.

Fetal heart rate monitoring has been found to be a difficult technique to which to apply mathematical or computer means for quantitating various parameters of fetal well being. Basically, this is because it is a study of pattern recognition; a process of evaluating multiple variables and determining from them the status of fetal oxygenation. With the basic understanding of the physiology and technology of electronic fetal heart rate monitoring behind us, this chapter will be devoted to basic pattern recognition.

Patient Information

A label is placed on the first page of the tracing for record identification and for future teaching and/or discussion purposes. One such label is shown in Figure 6.1. Should monitoring extend beyond one pack of paper, they are labeled as Part 1, 2, 3, etc. Monitors are numerically identified and tracings are labeled accordingly for several reasons. Should a technical problem occur it can be traced to the correct monitor. Also, certain monitors have different logic characteristics and should a hospital have various makes and models, one can better interpret the tracing.

BASELINE FETAL HEART RATE

The normal baseline fetal heart rate range is from 120 to 160 beats per minute (BPM). Changes of the

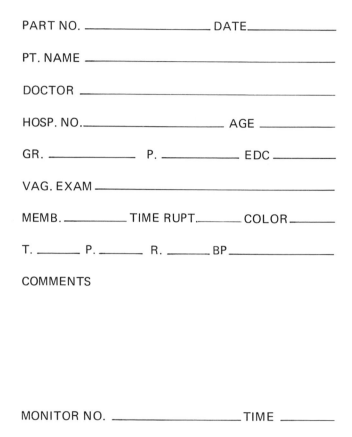

PART NO. _____ DATE _____

PT. NAME _____

DOCTOR _____

HOSP. NO. _____ AGE _____

GR. _____ P. _____ EDC _____

VAG. EXAM _____

MEMB. _____ TIME RUPT. _____ COLOR _____

T. _____ P. _____ R. _____ BP _____

COMMENTS

MONITOR NO. _____ TIME _____

Figure 6.1. Patient identification label placed on first page of fetal monitor tracing.

fetal heart rate that are considered baseline changes rather than periodic changes are those which last more than 15 min.

Fetal Tachycardia

This is defined as a baseline heart rate in excess of 160 BPM. Factors associated with or causing tachycardia are listed in Table 6.1. Since tachycardias represent increased sympathetic and decreased parasympathetic autonomic tone, there is generally a loss of variability associated with fetal tachycardias (Fig. 6.2).

Fetal Brachycardia.

Heart rates of less than 120 BPM are called bradycardias. A baseline fetal heart rate below 120 BPM with good variability is nearly always benign (Fig. 6.3). Fetal bradycardia first noted at the initiation of monitoring may be difficult to distinguish from a prolonged deceleration. Generally prolonged decelerations are associated with loss of variability. Baseline fetal heart rates of less than 70 BPM are generally seen without variability and may represent congenital complete heart block which is associated with a high incidence of congenital heart disease.[1] Mild degrees of baseline bradycardia are often seen in the second stage of labor. When fetal bradycardia occurs in the second stage it is generally reassuring if variability is maintained and the heart rate does not fall below 80 to 90 BPM.

Variability

The most important single fetal heart rate characteristic in predicting the status of the fetus at any given point is heart rate variability. The variability is a reflection of intact or normal neurologic modulation of the fetal heart rate and intact or normal cardiac responsiveness. There are two components of fetal heart rate variability—short-term and long-term variability (Fig. 6.4). Short-term variability is the beat to beat irregularity caused by the normal variance in intervals of cardiac electrical cycles. It is a consequence of the "push-pull" effect of sympathetic and parasympathetic nervous input. Long-term variability is the waviness of the fetal heart rate tracing. It generally has a frequency of 3 to 5 cycles/min. Fetal heart rate variability can only be accurately determined by direct fetal electrocardiogram (FECG) monitoring. Doppler external monitoring artifactually increases fetal heart rate variability due to the imprecision of the signal. With newer ultrasound/Doppler signals, however, long-term variability can often be fairly accurately assessed. Variability may become abnormal either by becoming increased or decreased. Increased variability has recently been shown to the earliest fetal heart rate sign of mild hypoxia.[2] As such, it is often seen early in the development of late

Table 6.1.
Causes of Fetal Tachycardia

Fetal Hypoxia
Maternal Fever
Parasympatholytic Drugs
Atropine
Vistaril/Atarax
Phenothiazines
Maternal Hyperthyroidism
Fetal Anemia
Fetal Heart Failure
Amnionitis
Fetal Cardiac Tachyarrhythmia
Beta-Sympathomimetic Drugs

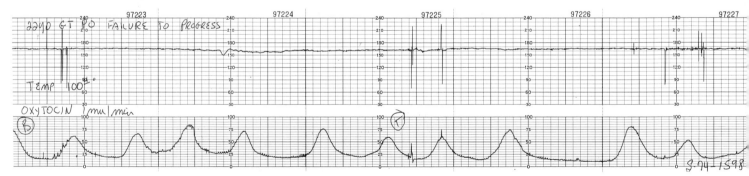

Figure 6.2. Fetal tachycardia, fetal heart rate 165 BPM. This tachycardia is associated with maternal fever (note temperature). Also note the associated loss of variability. The absence of associated decelerations and presence of an explanation (fever) makes hypoxia an unlikely cause.

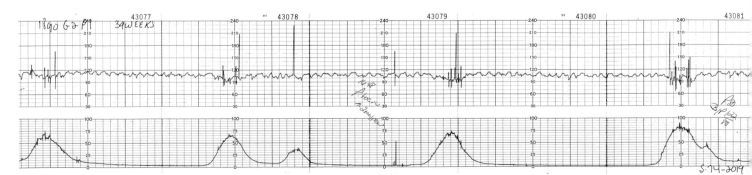

Figure 6.3. Fetal bradycardia. The heart rate is 110. There is normal variability present by direct (internal scalp electrode) monitoring. Four hours later, the patient delivered a 3025-g baby with Apgars 9 at 1 min and 10 at 5 min. Mother and baby did well.

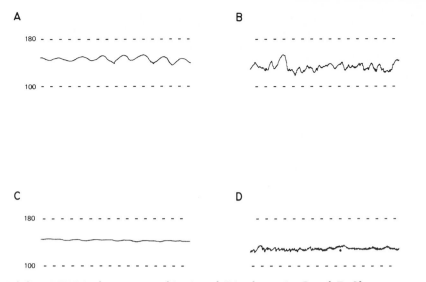

Figure 6.4. Long-term variability (LTV) is demonstrated in **A** and **B** is absent in **C** and **D**. Short-term variability (STV) alone is shown in **D** and its concurrent presence with LTV is shown in **B**. Absence of both LTV and STV is seen in **C**. (Reproduced with permission from Zanini B, et al: Am J Obstet Gynecol: 136:44, 1980.

Table 6.2.
Examples of Drugs Causing Decreased Fetal Heart Rate Variability

CNS Depressants
Analgesic/Narcotics
Demerol
Nisentil
Morphine
Barbiturates
Phenobarbital
Secobarbital
Tranquilizers
Diazepam
Phenothiazines
Largon
Phenergan
Parasympatholytics
Phenothiazines
Atropine
General Anesthetics

decelerations. When heart rate variability is normal or increased, fetal pH is probably normal. Decreased variability is generally seen with anything which causes fetal central nervous system (CNS) depression. As such, hypoxia/asphyxia is the most worrisome cause. However, any other condition that depresses the CNS will also decrease variability. Drugs are a common cause of decreased variability (Table 6.2). Two groups of drugs are known to cause decreased variability—those that cause CNS depression (Fig. 6.5) and those that have autonomic blocking effects. Parasympathetic blocking drugs decrease variability while increasing baseline heart rate. Sympatholytic drugs decrease variability while dropping heart rate.

Baseline heart rate variability also seems to be associated with fetal wakefullness. When the fetus is "asleep," there is decreased variability. This is often seen in labor with fetal sleep/wake cycles occurring in 20- to 30-min periods (Fig. 6.6). When fetal heart rate variability spontaneously decreases in labor but returns after a reasonable period of time, it is a benign finding. Stimulation of the fetus by manipulation of the uterus or noise may arouse the fetus and cause the variability to return.

The most ominous cause of decreased variability is fetal hypoxia/asphyxia. Generally, there are associated decelerations preceding the loss of variability. In the presence of nonreassuring heart rate patterns, such as persistent late decelerations, loss of variability is associated with a high incidence of fetal acidosis and low Apgar scores[3] (Fig. 6.7). A most difficult heart rate pattern to interpret is the persistently flat baseline (absent variability) seen in the fetus with a normal heart rate level and no decelerations. This may represent a previous insult to the fetus that has since been corrected but has caused neurologic damage. It may be seen in fetuses with significant congenital anomalies, especially of the central nervous and cardiac systems[4] or in extreme prematurity; or it may be idiopathic and be seen with a subsequently vigorous and healthy neonate. Table 6.3 is a list of the causes of decreased variability. It is important to emphasize that external monitors may mask poor variability (Fig. 6.8). However, if poor variability is seen on an external monitor, it is at least that bad and possibly worse.

PERIODIC CHANGES

Tachycardia, bradycardia, and alterations in variability are changes of the baseline fetal heart rate. Periodic changes are transient accelerations or decelerations of the heart rate of brief duration with return to the original baseline heart rate. Generally, these

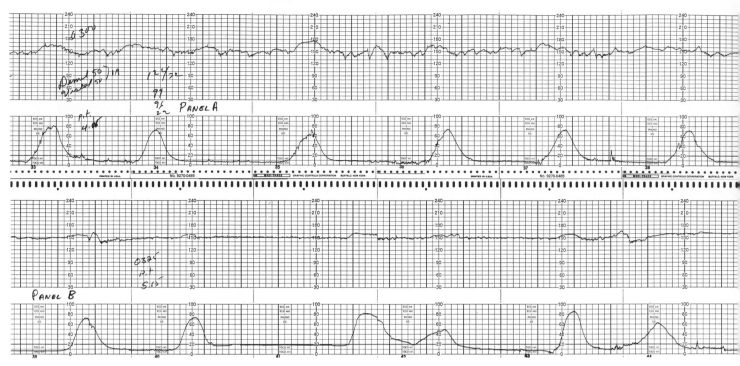

Figure 6.5. Narcotics are among the most frequent causes of decreased fetal heart rate variability in labor. In *A*, Demerol and Vistaril are given intramuscularly. At the beginning of *B*, about 20 min later, there is a noticeable decrease in variability without a change in baseline heart rate.

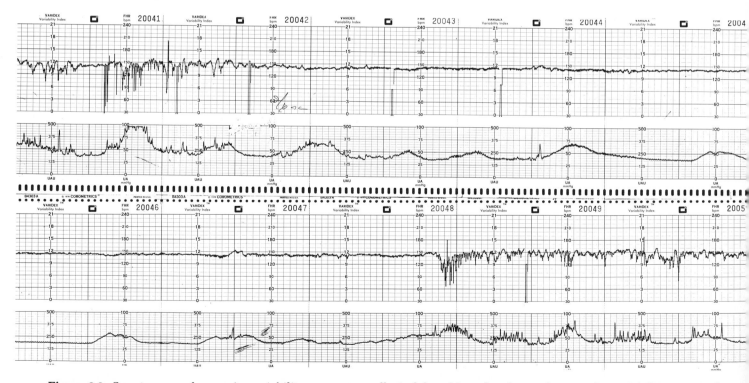

Figure 6.6. Spontaneous changes in variability occur normally in labor. Note the abrupt decrease in variability at *panel 20042* which again abruptly returns to normal at *panel 20048*. This decreased variability lasted 23 min. There were no medications used. A vigorous normal baby was subsequently delivered.

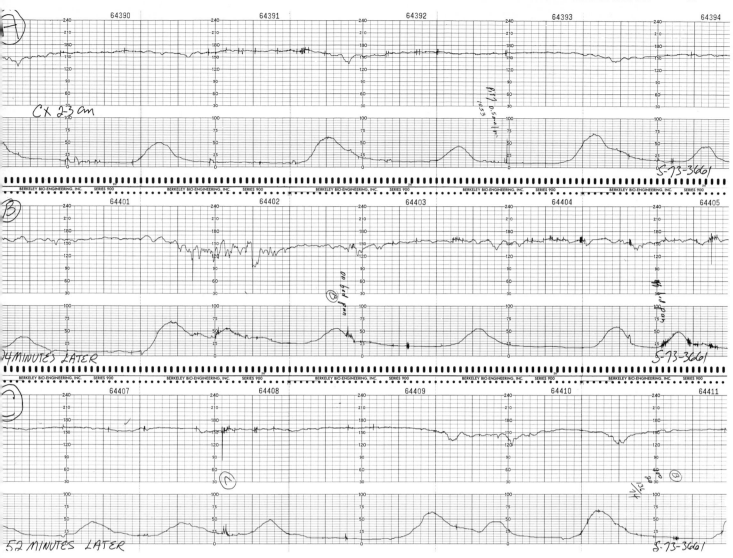

Figure 6.7. Persistent late decelerations are seen after most contractions. At **64407** and after, variability is notably decreased. There is an associated fetal tachycardia.

Table 6.3.
Causes of Decreased Fetal Heart Rate Variability

Hypoxia/Acidosis
Drugs
  CNS Depressants
  Parasympatholytics
Fetal Sleep Cycles
Congenital Anomalies
Extreme Prematurity
Fetal Tachycardia

periodic changes occur in response to contractions and are also seen in association with fetal movement.

DECELERATIONS

There are three principal types of deceleration named according to shape and temporal relationship to contractions. These are named early, late, and variable decelerations, and each represents a single basic pathophysiologic mechanism.

Early Decelerations

Early decelerations are uniform "U" shaped decelerations of slow onset and slow return to baseline (Fig. 6.9). They begin early in the uterine contraction cycle, have their nadir at the peak of the contraction and return to baseline before completion of the contraction. Acceleration of the heart rate generally does not precede or follow early deceleration. An important characteristic of early deceleration is the minimal amplitude. The degree of fetal heart rate slowing is generally proportional to the strength of the contraction but rarely falls below 100 to 110 or 20 to 30 BPM below baseline. Early decelerations are caused by fetal head compression and the altered cerebral blood flow causes cardiac slowing through a vagal reflex, thus may be eliminated with atropine. Early deceleration is generally seen in the early active phase of labor between 4 and 7 cm of cervical dilatation. It is not associated with tachycardia, loss of

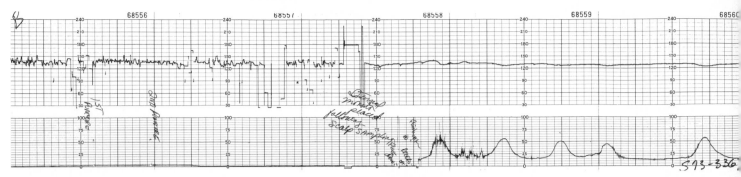

Figure 6.8. External Doppler ultrasound monitors may artifactally increase variability and mask smooth heart rates. Here with apparently normal variability on external monitoring, a flat (markedly decreased variability) heart rate is seen when direct monitoring is used.

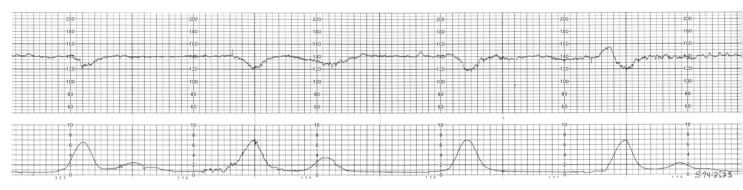

Figure 6.9. Early decelerations are seen with each contraction on this *panel.* They are uniform, mirror the contractions and decelerate only 10 to 20 BPM.

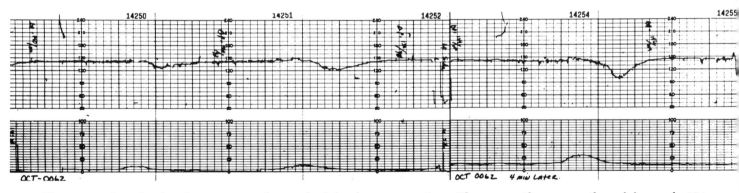

Figure 6.10. Late decelerations are seen after each of the three contractions. They are uniform, smooth, and drop only 20 to 30 BPM below baseline. There are no associated accelerations.

variability, or other heart rate changes. Early deceleration is a reassuring fetal heart rate pattern, not associated with fetal hypoxia, acidosis or low Apgar scores.

Late Decelerations

In shape and uniformity, late decelerations are similar to early decelerations, but the timing is delayed relative to the uterine contraction (Fig. 6.10). The onset of deceleration is usually seen 30 sec or more after the onset of the contraction; the nadir of the deceleration occurs well after the contraction peak; and usually the return to baseline occurs after the contraction is over. In recognizing late decelerations, several important characteristics in addition to

the timing are important. The descent and return are gradual and smooth. There are usually no accelerations seen preceding or following the deceleration. When late decelerations follow accelerations they are of questionable significance. The fetal heart rate rarely falls more than 30 to 40 BPM below baseline and usually not more than 10 to 20 BPM. Late decelerations are nearly always repetitive after each contraction. Often, variability is increased during the deceleration. Late decelerations are caused by fetal hypoxia usually from inadequate exchange within the placenta which is provoked by the uterine contraction. Therefore, late decelerations are proportional to the duration and strength of the contractions and often will be seen with the stronger contractions

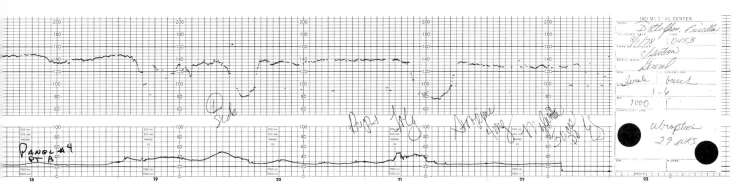

Figure 6.11. Late decelerations are seen occasionally only with the stronger contractions. In this *panel*, late decelerations are seen only with those contractions which exceed 70 mm Hg (internal pressure catheter and electrode).

Figure 6.12. Deep late decelerations are seen after each contraction on this externally monitored patient, a 29-week gestation admitted with vaginal bleeding. At ceasarean section, a large abruption was found subsequent to delivering an Apgar 1 at 1 min and 6 at 5 min, 1000-g female who survived.

and be absent with the weaker ones (Fig. 6.11). Also, the amplitude of the deceleration will usually be proportional to the pressure of the uterine contraction. There is generally a correlation between the magnitude of late decelerations (amount of slowing) and the degree of hypoxia, but occasionally the most depressed fetuses will have only shallow late decelerations. While not uniformly accepted, we will not use the terminology of mild, moderate and severe late decelerations but consider all late decelerations as significant and potentially ominous. Therefore, we must rely on other parameters of the fetal heart rate such as loss of variability and tachycardia to indicate fetal intolerance to this hypoxia.

Since the cause of late decelerations is uteroplacental insufficiency (UPI) elicited by intervillous stasis which occurs during uterine contractions, the factors that lead to this hypoxia may be intrinsic or extrinsic to the placenta. Decreased uterine blood flow is a much more common cause of late deceleration than impaired exhange from other causes. The most common cause of late deceleration is uterine hyperactivity/hypertonus usually as a result of excessive oxytocin stimulation.[5] Other causes of decreased flow would include supine hypotension, or other causes of local uterine hypotension such as epidural or spinal anesthesia. Late decelerations seen in association with vaginal bleeding and/or spontaneous uterine

hyperactivity are usually caused by abruptio placenta (Fig. 6.12). Several disease states including chronic hypertension, postmaturity, IUGR, diabetes mellitus, preecclampsia/ecclampsia, and collagen vascular disease may compromise placental exchange. The stress of labor may further aggravate exchange and produce late decelerations. Since each contraction will produce a repetitive hypoxic stress, with the persistence of late deceleration a metabolic acidosis may eventually develop. The most important two variables to watch for at this point are the development of fetal tachycardia and loss of variability (Fig. 6.13). These are important signs of developing acidosis and their development in the presence of persistent late decelerations correlate highly with neonatal depression.[3]

Variable Decelerations

The most frequently seen fetal heart rate deceleration pattern in labor is variable deceleration. This aptly named deceleration pattern is variable in nearly all respects. It is variable in duration, intensity, and timing relative to uterine contractions. It is probably caused by compression of the umbilical cord. Since cord compression during labor occurs most often during uterine contractions, variable decelerations most often coincide with uterine contractions (Fig.

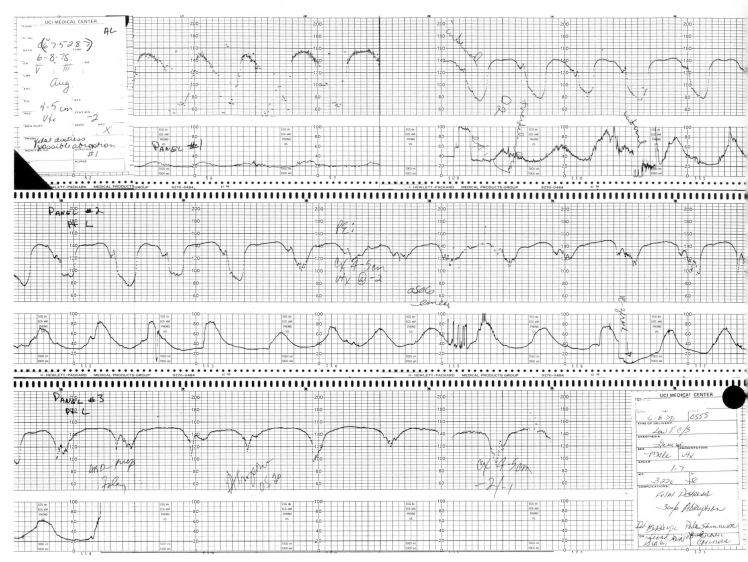

Figure 6.13. This is a gravida 5, para 3 admitted at term with contractions and minimal vaginal bleeding. On internal monitor (2nd half of *panel 1*) persistent late decelerations are noted which fail to respond to oxygen and position change. Variability is poor throughout and the baseline heart rate gradually increased from 140 to 155 BPM. In the presence of late decelerations, poor variability and rising baseline rate are signs of fetal intolerance to hypoxia and developing acidosis. In this case an Apgar 1 at 1 min and 7 at 5 min female was delivered. The 30% abruption is the etiology of the late decelerations.

6.14). But since this is an inconsistent occurrence, such decelerations may be seen with one but not the subsequent contraction. Characteristically these decelerations are very abrupt in both onset and return to baseline. Small abrupt accelerations of the fetal heart rate often precede and/or follow these decelerations.

In terms of fetal compromise, the insult will vary directly with the duration and degree of cord compression. With mild degrees of cord compression, a mild respiratory acidosis may develop from CO_2 retention. However, if placental function is adequate and contractions are not too frequent, this CO_2 retention should clear rapidly with reversal of the respiratory acidosis. Should cord compression be prolonged and/or repetitive, however, progressive fetal hypoxia and resultant metabolic acidosis may develop. For these reasons, variable decelerations are conveniently graded for severity as mild, moderate or severe. The more severe the variable deceleration pattern and the more prolonged and sustained it becomes, the more likely one is to deliver a depressed newborn. On the basis of the level and duration of decelerations without considering other parameters, Kubli et al.[6] graded variable decelerations as follows. Mild: duration less than 30 sec regardless of level or deceleration not below 80 BPM regardless of duration (Fig. 6.15). Moderate: level less than 80 BPM regardless of duration (Fig. 6.16). Severe: less than 70 BPM for greater than 60 sec (Fig. 6.17). To evaluate how a given fetus is responding to or tolerating these variable decelerations, one must look at other parameters of the fetal heart rate tracing. Loss of beat to beat variability and tachycardia suggest progressive neurologic depression from hypoxia and acidosis and therefore, it becomes important to watch these pa-

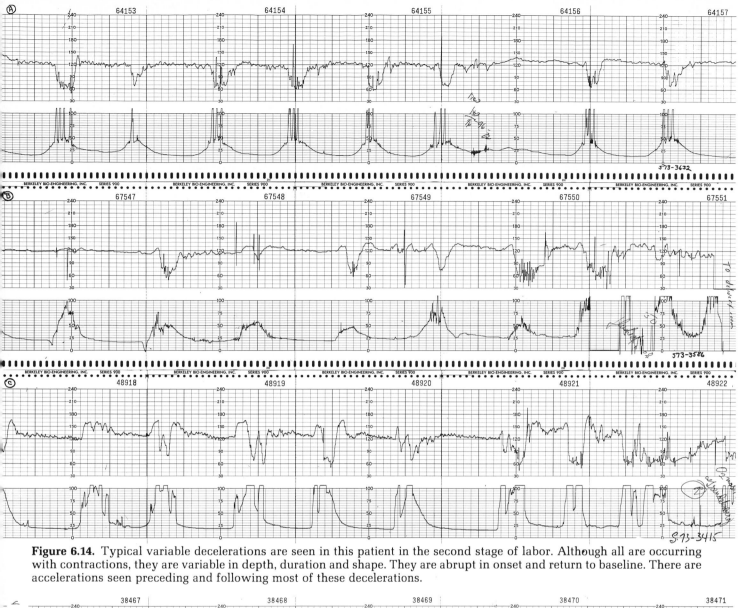

Figure 6.14. Typical variable decelerations are seen in this patient in the second stage of labor. Although all are occurring with contractions, they are variable in depth, duration and shape. They are abrupt in onset and return to baseline. There are accelerations seen preceding and following most of these decelerations.

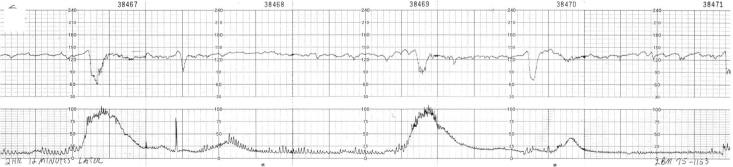

Figure 6.15. Mild variable decelerations are seen in this patient in early labor. They are occurring with contractions and probably with fetal movement. Baseline heart rate and variability are normal.

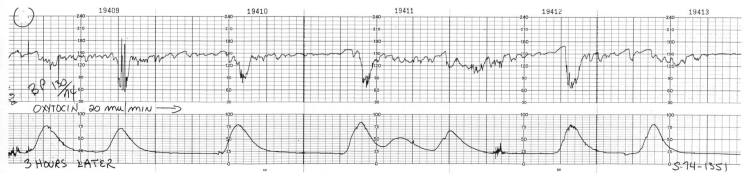
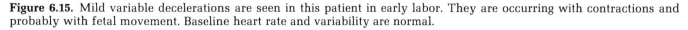

Figure 6.16. Moderate variable decelerations are seen in this panel. Baseline heart rate and variability are normal.

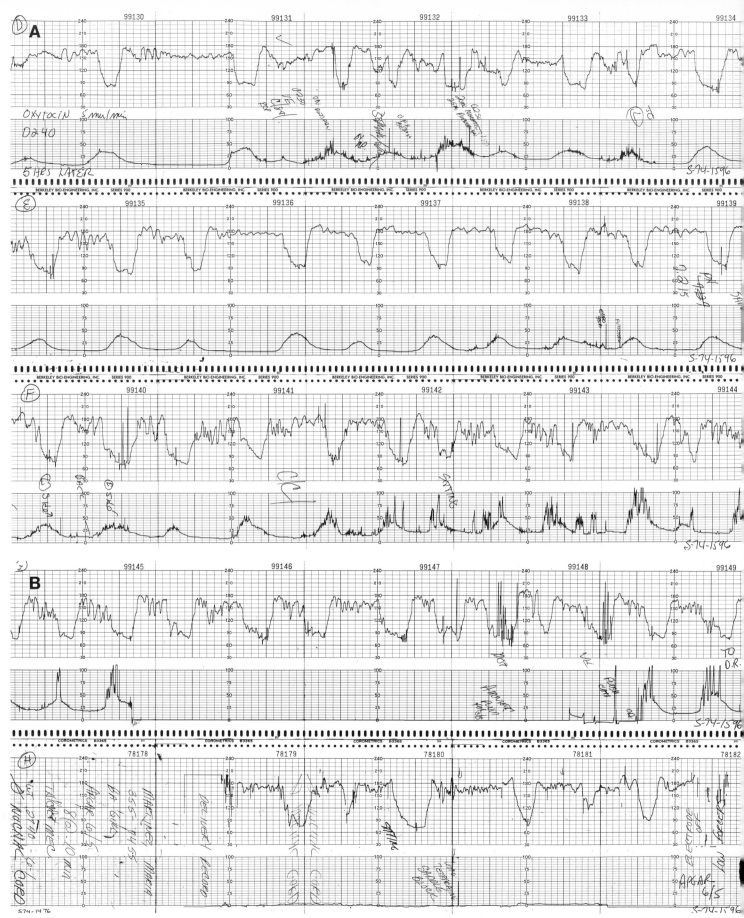

Figure 6.17. Severe variable decelerations are seen in a 14-year-old primagravida admitted at 43 weeks with meconium stained amniotic fluid. Variable decelerations are seen throughout, becoming progressively deeper and more prolonged. Baseline heart rate is somewhat erratic from 140 to 180. Increased heart rate variability seen in *G* and *H* probably represents early hypoxia between contractions. An Apgar 6 at 1 min and 5 at 5 min 2740-g infant was delivered. The low 5-min Apgar score may have been caused by meconium in the airway and difficult ventilation.

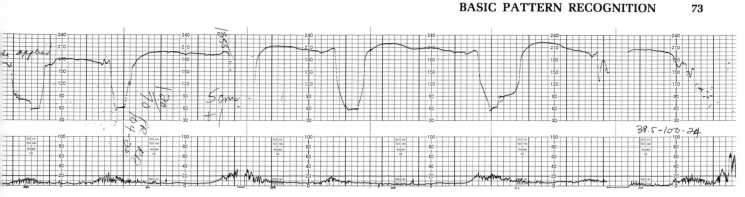

Figure 6.18. Severe ominous variable decelerations are seen with rising baseline heart rate to 210 BPM and virtually absent variability. A premature baby was delivered by cesarean section with Apgars of 1 at 1 min and 2 at 5 min.

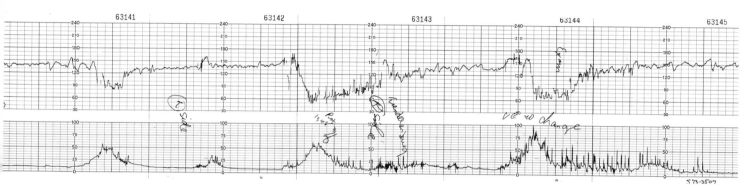

Figure 6.19. Severe variable decelerations are seen with slow return to baseline. Baseline heart rate and variability are normal.

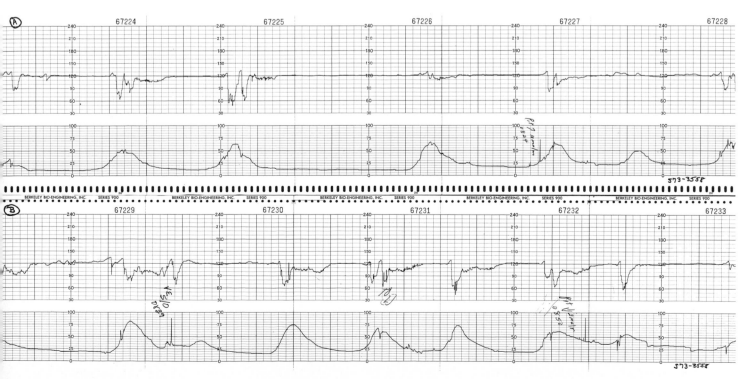

Figure 6.20. Mixed mild variable and late decelerations are seen with most contractions. With such mild variable decelerations it is unlikely that progressive cord compression has caused the hypoxia, but a coexistent UPI probably exists. Poor variability suggests acidosis may also be present.

rameters carefully (Fig. 6.18). Should these warning signs develop in the absence of other causes such as drugs, it is an important sign that the fetus is not tolerating the intermittent cord compression. The other sign of fetal intolerance to cord compression is a more gradual return of the variable deceleration pattern to baseline heart rate (Fig. 6.19). Usually variable decelerations are very abrupt in both their descent and return to baseline. Should the return to baseline become more gradual, the indication is that progressive hypoxia is developing. It is probable that this slow return represents a component of late deceleration which would be consistent with a developing fetal hypoxia. Sometimes there are distinct variable decelerations followed by distinct late decelerations where there is simultaneous but coincidental cord compression and primary UPI occurring (Fig. 6.20). With mild variable decelerations, especially without tachycardia or loss of variability, it is unlikely that the cord compression has caused the hypoxia and late deceleration; therefore, one must consider a placental perfusion or exchange problem coexists with cord compression.

As variable deceleration becomes more severe, there are additional fetal heart rate changes. The variable deceleration pattern will begin to appear smoother and rounded or blunted (Fig. 6.21). This change can be partially reproduced with atropine or may be seen in very premature infants. In extreme situations with severe and progressive variable deceleration, a blunt acceleration may follow the contraction. Goodlin described this as "overshoot."[7] It is a transient smooth acceleration lasting 30 to 90 sec occurring after severe variable decelerations. This is not the usual sharp acceleration that precedes and follows mild to moderate variable decelerations. The

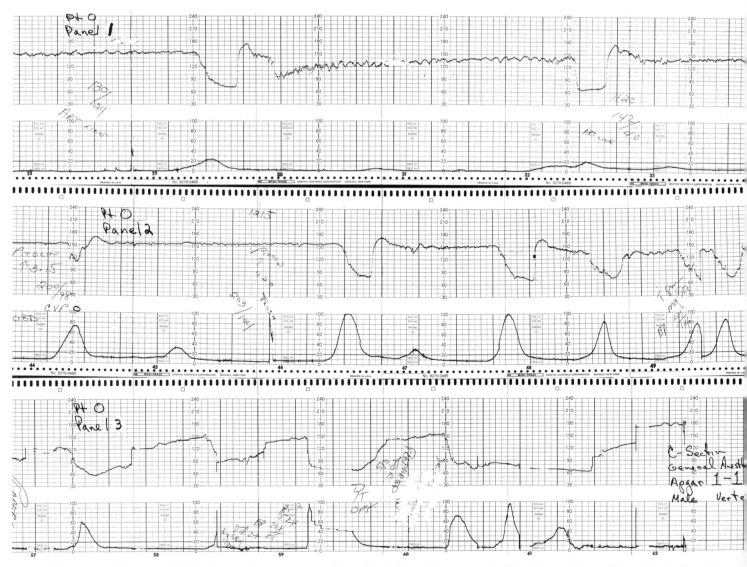

Figure 6.21. Severe variable decelerations are seen throughout these **three panels.** The blunted (rounded and not abrupt) accelerations seen following the decelerations is not the usual abrupt acceleration and may represent "overshoot". Variability is progressively lost and decelerations become ominously prolonged. Delivery in this 30-week severe preeclamptic was by cesarean section and a severely depressed neonate with Apgar scores of 1 at 1 min and 1 at 5 min was delivered.

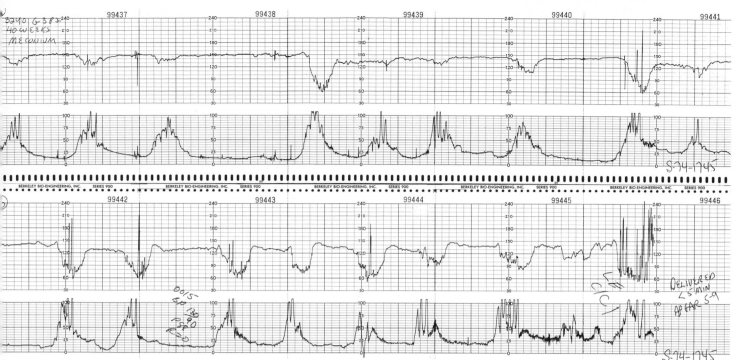

Figure 6.22. Variable decelerations here, as they often do, herald the onset of the second stage of labor in **A.** Maternal pushing can be detected by the short spikes on top of the contractions. Although the decelerations become larger and more regular, baseline heart rate and variability remain unchanged and reassuring. An Apgar 5 at 1 min and 9 at 5 min term size infant was delivered less than 5 min after the monitor was removed.

overshoot lacks the abruptness, is without short-term variability within the acceleration, and returns to baseline very gradually.

There is one other problem that may occur with variable deceleration. When variable decelerations approach 50 to 60 BPM, transient cardiac asystole may occur. Whether such asystole can result in fetal death is open to question and further study. Unusual cases of abrupt fetal death could possibly be explained by this mechanism. However, it has not been documented in monitored patients.

What makes variable deceleration so difficult to manage, therefore, is its unpredictability in contrast to late decelerations. This difficulty is best exemplified by variable deceleration occurring in the second stage of labor. Variable deceleration is most commonly seen in the second stage of labor as the cord is more likely to be compressed with descent of the fetus through the birth canal. In fact, the appearance of variable deceleration often heralds the onset of the second stage (Fig. 6.22). Since the second stage precedes delivery by only a relatively short time, and since intervention is usually immediately possible should truly ominous patterns develop, more prolonged and deeper variable deceleration can be tolerated. This is true as long as the baseline heart rate is not rising and variability is maintained. Since cord compression is more frequent in the second stage and is more likely to be more severe, this is a very common problem. To what extent head compression is

involved in the production of these decelerations is not totally clear. However, the depth and progression of many of these decelerations do make it clear that cord compression is the main component and referring to these second stage decelerations as early deceleration is inappropriate. Should loss of variability and/or a rising baseline develop with the more severe second stage variable decelerations, expediting delivery definitely becomes warranted (Fig. 6.23).

Prolonged Decelerations

Prolonged decelerations, i.e., isolated decelerations of greater than 60 to 90 sec are difficult to classify in terms of pathophysiology since they may be seen in a multitude of situations. As might be expected, cord compression can cause prolonged decelerations. This is generally seen in one of two situations: either with progression of severe variable deceleration, or with sudden occult or frank cord prolapse (Fig. 6.24). Profound placental insufficiency may cause prolonged decelerations. This is most characteristically seen with hypotension as in supine hypotension, or in epidural or spinal anesthesia (Fig. 6.25).

Paracervical anesthesia classically produces the most profound prolonged decelerations (Fig. 6.26). Whether this is from fetal uptake of local anesthetic, from local uterine hypotension (spasm of uterine arteries), uterine hypertonus, or all three is not totally clear. Other forms of UPI producing prolonged de-

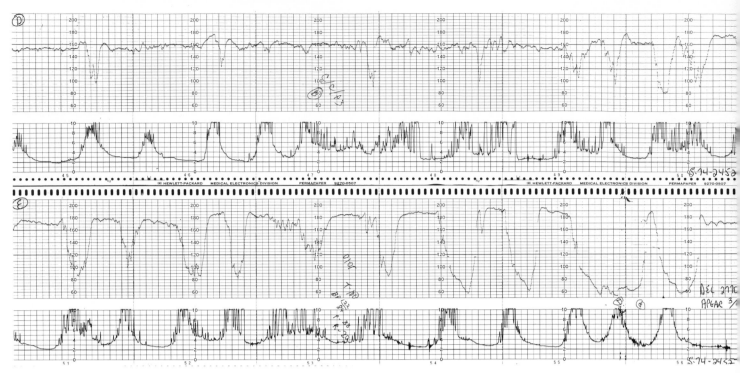

Figure 6.23. The patient is being monitored with an internal electrode and intrauterine catheter. There is a rapid progression of variable decelerations from mild to severe. The baseline heart rate rises from 150 at the beginning to 190. The heart rate variability is normal at the beginning of the tracing but is markedly decreased just prior to delivery. The patient was delivered by low forceps of a 2770-g male with Apgar scores at 3 at 1 min and 7 at 5 min and a single loop of tight nuchal cord.

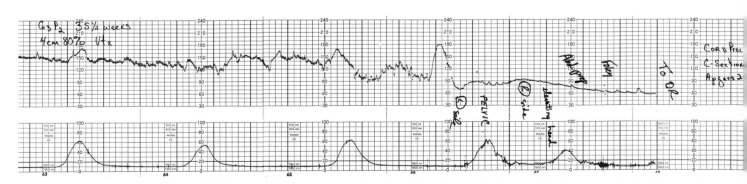

Figure 6.24. A sudden prolonged deceleration is seen in this patient in the early active phase of labor. Immediate pelvic exam revealed cord prolapse and cesarean section was performed.

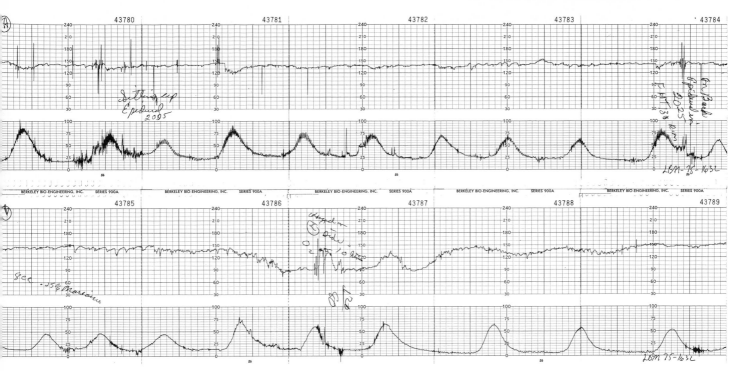

Figure 6.25. A prolonged deceleration is seen after injection of epidural anesthesia with Marcaine. This is followed by several late decelerations, often seen following such epidural induced decelerations. The pattern subsequently returned to normal and a vigorous newborn was delivered vaginally.

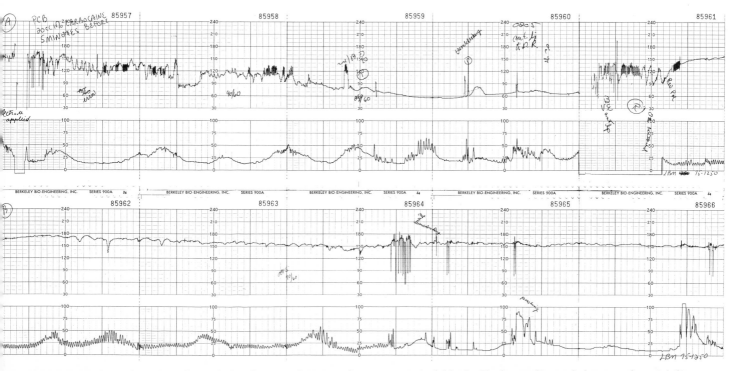

Figure 6.26. A profound prolonged deceleration is seen after paracervical block. Tachycardia and decreased variability follow the deceleration and the heart rate then returns to normal. Such transient rebound tachycardia and loss of variability is seen commonly following prolonged decelerations. An Apgar 9 newborn was delivered vaginally a short time later.

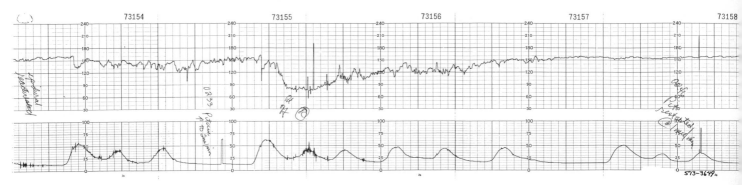

Figure 6.27. Here a prolonged deceleration is seen associated with excessive uterine activity secondary to oxytocin hyperstimulation. Again a rebound tachycardia with decreased variability follows the prolonged deceleration. Pitocin was stopped and restarted at a lower rate and the heart rate subsequently returned to normal.

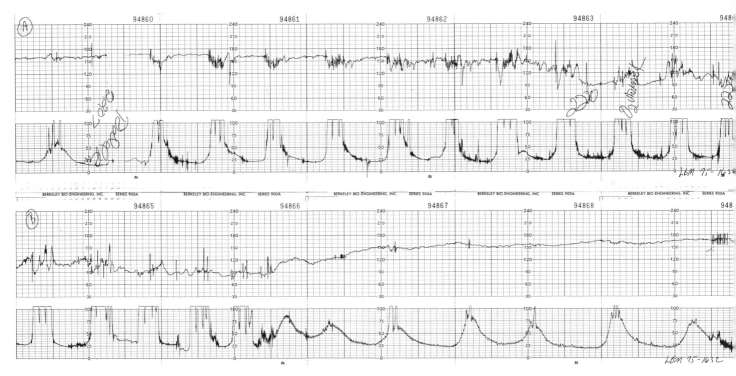

Figure 6.28. A prolonged deceleration from a baseline heart rate of 160 to 90 BPM is seen lasting 12 min in the second stage of labor. An apparent cause is not present. Tachycardia to 170 and decreased variability is seen after this deceleration. Also some subtle late decelerations are probably present during this time. Again, the heart rate pattern returned to normal. No further significant decelerations recurred and a vaginal delivery of an Apgar 7 infant occurred approximately 15 min later.

celerations may be caused by hypertonic or tetanic uterine contractions, (Fig. 6.27). Tetanic uterine contractions can be seen oxytocin hyperstimulation, abruptio placenta, and when large boluses of local anesthetics are delivered to the uterus as may be seen with paracervical block or inadvertent intravenous injection at the time of activation of an epidural block. Maternal hypoxia causing such decelerations might be seen in seizures or with respiratory depression that might be seen with a high spinal, overdose of narcotics, or magnesium sulfate. Generally, when one sees prolonged decelerations of the fetal heart rate, especially when the duration is more than 2 to 3 min, a rebound tachycardia and loss of variability of the fetal heart rate is seen (Fig. 6.28). This is probably due to release of fetal epinephrine but may

in addition be caused by the resulting CNS depression. If the original insult does not recur immediately, the placenta is very effective in "resuscitating" the fetus, and generally in these situations, this is a better choice than intervention. The loss of variability and tachycardia are not necessarily prognostically ominous since the pathology may no longer be present and the placenta can effectively restore the fetus to its normal state. Occasionally in addition to the loss of variability and tachycardia seen after such prolonged decelerations, one sees a period of late decelerations that usually clears spontaneously also. The prolonged decelerations may not always return to baseline. When seen late in the course of severe variable deceleration or prolonged and recurrent late decelerations, such a deceleration may occur just

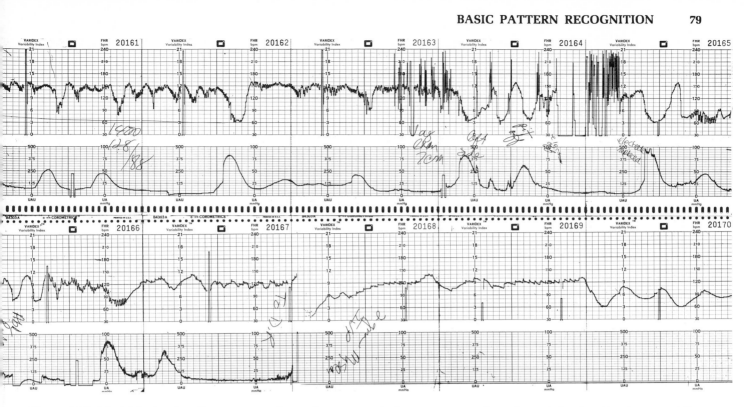

Figure 6.29. Variable decelerations are seen becoming progressively more severe. A prolonged deceleration is seen at the end of the *2nd panel.* An immediate cesarean section was performed but an Apgar 0 unresuscitable stillborn infant was delivered. This is an extremely atypical pattern. Note the bizarre variability that is seen in the last 8 min preceding the prolonged deceleration. The significance of the unusual variability is unclear.

before fetal death (Fig. 6.29). Recurrent prolonged decelerations without apparent etiology probably represent cord compression and are the most difficult of all patterns to manage. This is because one cannot prognosticate fetal tolerance based on previous performance of the fetal heart rate in labor or based on other parameters of the fetal heart rate such as variability. Such prolonged decelerations may just continue and prolonged cord compression may cause fetal death or may be associated with fetal asystole which may or may not be a cause of sudden fetal death as previously discussed. There are, however, a few other more benign causes of prolonged decelerations which merely represent a reactive fetal vagus nerve and not fetal distress. Occasionally one will see such decelerations associated with pelvic examination, application of a scalp electrode, rapid descent of the fetus through the birth canal, or with sustained maternal valsalva (Fig. 6.30). Such decelerations generally do not last more than 1½ to 2 min and are not usually followed by tachycardia or loss of variability. These probably represent vagal reflex decelerations.

ACCELERATIONS

Since periodic changes are defined as transient changes above and below the baseline, the counterpart of decelerations are accelerations. Accelerations of the fetal heart rate seem to occur most commonly in the antepartum period, in early labor, and in as-

sociation with variable decelerations. There are probably at least two physiologic mechanisms responsible for accelerations. Those seen in response to fetal movement or contractions (Fig. 6.31) seem to have the same significance as fetal heart rate variability, i.e., their presence represents fetal alertness or arousal states. The other cause of accelerations seems to be partial umbilical cord occlusion. If the low pressure umbilical vein is compressed and the higher pressure umbilical artery remains patent, a period of decreased placental return and fetal hypotension results in a baroreceptor response. The normal baroreceptor response to hypotension or decreased cardiac return is an increase in heart rate, hence the acceleration.

The presence of fetal heart rate accelerations in the intrapartum period, as in the antepartum period, is reassuring. These accelerations may occur with contractions, fetal movement, or without apparent stimulus. In addition, as with decelerations, accelerations may be seen in response to pelvic examination and stimulation of the fetal head (Fig. 6.32). The absence of fetal heart rate accelerations in the intrapartum period is not of itself alarming as long as variability is normal. The biggest problem created by accelerations of the fetal heart rate is that at times it is difficult to be sure if one is dealing with decelerations or accelerations with return to baseline (Fig. 6.33). This is especially true in the beginning of the monitoring period when the baseline has not been

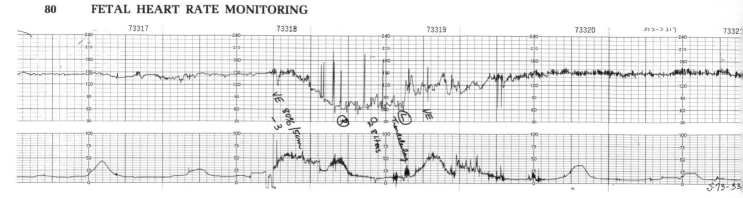

Figure 6.30. A, A prolonged deceleration is seen after pelvic exam. Also note the uterine hyperactivity commonly seen following pelvic exam (Ferguson reflex?). This probably represents a fetus with an active vagal reflex.

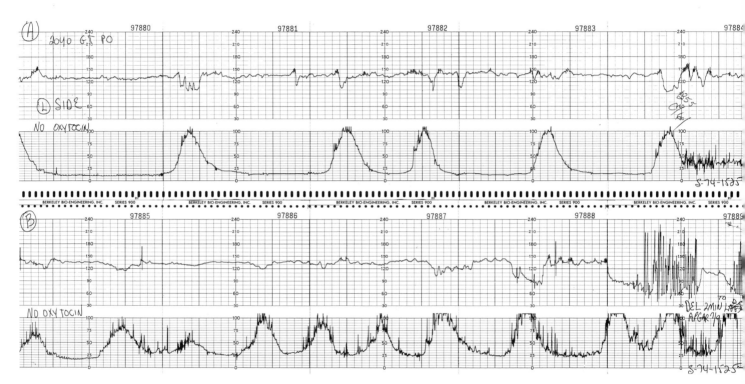

Figure 6.30. B, In this case, a prolonged deceleration is seen at the end of *B*. This patient progressed rapidly from 6 cm at the end of *A* to delivery 2 min after the end of *B*. Such prolonged decelerations should incite pelvic exam, not only to rule out cord prolapse, but as is often the case to check for rapid descent as occurred in this case.

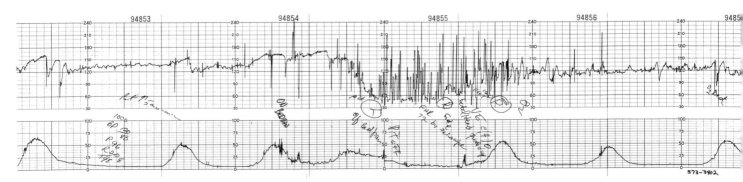

Figure 6.30. C, Here a prolonged deceleration occurs while the patient was on a bedpan. Again a fetal vagal reflex may cause decelerations with maternal valsalva.

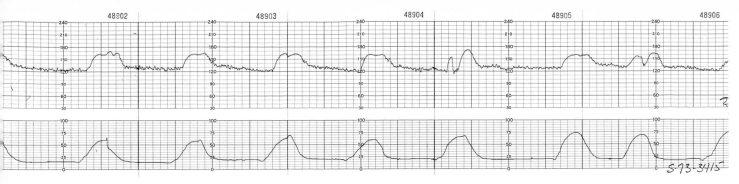

Figure 6.31. Accelerations of the fetal heart rate are seen with each contraction. Baseline heart rate and variability are normal. Such a pattern is reassuring.

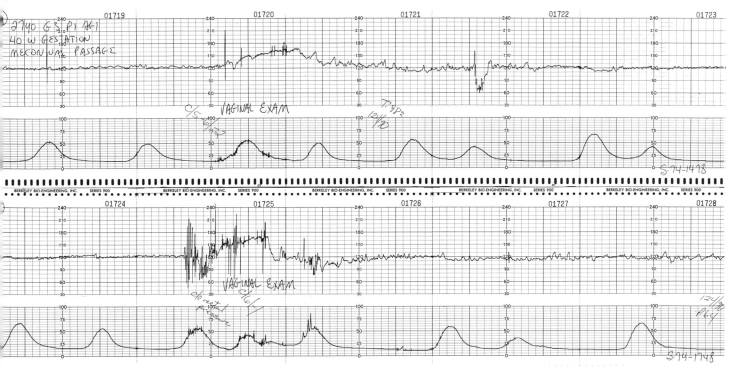

Figure 6.32. Just as vaginal exam may precipitate prolonged deceleration (Fig. 6.30A), vaginal exam may stimulate the fetal heart rate to accelerate as occurs with exam in both *panels.*

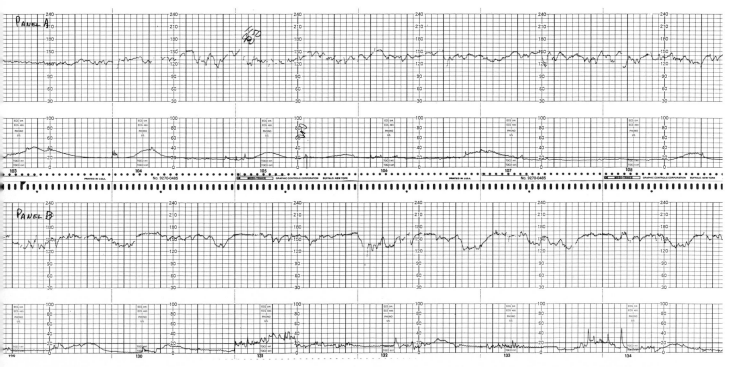

Figure 6.33. In *B* accelerations with return to baseline could easily be confused for late decelerations. Looking back at *A*, it can be seen that the real baseline heart rate is 120 to 130. Also, note that the return to baseline tends to be flat rather than rounded at the nadir as would be late decelerations.

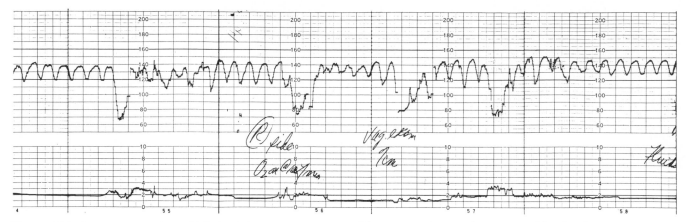

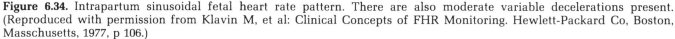

Figure 6.34. Intrapartum sinusoidal fetal heart rate pattern. There are also moderate variable decelerations present. (Reproduced with permission from Klavin M, et al: Clinical Concepts of FHR Monitoring. Hewlett-Packard Co, Boston, Masschusetts, 1977, p 106.)

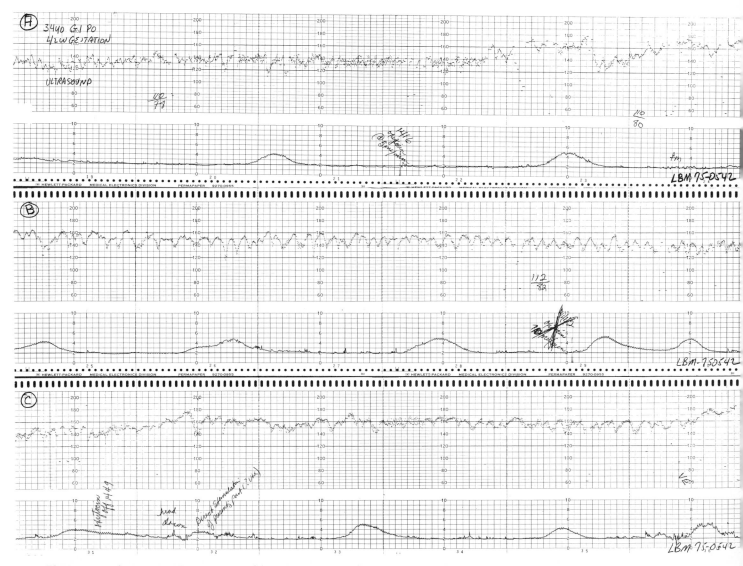

Figure 6.35. As seen in *B*, exaggerated long-term variability may resemble sinusoidal heart rate patterns. The presence of short-term variability within the pattern and the normal patterns before and after *B* distinguish this "pseudosinusoidal" pattern from a true sinusoidal one.

established. This is an important practical problem because there may be cases of misinterpretation with intervention for fetal distress when in reality there were no decelerations, but accelerations mistaken for baseline heart rate and return to baseline mistaken for decelerations. There are two clues to help avoid this difficulty. First, accelerations and decelerations are rounded at their peak, whereas the baseline tends to be flat. Next, with accelerations especially, there is usually a period preceding or following without periodic changes where the baseline may be more clearly determined, from which one then may distinguish changes above or below the baseline.

UNUSUAL PATTERNS

Sinusoidal patterns have been most frequently described and seen in antepartum heart rate testing. They may, however, rarely be seen in the intrapartum period. A sinusoidal pattern is one with a sine wave pattern above and below the baseline with a cyclicity of about 4 to 8/min (Fig. 6.34). What one is looking at is increased long-term fetal heart rate variability in the absence of short-term variability. This has been most often described in severe fetal anemia and can be rarely seen in conjunction with late decelerations. In addition, sinusoidal patterns may be seen with severe hypoxia alone, and has also been described with parenteral alphaprodine (Nisentil). Many times, benign fetal heart rate patterns with increased long-term variability may be easily confused with sinusoidal patterns (Fig. 6.35). These benign patterns may be distinguished by the lack of uniformity of the sine wave pattern, the fact that the variability is not equally distributed above and below the baseline and most importantly the presence of short-term variability.

ARRHYTHMIAS

Fetal cardiac arrhythmias are not uncommon in the intrapartum period. They are easily confused on fetal heart rate tracings with artifact and signal loss. The patterns seen with arrhythmias are described in Chapter 4. Nearly always, the arrhythmias do not signify fetal hypoxia and they are not significantly correlated with congenital heart disease except with complete heart block.

A knowledge of the physiology and pathophysiology of the fetal heart rate coupled with experience in pattern recognition is essential in the appropriate utilization of electronic fetal heart rate monitoring. Pattern recognition is a process of recognizing fetal heart rate changes, such as decelerations, which suggest the type of pathophysiologic process occurring; of determining how the fetus is tolerating that process at any given moment by such parameters as variability and baseline heart rate; and of prognosticating how long such a process might be allowed to continue without significant fetal depression or damage by the severity, repetitiveness, and duration of the pattern. Unfortunately, such a process is difficult to analyze quantitatively making the processes of pattern recognition and integration all important.

REFERENCES

1. Shenker L: Fetal cardiac arrhythmias. Obstet Gynecol Survey 34:561, 1979
2. Druzin ML, Ikenoue T, Murata Y, et al: A possible mechanism for the increase in fetal heart rate variability following hypoxemia. Presented at the Society for Gynecologic Investigation, San Diego, California, 1979
3. Paul RH, Suidan AK, Yeh SY, et al: Clinical fetal monitoring VII: The evaluation and significance of intrapartum baseline FHR variability. Am J Obstet Gynecol 123:206, 1975
4. Garite TJ, Linzey EM, Freeman RK, et al: Fetal heart rate patterns and fetal distress in fetuses with congenital anomalies. Obstet Gynecol 53:716, 1979
5. Shenker L: Clinical experience with fetal heart rate monitoring of 1000 patients in labor. Am J Obstet Gynecol 115:1111, 1973
6. Kubli FW, Hon EH, Khazin AE, et al: Observations on heart rate and pH in the human fetus during labor. Am J Obstet Gynecol 104:1190, 1969
7. Goodlin RC, Lowe EW: A functional umbilical cord occlusion heart rate pattern. The significance of overshoot. Obstet Gynecol 42:22, 1974

CHAPTER 7

Fetal Acid Base Monitoring

Although this text is principally concerned with electronic fetal heart rate (FHR) monitoring, one must include a discussion of fetal acid base monitoring because it is an important adjunct to electronic fetal heart rate monitoring.

In the absence of oxygen, the fetus will be restricted to anaerobic metabolism with the production of lactic acid and it is for this reason that fetal pH can be used as an indirect measure of fetal oxygenation. A brief review of glucose metabolism will serve to remind the reader that glucose is first broken down to lactic acid during the anaerobic phase of the carbohydrate metabolic pathway. There is only a minimal amount of energy produced at this point, but when lactic acid is converted to CO_2 in the presence of oxygen there is a large amount of energy produced by this more efficient aerobic phase of glucose metabolism. When oxygen is absent, the lactic acid cannot be broken down and it accumulates, causing a retention of hydrogen ion, resulting in metabolic acidosis. In the presence of oxygen, the lactic acid is converted to CO_2 which is easily transferred across the placenta to the maternal circulation. When there is umbilical cord occlusion, however, the CO_2 being produced by the fetus cannot be transferred to the maternal circulation with a resulting CO_2 accumulation in the fetal compartment. The excess CO_2 is hydrolyzed and carbonic acid (H_2CO_3) is formed. The increase in H_2CO_3 forces the equilibrium toward the dissociated H+ and HCO3− components, resulting in fetal acidosis. Of course, this is respiratory acidosis and it can be easily reversed when the umbilical cord occlusion is released and CO_2 is equilibrated, across the placenta, with maternal circulation (Fig. 7.1).

During periods of metabolic acidosis resulting from fetal hypoxia with production of lactic acid, there is a decrease in the buffer base as the various components (bicarbonate, phosphates, hemoglobin, and protein) absorb the excess hydrogen ions being produced. The normal fetal base deficit runs about 7 meq/liter, but when fetal metabolic acidosis occurs, it may exceed 10 or 15 meq/liter.[1] The pCO_2 may be mildly elevated and of course the fetal pH will be decreased.

Fetal respiratory acidosis is characterized by a high pCO_2. The normal fetal pCO_2 is usually in the 40 to 50 mm Hg range. With prolonged umbilical cord occlusion, it may get up to 60 or 80 mm Hg and of course will result in a respiratory acidosis characterized by very little change in the base deficit but a decrease in pH and an elevated pCO_2.

Normal values for fetal scalp capillary pH are in the range of 7.25 to 7.35.[2] The scalp values usually fall between the umbilical artery that has a lower pH and the umbilical vein that has a higher pH because it is carrying freshly oxygenated and decarbonated blood from the placenta. Fetal scalp pH values between 7.20 and 7.25 are considered preacidotic and values below 7.20 are considered frank acidosis[3] (see Table 7.1).

When a fetus is hypoxic, the resulting metabolic acidosis can really only be reversed by adequate fetal oxygenation since we lack the ability to directly administer fixed base to the fetus as we can to the neonate in the form of bicarbonate. The process for reversing fetal metabolic acidosis usually takes 20 or 30 min, depending on the degree.[4] Thus, if one were to recognize a remedial cause for hypoxic fetal metabolic acidosis, the trend of serial fetal pH values would be more important than the absolute value if one is trying to assess recovery. This concept of intrauterine resuscitation is important to consider because hasty intervention with an acidotic fetus may result in an acidotic neonate that will have compromised pulmonary blood flow due to the acidosis and the reoxygenation of this neonate may be more difficult than to have allowed more time for "intrauterine resuscitation". Of course, the validity of this concept is dependent on the remedial character of the fetal hypoxia and if the fetal hypoxia is not remedial, delay could be detrimental.

Thus, if the cause of the fetal hypoxemia were an abruption, delay would be deleterious, but if the cause were oxytocin hyperstimulation, delay with

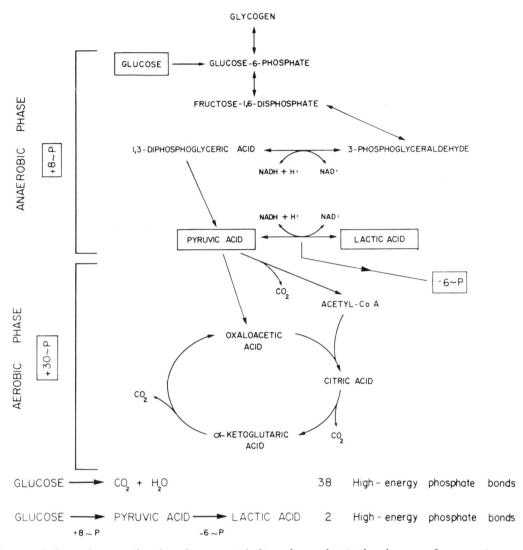

GLYCOGEN

GLUCOSE → GLUCOSE-6-PHOSPHATE

FRUCTOSE-1,6-DISPHOSPHATE

1,3-DIPHOSPHOGLYCERIC ACID ← → 3-PHOSPHOGLYCERALDEHYDE

NADH + H⁺   NAD⁺

NADH + H⁺   NAD⁺

PYRUVIC ACID ← → LACTIC ACID

CO_2

ACETYL-Co A

OXALOACETIC ACID

CITRIC ACID

CO_2

α-KETOGLUTARIC ACID

CO_2

ANAEROBIC PHASE   +8~P

AEROBIC PHASE   +30~P

-6~P

GLUCOSE → CO_2 + H_2O 38   High-energy phosphate bonds

GLUCOSE → PYRUVIC ACID → LACTIC ACID   2   High-energy phosphate bonds
+8~P   -6~P

Figure 7.1. The metabolic pathway utilized in glucose catabolism shows that in the absence of oxygen (anaerobic phase) the end product is lactic acid which will produce metabolic acidosis if not metabolized to CO_2 via aerobic metabolic pathways. (Reproduced with permission from Hon E, Khazin A: Obstet Gynecol 33:220, 1969.)

Table 7.1.

Fetal Scalp Blood Normal Values

pH	7.25–7.35
pCO₂	40–50 mm Hg
pO₂	20–30 mm Hg
Base Deficit	<10 meq/liter

Metabolic Acidosis (UPI—Late Deceleration)

pH	<7.25
pCO₂	45–55 mm Hg
pO₂	<20 mm HG
Base Deficit	>10 meq/liter

Respiratory Acidosis (Umbilical Cord Compression—Variable Deceleration)

pH	<7.25
pCO₂	>50 mm Hg
pO₂	Variable
Base Deficit	<10 meq/liter

discontinuation of the oxytocin, position change and administration of oxygen could clearly benefit the fetus more than a cesarean section.

Fetal respiratory acidosis due to umbilical cord occlusion will clear very rapidly if the cord occlusion is released. The main significance of fetal respiratory acidosis is that if one is not aware of its possibility, it may be misinterpreted as fetal metabolic acidosis and could lead to inappropriate intervention. Clinically, it is important to understand that if a fetal scalp sample is taken during or soon after a variable deceleration pattern in the FHR, one may get a low fetal pH because of cord occlusion and respiratory acidosis (Fig. 7.2). For this reason, it is usually valuable to measure a pCO₂ and/or a base deficit on the scalp blood in order to know the respiratory component. Saling and Schneider[3] equilibrates the fetal scalp blood with a gas mixture containing a pCO₂ of 40 mm Hg and then eliminates the respiratory component.

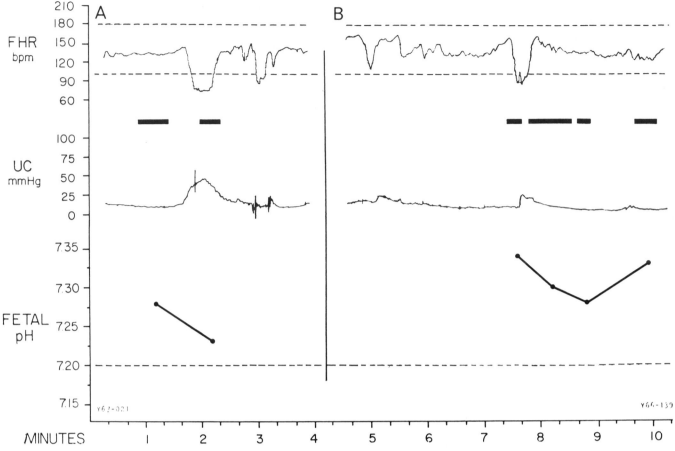

Figure 7.2. Fetal scalp blood pH changes during variable deceleration. Note the rapid fall and rise in pH associated with variable deceleration of the FHR. (Reproduced with permission from Hon E, Khazin A: Obstet Gynecol 33:20, 1969.)

At the time of the first fetal scalp blood sample, one should also measure the maternal venous blood pH in order to rule out significant maternal acid base imbalance.[4] The fetal pH usually runs about 0.1 pH unit below the maternal and one may use this as a guideline in interpreting fetal scalp pH values in association with a significant maternal acidosis or alkalosis. Especially during late labor, one may see maternal metabolic acidosis in association with dehydration and exhaustion. Maternal respiratory alkalosis has been reported in association with hyperventilation[5] and may be significant in patients instructed in breathing aids to labor where hyperventilation is prominent.

During late labor, caput formation and stasis of blood in the fetal scalp may produce local acidosis, resulting in a fetal scalp blood pH below that of the central fetal circulation.[2, 6] There is no way to be certain that this is the case until after delivery where a fetal scalp blood pH lower than the umbilical artery pH would clearly indicate a local cause of the fetal scalp blood acidosis.

EQUIPMENT NECESSARY FOR FETAL SCALP BLOOD SAMPLING

Before sampling fetal blood, one must be sure to have the correct equipment available and there must

also be an assistant to help hold the patient in position, to make notations on the monitor, to connect the light source to the battery and to accept the filled capillary tubes from the physician and prepare them properly for the laboratory.

A sterile tray (now available with disposable items) should contain the following: (1) four or five 200-μliter heparinized capillary tubes; (2) a conical endoscope with light source; (3) a 2-mm blade on a long handle; (4) silicone grease; (5) 10 or 15 sponges and a long-handled sponge holder.

The physician should wear sterile gloves and the patient should be prepped and draped in a sterile manner.

TECHNIQUE OF FETAL SCALP BLOOD SAMPLING

The optimum position of the patient for fetal scalp blood sampling is very important. This technique is difficult in early labor and without proper patient positioning it is impossible.

The lithotomy position with a patient in stirrups and the maternal buttocks extending over the edge of the table is preferred by most. This can be done in most convertible labor beds but if not available, it is easily accomplished in the delivery room. The lateral Sims' position is also satisfactory, requires less patient movement and allows the patient to remain in the lateral position. When using the lateral Sims's position, it is important that the patient be well flexed at the hip with the lower leg extended. The upper leg should be flexed and held by an assistant with the patient's buttocks extending well over the edge of the bed to allow the person taking the scalp sample to be positioned below the level of the maternal vagina. With both lithotomy and Sims' techniques, the most important factor is for the scalp sampler to be able to angle the cone downward below the horizontal.

With the patient in position, the cone (with light source) is inserted into the posterior fornix under direct visualization. Once the cone is inserted past the anterior lip of the cervix, the cone is angled anteriorly into the cervix and the presenting part is visualized. A sponge is used to wipe the scalp surface clean and then silicone grease is applied to form a nonwetable surface which will allow the fetal scalp blood to form in easily accessible beads. A standard fetal scalp blade with a depth of 2 mm is then used with a quick "stab" to make a clean incision and blood will appear. A 200-μliter heparinized capillary tube is then inserted to touch the drop of blood, and keeping the tube angled downward, the blood is allowed to flow by gravity. One needs about a quarter of a tube of blood without bubbles for a pH, but for complete fetal scalp blood gases (pH, pCO_2, pO_2, and base deficit) one needs about ¾ of the tube filled. After taking the sample, the capillary tube should be immediately handed to an assistant for proper scaling and mixing with a magnetic "flea". Pressure with a sponge should be kept on the scalp wound through the next two contractions and it should then be observed during another contraction to be sure the bleeding has stopped. Sometimes more pressure is required and other times (rarely) one may need to put a skin clip on the wound to stop the bleeding. Once fetal scalp blood sampling has been done, continued observation of the patient must be carried out, as even what appears to be "heavy show" during labor may be significant fetal hemorrhage if it is fetal scalp bleeding from the previous puncture site.[7]

INDICATIONS FOR FETAL SCALP BLOOD SAMPLING

There is not total agreement on the indications for fetal scalp blood sampling. Certainly if an institution does not have 24-hr ready access to accurate micro-blood gas analysis with a 10- to 15-min turn-around time, one should not utilize fetal scalp blood sampling. The ability to implement decisions for rapid operative intervention is also necessary to effectively utilize this technique.

Given the necessary logistical support, the indications for fetal scalp blood sampling should be limited to patients who are in labor with membranes ruptured and cervical dilatation sufficient to allow introduction of the cone (usually 2 to 3 cm) and with the

fetal head at a station that is within 2 cm of the spines. It is this author's opinion that fetal scalp blood sampling for acid base studies should be limited to patients who have electronic FHR tracings suggestive of hypoxia. The better one understands FHR monitoring, the less necessary fetal scalp blood sampling will be. On our service, fetal scalp sampling is used in the following situations.

1. When a confusing FHR pattern is present with elements that suggest fetal hypoxia,
2. When there is a sustained flat FHR without ominous periodic changes.
3. When uncorrectable late deceleration with good variability is present in a patient where vaginal delivery is anticipated within 60 to 90 min.

CORRELATION BETWEEN FHR PATTERNS, FETAL PH, AND OUTCOME

In the 1960's, there was a raging debate as to whether continuous electronic fetal heart rate monitoring or intermittent fetal scalp blood pH was superior for monitoring the human fetus during labor. As things have evolved, most authorities have come to the conclusion that continuous electronic FHR monitoring provides the best "front line screen" for monitoring the fetus during labor because the technique is easy, it can be done with intact membranes, and most importantly because it gives continuous data. Fetal scalp blood sampling will only give information about the time the sampling occurred, it cannot be done until labor is well under way with ruptured membranes, and the technique is much more difficult than the application of the electronic monitoring device. Therefore, today, electronic FHR monitoring is used as the primary means of surveillance with fetal scalp blood pH sampling used as the back-up technique to comment on the hypoxic significance of the electronically-derived FHR pattern.

Early studies on the correlation between FHR patterns and fetal scalp blood pH revealed that there was at least a general correlation.[1, 4, 8, 9] Kubli et al.[2] showed that it was indeed rare to have a fetal scalp blood pH value below 7.20 with an innocuous FHR pattern. However, many patterns of late deceleration and moderate-to-severe variable deceleration were often associated with fetal scalp blood pH values above 7.20. Furthermore, about 10% of fetal scalp blood pH samples obtained at the time of delivery were found to be below the values found in the umbilical artery.[6] This suggests that local factors in the fetal scalp may frequently be responsible for a falsely low fetal scalp blood pH value.

The correlation between fetal scalp blood pH measurements and neonatal Apgar score increases as the sample is taken closer to the time of birth. With samples taken within 5 min of delivery, Hon and Khazin[10] and Modanlou et al.[11] showed that the correlation between low pH and low Apgar scores at both 1 and 5 min was very high. However, there appears to be a rather poor correlation between fetal pH and Apgar scores between 7 and 10. This may be accounted for partially by local factors that may make the fetal pH low at the scalp when the central fetal circulation is normal, especially at the time of delivery when caput formation is the greatest.

Finally, one must keep in mind the fact that changes in fetal scalp blood pH occur only after significant anaerobic metabolism has occurred, whereas FHR changes of late deceleration may occur with early hypoxemia before metabolic acidosis has developed. This probably accounts for the higher correlation between low pH and low Apgar scores with scalp sampling,[10] and the high correlation between normal FHR patterns and high Apgar scores with electronic FHR monitoring.[12] It also raises the question of whether one best serves his patient by achieving higher correlation by awaiting the fall in fetal scalp blood pH in patients with uncorrectable late deceleration, or whether one should intervene on the basis of the FHR pattern alone to achieve higher Apgar scores but probably higher operative delivery rates. The truth probably lies somewhere between.

CLINICAL INTERPRETATION OF FETAL SCALP PH VALUES

If the fetal scalp blood pH is above 7.25, it is reasonable to continue to observe the patient. If the ominous FHR pattern persists, however, one is then obliged to resample at appropriate intervals not to exceed 30 min, but sometimes less, depending on other findings and the evolution of the FHR pattern.

If the fetal scalp pH is between 7.20 and 7.25, it is necessary to resample immediately in order to confirm the value and to determine if there is a trend. One should also rule out a significant respiratory component to the acidosis and be sure the mother is not acidotic. Unless vaginal delivery was very near, with a "metabolic" pH confirmed in this range, operative delivery would be indicated on our service, although some would wait for the value to be 7.20 or below.

If the initial sample was below 7.20, intevention is clearly indicated, providing respiratory and maternal contributions were ruled out.

Since changes in fetal scalp blood pH occur later than late deceleration during the development of fetal hypoxia, the question of the appropriate point for intervention is under active debate among authorities. If one responds to all uncorrectable late decelerations with operative delivery, it is clear that in terms of Apgar scores there will be a very high incidence of good scores and possibly some unnecessary intervention.

However, if one were to wait for the pH to fall, there would undoubtedly be fewer operative interventions,[14] but by the time intervention occurred there would be more acidotic neonates with low Apgar scores and possibly other sequelae of neonatal asphyxia with acidosis.[13] It is thus left for the clinician to use electronic FHR monitoring and fetal scalp blood sampling as complementary methods that are still only parts of the whole clinical picture that he must appreciate in order to make appropriate decisions for intervention or nonintervention.

REFERENCES

1. Hon EH, Khazin AF: Observations on fetal pH and fetal biochemistry. I. Base deficit. Am J Obstet Gynecol 105:721, 1969
2. Kubil EW, Hon EH, Khazin AF, et al: Observations on heart rate and pH in the human fetus during labor. Am J Obstet Gynecol 104:1190, 1969
3. Saling E, Schneider D: Biochemical supervision of the foetus during labour. J Obstet Gynecol Br Commonw 74:799, 1967
4. Hon EH, Khazin AF: Biochemical studies of the fetus. I. The fetal pH monitoring system. Obstet Gynecol 33:219, 1968
5. Miller F, Petrie R, Arce J, et al: Hyperventilation during labor. Am J Obstet Gynecol 120:489, 1974
6. Kubil F: Influence of labor on fetal acid-base balance. Clin Obstet Gynecol 11:155, 1968
7. Mondanlou H, Smith E, Paul RH, et al: Complications of fetal blood sampling during labor. Clin Pediatr 12:603, 1973
8. Wood C, Lumbley J, Renou P: A clinical assessment of foetal diagnostic methods. J Obstet Br Commonw 74:823, 1967
9. Tejani N, Mann L, Bhakthavathsalan A, et al: Correlation of fetal heart rate-uterine contraction patterns with fetal scalp blood pH. Obstet Gynecol 46:392, 1975
10. Hon EH, Khazin AF: Biochemical studies of the fetus. II. Fetal pH and Apgar scores. Obstet Gynecol 33:237, 1969
11. Modanlou H, Yeh SY, Hon H, et al: Fetal and neonatal biochemistry and Apgar scores. Am J Obstet Gynecol 117:942, 1973
12. Schifrin B, Dame L: Fetal heart rate patterns prediction of Apgar score. JAMA 219:322, 1973
13. Tejani N, Mann L, Bhakthavathsalan A: Correlation of fetal heart rate patterns and fetal pH with neonatal outcome, Obstet Gynecol 48:460, 1976
14. Quilligan EJ: Identifying true fetal distress. Cont Ob-Gynecol 13:89, 1979

CHAPTER 8

The Clinical Management of Fetal Distress

It is unfortunate that the term "fetal distress" has been applied to all forms of poor fetal outcome. The precise definition of fetal distress is impossible because the term means so many different things to different people. When the outcome is fetal death, there is general agreement that fetal distress preceded that event. Because fetal death is the only clearly defined outcome parameter, all discussions of fetal distress are hampered by the fact that sublethal distress is a vague term. There are many findings that most experts would agree are often found in association with fetal hypoxia. The following is a list of such findings.

1. Abnormal nonstress test (NST)/contraction stress test (CST).
2. Low estriol.
3. Oligohydramnios.
4. Intrauterine growth retardation.
5. Abnormal fetal heart rate patterns during labor.
6. Fetal acidosis.
7. Low Apgar scores.
8. Umbilical cord damage.
9. Small infarcted placenta.
10. Persistent fetal circulation in the neonate.
11. Neonatal seizures.

It should be noted, however, that none of the above findings is always due to fetal hypoxia. Since the goal of intrapartum fetal heart rate (FHR) monitoring is to detect fetal hypoxia at its earliest stage and to prevent the severe consequences of prolonged and severe hypoxia, a discussion of the management of intrapartum fetal distress is really directed at the detection of mild fetal hypoxia and the prevention of severe fetal hypoxia. One must then always be thinking of FHR patterns in terms of whether they are reassuring of adequate fetal oxygenation or whether one can no longer be assured of adequate fetal oxygenation. Reassuring FHR patterns include those with no periodic changes, acceleration, early deceleration and mild variable deceleration. These patterns have not been associated with an increased risk of fetal acidosis, low Apgar scores or other parameters of poor outcome due to fetal hypoxia.[1,2]

Nonreassuring patterns include the more severe forms of variable deceleration, any degree of late deceleration and various atypical or preterminal patterns. Prolonged decelerations are often a variation of severe variable deceleration but because they occur under special circumstances and have specific management implications, they should be considered separately from a therapeutic standpoint. Nonreassuring patterns are often associated with good Apgar scores but low Apgar scores are common.[3]

Baseline FHR changes of tachycardia and loss of variability should be interpreted in light of the clinical situation and the associated periodic changes that are present. Sinusoidal patterns are a rare form of baseline FHR fluctuation and sinusoidal patterns will be discussed separately under antepartum monitoring with only brief mention in this chapter.

LATE DECELERATION

We have already pointed out that late deceleration is found in association with uteroplacental insufficiency and probably implies some degree of fetal hypoxia.[4] The appearance of late deceleration is the earliest marker we now have for fetal hypoxia. In its mildest form, late deceleration is usually associated with normal or increased FHR variability. The pattern is characteristically described as uniform, appearing consistently from one contraction to the next with the depth of the deceleration corresponding to the magnitude of each contraction. This rule probably is more applicable once fetal hypoxia is established, but in the earliest phases of developing fetal hypoxia one may see the pattern occurring only intermittently (Fig. 8.1). While it would seem prudent to take measures to optimize uterine blood flow at this stage, intermittent late deceleration with good or increased FHR variability probably only bares watching and often will not become any more severe. In this situation, the patient should be laboring in the lateral position, she should be well hydrated, the oxytocin should be turned off, and she should be receiving oxygen (Fig. 8.2). If the late deceleration has occurred in association with a hypotensive episode after conduction anesthesia or with a relative hypotensive episode as following the administration of an anti-

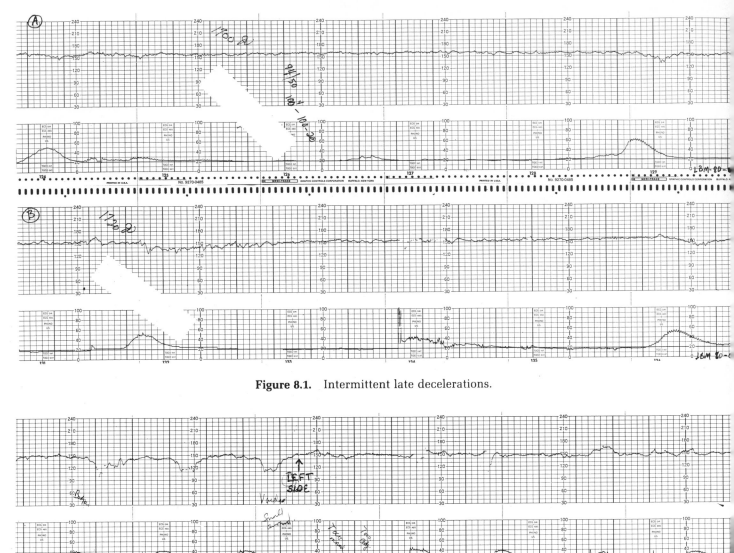

Figure 8.1.   Intermittent late decelerations.

Figure 8.2.   Late deceleration corrected by turning patient on her side.

hypertensive agent in a patient with hypertension, appropriate measures should be taken to restore blood pressure (see Table 8.1).

Assuming that this patient goes on to develop persistent late deceleration despite maximizing uterine blood flow as noted above, one is then faced with the decision of whether to deliver the patient by the most expeditious means or to get a fetal scalp blood sample with a plan to serial sampling at least every 30 min as long as the pattern persists and the patient has not delivered. Generally, I would reserve the scalp sampling approach to a patient who is making good progress, still has FHR variability (Fig. 8.3A) that is in the normal range, and is expected to deliver within the hour. Sometimes fetal scalp blood sampling may be used for a longer period where there is a great risk to the mother from operative intervention and one is willing to embark on a longer period of serial scalp sampling. If one waits until the fetus is clearly acidotic, one will expect to have a greater chance of a

Table 8.1.
Medical Management of Late Deceleration

1. Place Patient on Side.
2. Administer O_2 (100%) by Tight Face Mask.
3. Discontinue Oxytocin.
4. Correct Any Hypotension.
   (a) Appropriate Position Change.
   (b) IV Hydration with Appropriate Fluid.
   (c) Reserve Pharmacologic Pressor Treatment (Ephedrine) for Severe or Unresponsive Hypotension due to Conduction Anesthesia.

low Apgar score and perhaps other sequelae of fetal hypoxia and acidosis.[5] If one opts to use serial fetal scalp blood sampling, he may probably safely avoid operative delivery as long as the pH stays above 7.25. If there is a downward trend between 7.25 and 7.20, or the absolute value is below 7.20, one should abandon scalp sampling and deliver the patient by the most expeditious means.

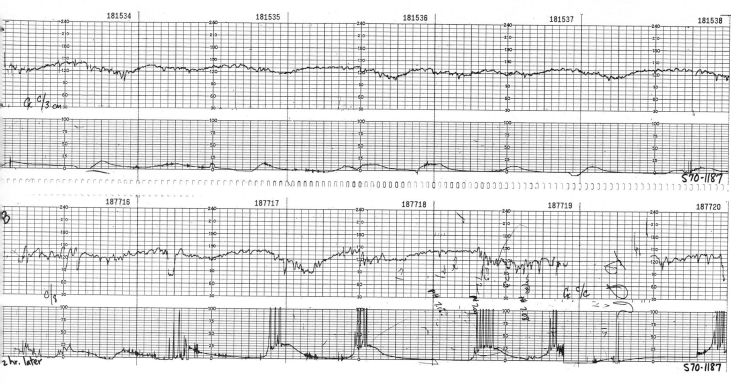

Figure 8.3A. Late deceleration with good variability is seen in the ***upper panel***. The ***lower panel*** is 1½ hr later, showing a continuation of late deceleration with good variability. The pH taken at this time is 7.08, suggesting that earlier intervention might have been advisable.

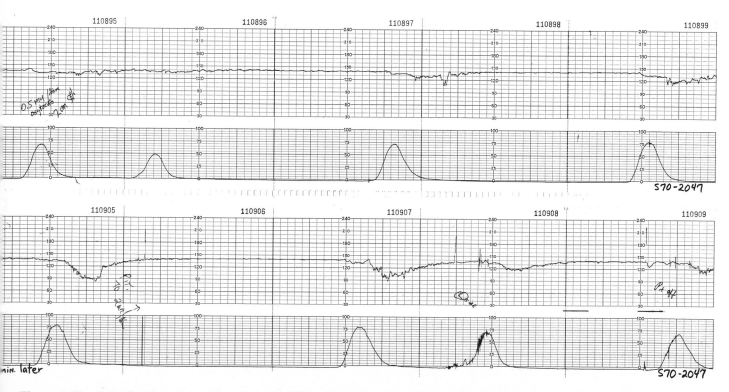

Figure 8.3B. Late deceleration with poor variability. (Reproduced with permission from Paul R, Freeman R: Selected Records of Intrapartum Fetal Monitoring with Self Instruction. Los Angeles, USC Publishers, 1971.)

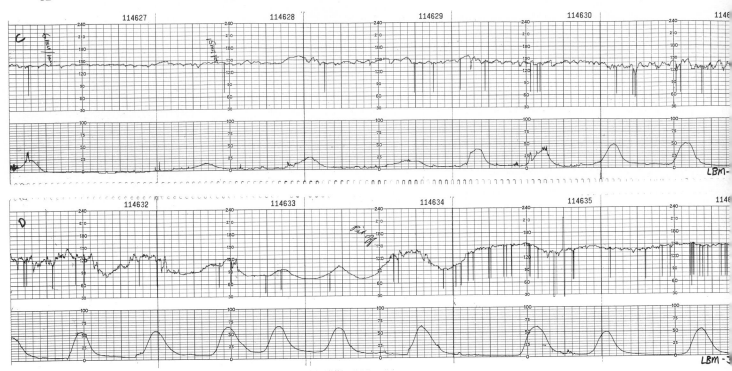

Figure 8.4. Late deceleration due to oxytocin hyperstimulation and corrected by stopping the oxytocin infusion when it says "Pit off" in *section 114634*. (Reproduced with permission from Paul R, Freeman R: Selected Records of Intrapartum Fetal Monitoring with self instruction. USC Publishers, 1971.)

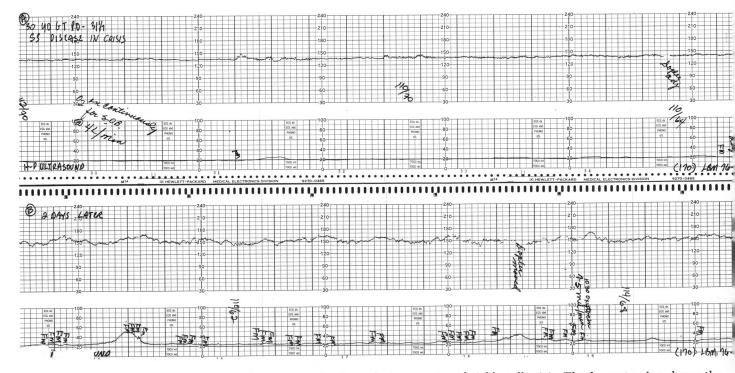

Figure 8.5. The *upper tracing* reveals a nonreactive fetus during a maternal sickle cell crisis. The *lower tracing* shows the same fetus demonstrating reactivity (acceleration of the FHR with fetal movement) after maternal recovery from the crisis.

So far the discussion has concerned the management of late deceleration when there is still good variability. Sometimes the initial recording will show uncorrectable late deceleration with a complete absence of variability (Fig. 8.3B). Since this pattern is almost always associated with severe fetal acidosis, it is our approach to move straight to expeditious delivery without a further trial of labor in such situations as the delay involved in scalp sampling would not seem justified.

When one is using oxytocin, it may be possible to alleviate the late deceleration by discontinuing the drug (Fig. 8.4), but if one cannot achieve adequate progress without contractions that produce consistent uncorrectable late deceleration, it would appear that delivery by cesarean section would be indicated. Often, however, by using an infusion pump with slowly increasing incremental doses of oxytocin, one may achieve a labor pattern sufficient to produce progress without producing late deceleration.

Occasionally, one may see a patient who is severely anemic, either from blood loss or from maternal disease such as sickle cell disease (Fig. 8.5), leukemia, or chronic renal failure. Such patients have been transfused on our service, and after transfusion the fetus has been able to tolerate labor without late deceleration, whereas before transfusion it was not possible to push the oxytocin hard enough to get productive contractions without late deceleration. We have seen an occasional patient with respiratory failure and low maternal pO_2 levels, who was having late deceleration, but after improvement in the maternal blood gas levels with respirator adjustment or with the institution of positive pressure breathing, such patients have tolerated labor without late deceleration. Similarly, patients with severe asthma and low maternal pO_2 values have been seen to benefit from pharmacologic treatment of their asthma with correction of late deceleration as the maternal pO_2 improves. The fetal response to contractions in diabetics in ketoacidosis may show late decelerations that clear as soon as the mother is properly hydrated, put on an insulin infusion, and had her electrolytes

replaced. As one can see, the total clinical picture is important when deciding how to manage a patient with late deceleration. It is also important to have a good understanding of the pathophysiology involved in any given patient where late deceleration is present in order to individualize that patient's care.

VARIABLE DECELERATION

Variable deceleration is believed to be caused by umbilical cord compression. It is the most common periodic change observed in laboring patients, being present in over 50% at one time or another. The pattern is characterized by abrupt falls in FHR to levels as low as 50 beats per minute (BPM). The pattern varies from one contraction to the next and is influenced a great deal by maternal position change. While the pattern is the most profound of the periodic FHR changes, the vast majority of the time it cannot be considered true fetal distress because unless the cord occlusion is frequent, prolonged and severe, there is no increased risk of low Apgar scores, fetal metabolic acidosis, or other significant neonatal morbidity. The problem with variable deceleration is that it may suddenly get much more severe, or it may also suddenly go away. It is much less predictable from one minute to the next than late deceleration which tends to follow a slowly deteriorating course, allowing one to watch its development over a period of time. Also because variable deceleration can change from one contraction to the next, it is hard to know what to expect in the near future. This makes the management of this pattern especially difficult when one is working in a hospital without rapid capability to move to operative delivery.

We have found that it is much easier to define the limits of reassuring variable deceleration than it is to give absolute criteria for when variable deceleration represents sufficient evidence of asphyxia to demand operative intervention. The following four criteria may be used as a guide to the limits of reassuring variable deceleration (Fig. 8.6).

1. The FHR deceleration is lasting no more than 30 to 45 sec on a repetitive basis.

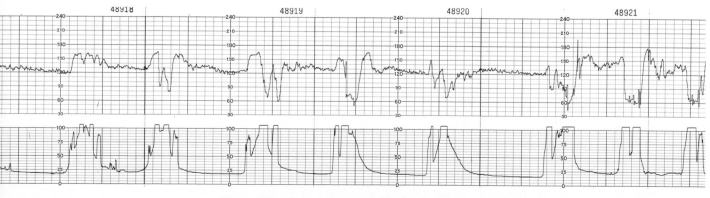

Figure 8.6. Reassuring variable deceleration.

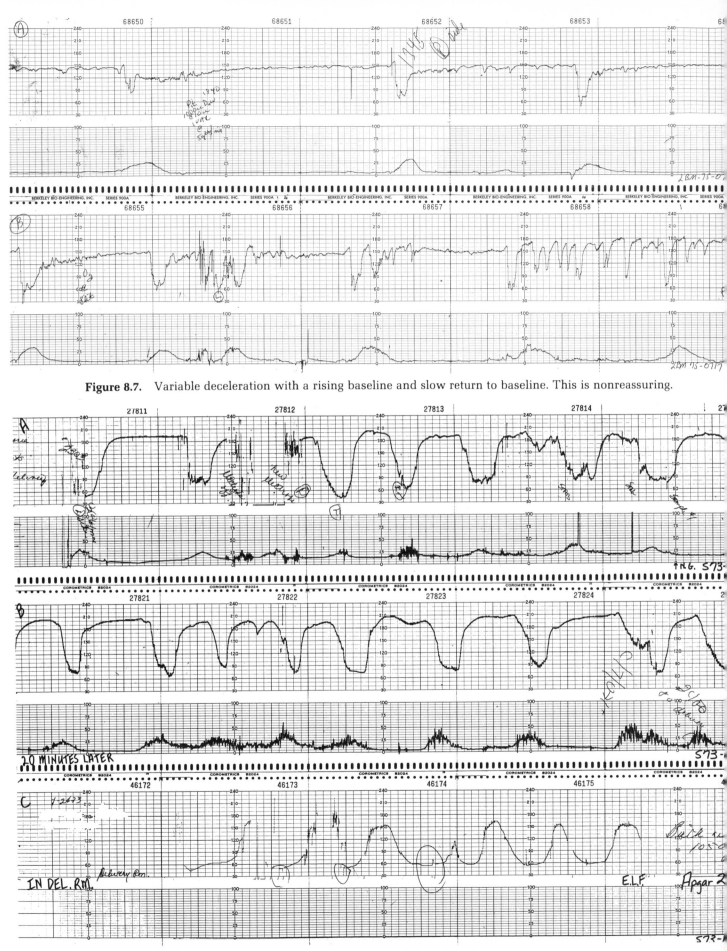

Figure 8.7. Variable deceleration with a rising baseline and slow return to baseline. This is nonreassuring.

Figure 8.8. Variable deceleration with tachycardia and loss of FHR variability. This pattern is nonreassuring. (Reproduced with permission from Paul R, Petrie R: Fetal Intensive Care Current Concepts. USC Publishers, 1973.)

2. The return of the FHR to the baseline is abrupt. There is no "late component" manifested by a slow return or a late deceleration after the return.

3. The baseline FHR is not increasing.

4. The baseline FHR variability is not decreasing.

When these limits are exceeded (Figs. 8.7 and 8.8), it does not necessarily mean that operative delivery is indicated, especially if one can move quickly to delivery by cesarean section, should the pattern deteriorate further.

If the patient is a primagravida in the early part of the first stage of labor and she is having variable deceleration that exceeds these criteria, it would not be likely to expect things to improve as labor progresses since variable deceleration tends to worsen as labor progresses and descent of the fetus puts more traction on the umbilical cord if it is entrapped or wound around the baby's neck. Generally, then, severe, uncorrectable, variable deceleration occurring in early labor is best managed by delivery by cesarean section. However, if a patient is in the second stage of labor and is having variable decelerations that exceed the stated criteria in severity, it is reasonable to wait as long as the baseline variability is not decreasing or a progressive rise in the fetal heart rate is occurring. It is common to see variable deceleration lasting more than a minute at 2-to-3-min intervals during the second stage of labor (Fig. 8.9), but if progress is occurring it is best to avoid a difficult forceps delivery as long as the baseline FHR is remaining unchanged with respect to variability and tachycardia. Fetal scalp blood sampling is generally of very little use in patients with variable deceleration

but if one anticipates delivery in 30 to 60 min in a patient with severe variable deceleration where the baseline heart rate is beginning to rise and/or the variability is beginning to decrease, a fetal scalp blood pH sample (corrected for respiratory acidosis) that is above 7.25 would be a way to delay or avoid intervention in certain such situations.

The clinical guideline to management of patients with variable deceleration is then to be reassured by the pattern if it does not exceed the stated criteria and to manage the patient with the clinical data available if those criteria are exceeded following the general rule that the closer one estimates vaginal delivery to be, the higher will be the threshold for intervention (Table 8.2). Using this policy on our clinical service has allowed us to avoid safely intervention in the vast majority of patients with variable deceleration without apparent undue jeopardy to the fetus. It is variable deceleration that is responsible for most unnecessary cesarean sections that are done when the physician is not experienced with fetal monitoring and certainly must have been the major reason for operative intervention when only ausculatory FHR monitoring was available.

Table 8.2.
Medical Management of Severe Variable Deceleration

1. Change Position to Where FHR Pattern is the Most Improved. Often Trendelenberg is Helpful.
2. Discontinue Oxytocin if Running.
3. Check for Cord Prolapse or Imminent Delivery by Vaginal Examination.
4. Administer 100% O_2 by Tight Face Mask.

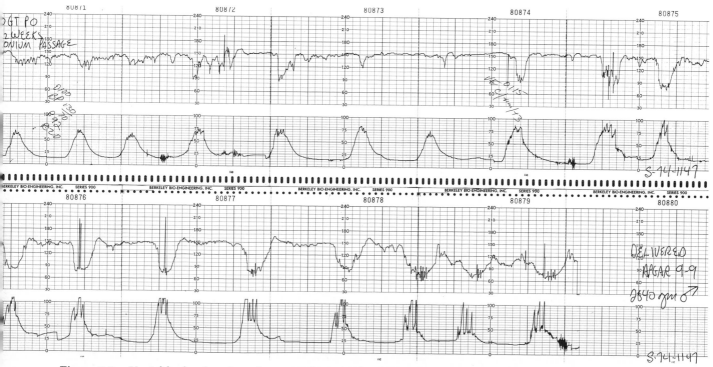

Figure 8.9. Variable deceleration of progressive severity occurring at the end of the second stage of labor.

PROLONGED DECELERATIONS

Rarely, prolonged decelerations lasting several minutes and occurring as more or less isolated events may be observed either in association with identifiable causes or without apparent etiology. If there is no known cause, prolonged decelerations are more ominous as they may represent umbilical cord compression of a severe degree or they may represent a catastrophic event such as a sudden abruption or a ruptured uterus. The following is a list of known causes of prolonged decelerations that may be identified and managed during the intrapartum period.

1. Tetanic contraction (spontaneous or oxytocin induced) (Fig. 8.10).
2. Vaginal examination (Fig. 8.11).
3. Application of an internal fetal scalp electrode.
4. Fetal scalp blood sampling.
5. Prolapsed umbilical cord (Fig. 8.12).
6. Maternal convulsion.
7. Paracervical block (Fig. 8.13).
8. Epidural block (Fig. 8.14).
9. Supine hypotension.
10. Central nervous system (CNS) anomalies.
11. Prolonged umbilical cord compression often associated with rapid descent of the fetus during expulsion.
12. Maternal respiratory arrest (high spinal, IV narcotic)

If the prolonged deceleration is temporarily related to an identifiable event, it is best to correct the situation and allow labor to continue if the clinical

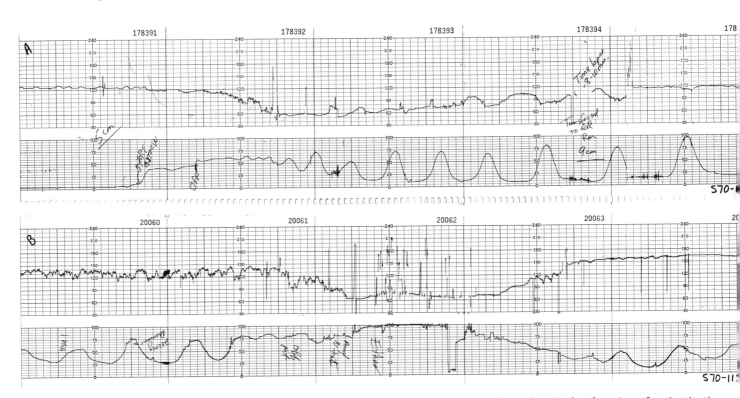

Figure 8.10. The **upper panel** represents a tetanic contraction with a severe prolonged FHR deceleration after institution of oxytocin. The lower panel represents a tetanic contraction with a severe prolonged FHR deceleration after IV Dramamine. (Reproduced with permission from Paul R, Freeman R: Selected Records of Intrapartum Fetal Monitoring with self instruction. USC Publishers, 1971.)

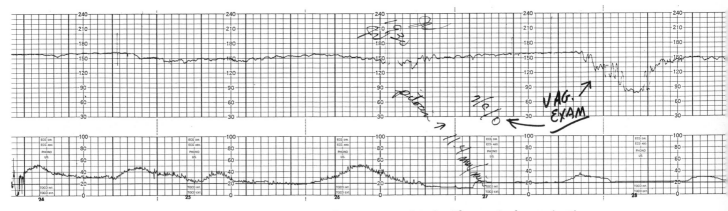

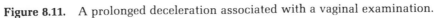

Figure 8.11. A prolonged deceleration associated with a vaginal examination.

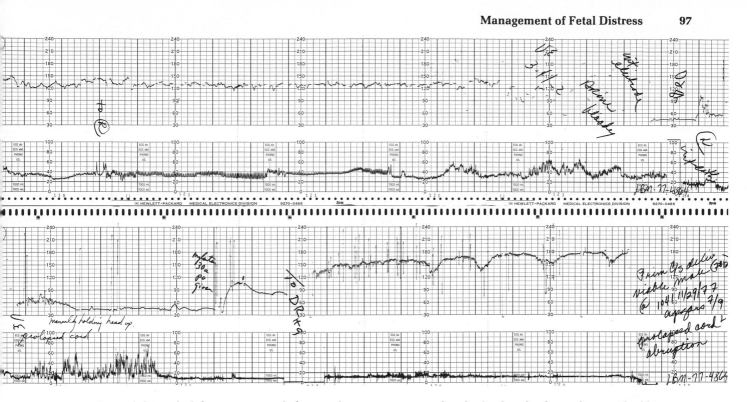

Figure 8.12. Toward the end of the ***upper panel***, the membranes are ruptured and a fetal scalp electrode is applied because of severe vaginal bleeding. The FHR is noted to be 40 BPM following the previous 130 BPM rate from the prior Doppler recording. Reexamination at the beginning of the ***lower panel*** reveals a prolapsed umbilical cord. After elevating the presenting part, the FHR shows a marked tachycardia just before a cesarean section is done which revealed an abruption. The Apgar scores were 7 at 1 min and 9 at 5 min.

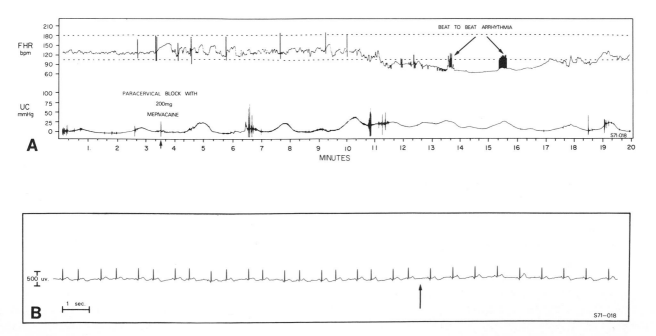

Figure 8.13A. ***A***, A prolonged FHR deceleration after a paracervical block. Note the uterine hypertonus and the beat-to-beat fetal arrhythmia. ***B***, The fetal electrocardiogram tracing during the beat-to-beat fetal arrhythmia from the paracervical block induced fetal bradycardia shown in Figure 8.13A. Note the rate reverts to a normal sinus rhythm at the ***arrow***.

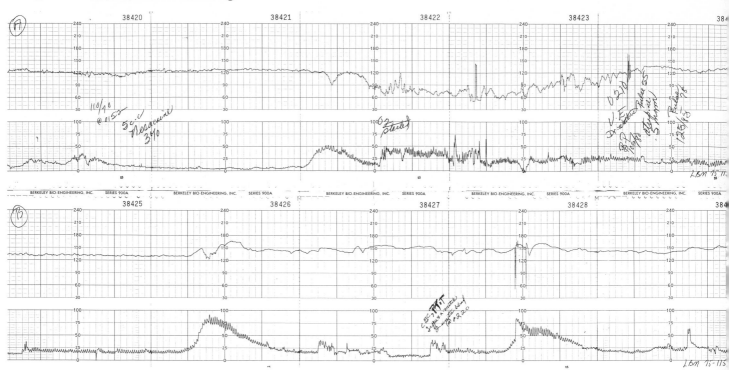

Figure 8.14. A prolonged FHR deceleration after activation of an epidural block. During the deceleration the mother's BP was not low but her pulse rate was only 55 so the anesthesiologist gave 0.5 mg atropine IV. Note the subsequent rise in the FHR and the loss of short-term variability.

picture would allow it. If, however, a prolonged deceleration occurs and there is no obvious cause, it has been our policy to observe the patient after recovery with immediate readiness to proceed to operative delivery in case the deceleration recurs. There are no clinical studies to validate this approach, but we have reasoned that if a profound deceleration occurs repetitively, there must be a recurrent cause, such as occult cord prolapse, and if delivery is not imminent, cesarean section seems reasonable. Clearly, if the prolonged deceleration is not recovering by 4 or 5 min, one should move toward rapid intervention as recovery may not be going to occur. When intervention is decided upon, it is usually best to wait 10 to 15 min in the cesarean section room after recovery of the FHR in order to maximize fetal oxygenation and clear any acidosis before delivery. This intrauterine resuscitation is usually quite effective but one must be ready to intervene while awaiting complete recovery in case the deceleration recurs during this period. If significant hypoxia did occur during the deceleration, there will usually be a fetal tachycardia which follows. When the FHR has returned to the previous baseline with restoration of the previous variability, there is probably no need to delay further. It should also go without saying that when the prolonged deceleration is recognized, one should immediately put the patient on her side, administer oxygen, turn off the oxytocin if it is running, correct any hypotension that may have occurred, and do a vaginal examination. These measures should also be continued throughout the recovery phase.

When late or prolonged decelerations occur in patients soon after receiving a conduction anesthetic, one should correct the maternal hypotension by positioning the patient either in the lateral position or even more effectively by leaving her supine, instituting sustained left uterine displacement, and raising her legs in the air. These measures will give the patient an "autotransfusion" of several hundred milliliters of blood. In addition, the patient should receive a rapid infusion of IV fluids (preferably she would have been prehydrated before the block) and be started on oxygen inhalation. In the very rare event that these measures do not restore the blood pressure and the FHR, the use of ephedrine is indicated. Since this drug has both alpha and beta adrenergic effects, it appears to restore blood pressure and uterine blood flow, whereas the conventional pressors such as norepinephrine are pure alpha adrenergic agents that will restore blood pressure but because of uterine vasoconstriction, the uterine blood flow may not be adequately restored.[6]

PRETERMINAL PATTERNS

The dying fetus will usually not have a FHR pattern that is a classical example of those patterns commonly associated with fetal distress. However, before death, we have not observed a fetus that did not show a loss of variability. In addition, most fetuses will have a period of profound bradycardia as a terminal event. Periodic changes may resemble variable deceleration but the patterns are very rounded

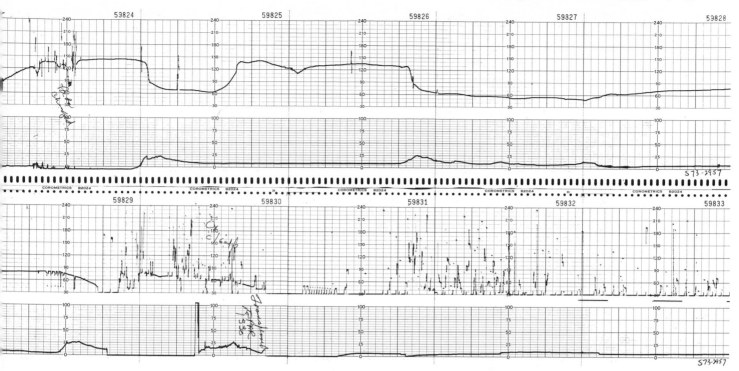

Figure 8.15. A terminal FHR pattern with a "blunted" variable deceleration pattern.

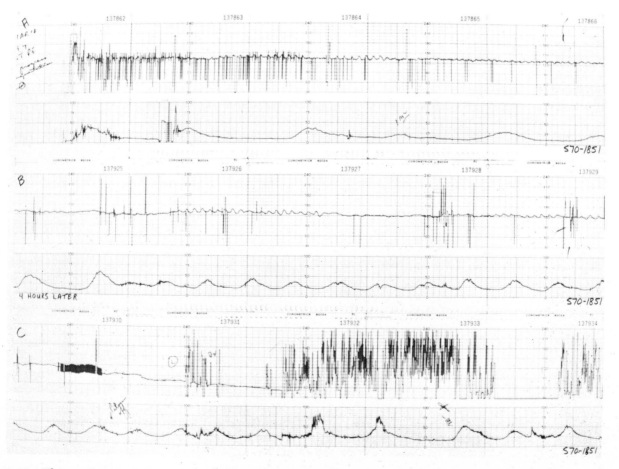

Figure 8.16. This tracing represents a terminal fetus. Note absent short-term variability and intermittent sinusoidal pattern. Just before the final terminal bradycardia there is an apparent beat-to-beat arrhythmia.

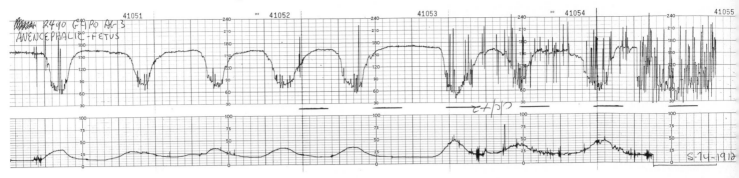

Figure 8.17. This pattern shows absent FHR variability, "blunted" variable deceleration and fetal tachycardia. This was an anencephalic fetus with fetal death occurring at the end of the tracing just before delivery.

and "blunted" (Fig. 8.15). Tachycardia may or may not precede fetal death. Rarely sinusoidal patterns have been seen in terminal fetuses. Although the baseline FHR in the terminal fetus is usually unstable and characterized by a blunted slow wandering, some terminal fetuses will have an absolutely fixed heart rate that looks like it was drawn with a ruler. Intermittent premature beats are frequently seen, and on one occasion a rapid beat-to-beat alternating atrial pacemaker was seen in a severely hypoxic fetus just preceding death (Fig. 8.16). Finally, one must be aware that these "preterminal" patterns may be seen in fetuses with major congenital anomalies (Fig. 8.17).[7]

The implications for intervention become very difficult when one is dealing with one of these profoundly severe patterns because some interventions have occurred with salvage of apparently normal neonates. However, too often the neonate is either severely damaged or does not survive. In some instances, the severe fetal anomaly is not confirmed until after cesarean section for fetal distress has occurred. Until we can be more knowledgeable about the predicted outcome in such fetuses, I think we are forced to intervene with the full knowledge that we may be doing more harm than good.

Clearly the most reliable thing about electronic FHR monitoring is identifying the great majority of fetuses that are not in jeopardy during labor. Prediction of high Apgar scores with reassuring fetal heart rate patterns is nearly 100% if one excludes nonhypoxic causes and intervening events such as mechanical injuries during birth.[3] The following is a list of those factors that may give rise to low Apgar scores in patients with normal FHR patterns just preceding delivery.

1. Birth trauma (breech, midforceps, shoulder dystocia).
2. Drugs (general anesthesia with prolonged induction delivery time).
3. Infection (chorioamnionitis, TORCH, group B strep).
4. Meconium aspiration.
5. Congenital malformations.
6. Extreme prematurity.
7. Fetal hemorrhage from an anterior placenta at cesarean section.
8. Upper airway obstruction in the newborn.

Sometimes we have seen instances where a physician indicated that the FHR pattern was completely normal and there was an unexplained low Apgar score. In this situation it is common to find either that the FHR pattern was a poor quality external tracing without sufficient clarity to define the FHR pattern or that there was late deceleration present of a subtle nature and it was missed by the clinician. Finally, a common cause for poor correlation with outcome is that the monitoring is stopped when the patient is moved to the delivery room and 45 to 60 min pass before delivery.

So while there is a very high correlation between reassuring FHR patterns and Apgar scores, there is a rather poor correlation between nonreassuring patterns and Apgar scores. Fewer than half of patients with nonreassuring FHR patterns will have neonates with 5-min Apgar scores below 7.[3] This supports the concept that FHR changes are early warning signs and lends rationale to the notion that no patient should have intervention for abnormal FHR patterns without the "validating" low fetal scalp blood pH measurement being first recorded. However, since we are not yet aware of where the point of permanent sequellae to intrapartum fetal hypoxia lies, the best approach should be one where the end point is for the best outcome rather than for the highest correlation, provided the incidence of intervention is not excessive. On our service at Women's Hospital in Long Beach where there is a very high risk population served, the incidence of cesarean section for intrapartum fetal distress is 1.9% and fetal scalp blood sampling is only done once or twice in every 300 deliveries. With continuous electronic FHR monitoring of all patients during labor at Women's Hospital in Long Beach, there has only been one intrapartum death in 12,000 deliveries in fetuses more than 1,000 g. The one intrapartum death had classical late deceleration for hours, but this was not recognized. During that time we did observe several immature monitored fetal deaths where intervention was intentionally denied because of the immaturity, and all those fetal deaths were preceded by ominous FHR patterns, often for hours before death. The approach herein described for the management of fetal distress was generally in use during this time period and these figures appear to support the value of continuous intrapartum FHR monitoring for all patients. The rest of this chapter will be devoted to case examples of the clinical management of fetal distress.

CASE EXAMPLE

The following cases are included in order to illustrate some interesting problems of management where fetal distress occurred.

Case 1

This case illustrates an example of vasa praevia (Fig. 8.18). In panel A the patient was first monitored externally after admission with a history of irregular contractions, questionable leakage of fluid vaginally, and mild vaginal bleeding. She was at term. The initial pattern revealed a prolonged deceleration followed by tachycardia and variable deceleration with minimal uterine activity. The patient was taken to double set up examination and no placenta praevia was identified with a cervix 4 cm and vertex at −1 station. Because of the decelerations and tachycardia, a cesarean section was done. An anemic fetus was delivered with Apgar scores of 4 and 7. The neonate did well after transfusion. Examination of the placenta and membranes revealed a ruptured fetal vein in an area of velamentous cord insertion at the site of membrane rupture.

Retrospectively, the case should have been suspicious for the diagnosis of fetal hemorrhage from a vasa praevia. The tachycardia was probably due to fetal hypovolemia and the variable deceleration can be explained by the funic presentation represented by the vasa praevia being compressed over the cervical os.

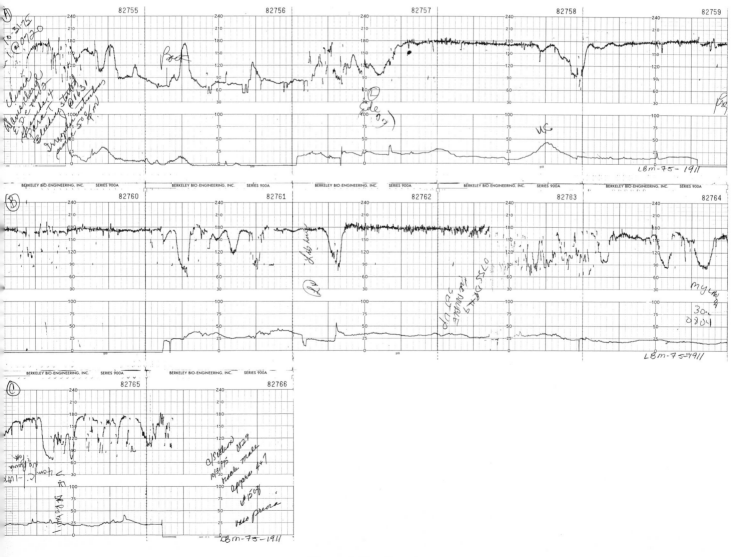

Figure 8.18.   Case 1.

Case 2

This case represents an example of a patient who was inappropriately treated with ephedrine for hypotension following an epidural (Fig. 8.19). In the middle of panel A, the epidural is activated with 6 ml of 1½% xylocaine. Her baseline blood pressure was 100/60. In panel B, her blood pressure is 90/60. The FHR pattern to this point is perfectly normal. At the beginning of panel D, approximately 50 min after activation of the epidural, the blood pressure (BP) is

noted to be 80/50. The patient is on her side and oxytocin is running at 3 munits/min. Even though the patient was asymptomatic, and the FHR was normal, 10 mg of ephedrine was given IV. There is a prompt FHR deceleration followed by a rise in the maternal BP to 140 systolic. The mother is placed in trendelenberg position, oxygen is started and the oxytocin is discontinued. The FHR recovers but the recovery is characterized by a tachycardia of 180 BPM.

Retrospectively, the patient had had a BP of 90 to

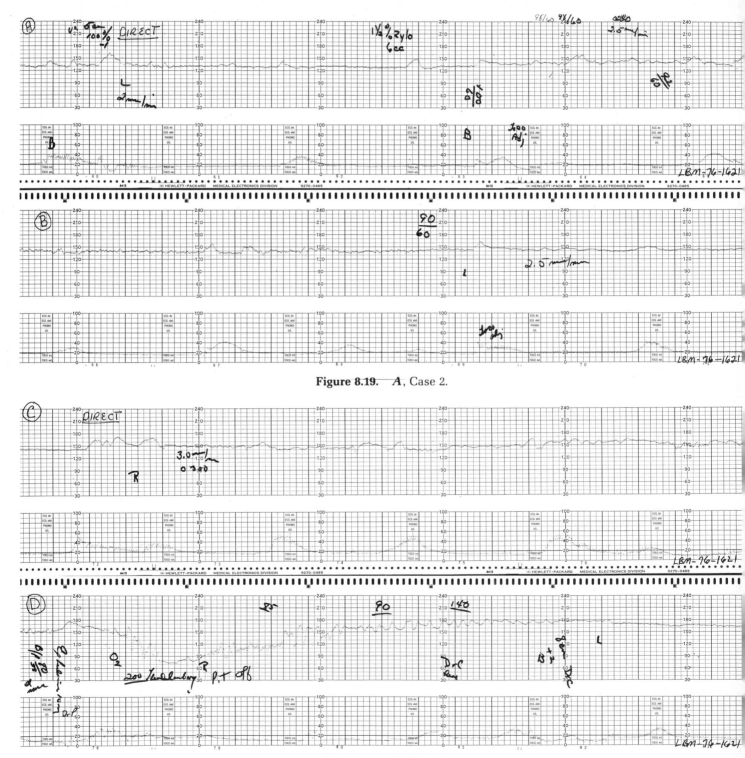

Figure 8.19.   *A*, Case 2.

Figure 8.19.   *B*, Case 2.

100 systolic throughout gestation, and she was not prehydrated adequately. The ephedrine certainly corrected her brachial blood pressure but apparently caused decreased uterine blood flow as shown by the FHR response. The alpha adrenergic effects of ephedrine may have caused this. The problem probably could have been averted if the patient had been adequately prehydrated.

Case 3

This case illustrates the FHR-uterine contraction (UC) pattern while a patient's uterus is rupturing (Figs. 8.20 A and B). The patient entered in labor with a known previous cesarian section at 40 weeks' gestation. She was monitored with a scalp electrode and uterine pressure catheter. She was fully effaced, 6 cm dilated and at 0 station when monitoring began. In Figure 8.20A there is a mild tachycardia of 160 BPM with good variability and mild variable deceleration. Beginning about half way through Figure 8.20A for the first time there is noticed some added late decel-

eration and at the end of Figure 8.20A there is a fetal tachycardia of 180 BPM. Figure 8.20B shows further progression of the late component mixed with moderate variable deceleration. A decision to do a cesarean section was made in the last panel of Figure 8.20B and the uterine catheter was removed. The severe decelerations can be seen to merge during the last half of Figure 8.20B and the baseline FHR continued to rise. A cesarean section was done soon after the end of this tracing and a ruptured lower segment transverse incision was encountered. The fetus weighed 3840 g and was moderately depressed but did well. The uterus was repaired.

This case indicates that there was no evidence of a loss of uterine pressure, even though the rupture was probably present during monitoring. The fetus probably fills the defect and keeps the uterine cavity effectively a closed space. Fetal distress appears to be the most sensitive warning sign of such catastrophies, and in this case earlier intervention probably would have been wiser. Clearly, if one is to allow labor after a previous cesarian section, it would be wise to electronically monitor the labor.

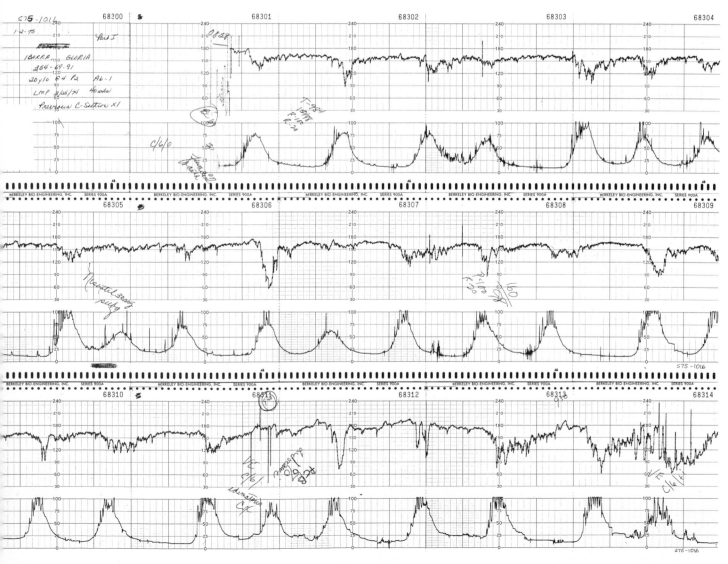

Figure 8.20. *A*, Case 3.

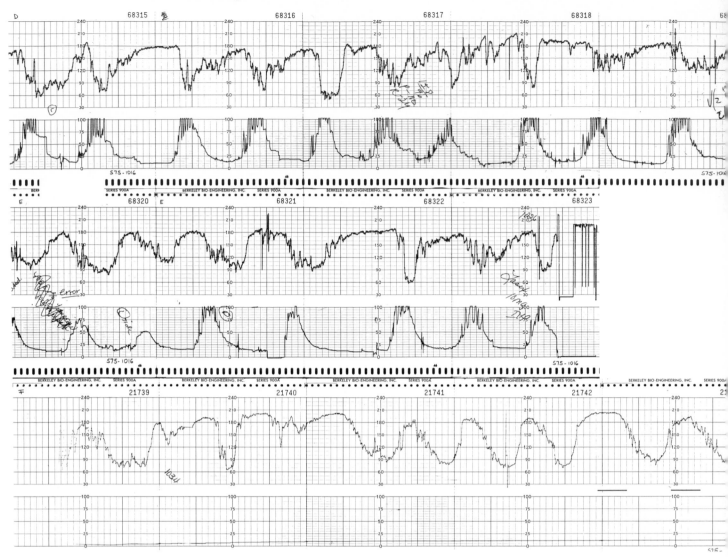

Figure 8.20. *B*, Case 3.

Case 4

This case illustrates a case of fetal distress that was not recognized for technical reasons (Fig. 8.21). The patient was a primagravida with eclampsia who was admitted at 29 weeks' gestation and treated with Apresoline and $MgSO_4$. She was monitored with Doppler for heart rate and an external toco while oxytocin was being administered. This recording begins several hours after she had been admitted and the tracing you see in the first half of the upper panel is representative of the previous several hours.

The FHR from Doppler is of very poor quality but one can see evidence of small decelerations that were missed because of artifact. In the lower panel the scalp electrode was applied in the middle of section 63827. A smooth heart rate with small decelerations is noted and then it was recognized that the paper speed was only 1 cm/min. At the end of section 63828, the paper speed was increased to 3 cm/min. An internal catheter was placed at the same time as

the scalp electrode and the last 3 sections of the lower panel show obvious late decelerations with absent variability which had been present all along but was not recognized because of poor data acquisition. A cesarean section was done but a very depressed baby was born that has a guarded prognosis.

Case 5

This case illustrates the effect of lowering maternal blood pressure on the FHR and fetal pH (Fig. 8.22). The patient was a severe preeclamptic with BP 172/120 after full treatment with $MgSO_4$. The tracing in the upper panel shows a normal FHR-UC tracing with good variability and a baseline rate of about 135 BPM. There are no periodic decelerations. The middle panel shows the FHR tracing after the maternal BP was dropped to 140/104 with Diazoxide. Note the decreased variability, rise in baseline FHR to about 160 BPM, and the presence of late decelerations. At the beginning of the bottom panel, oxygen is started,

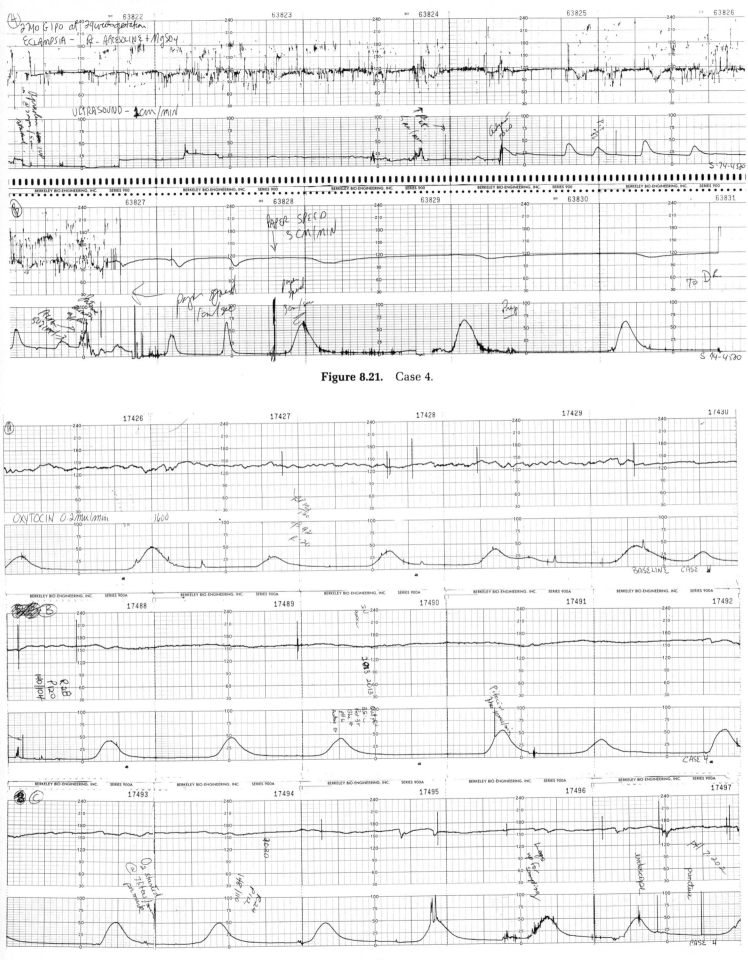

Figure 8.21. Case 4.

Figure 8.22. Case 5.

the baseline FHR remains elevated, and late decelerations are still present. At the end of the bottom tracing, a fetal scalp pH was 7.20, indicating moderate fetal acidosis. The FHR pattern persisted and the patient was delivered by Cesarean section and the baby had normal Apgar scores.

This case illustrates that even though blood pressure lowering may be indicated for maternal reasons, one must be careful to watch the fetal response. Even though the maternal pressure was still elevated after the diazoxide treatment, the decrease from 172/120 to 140/104 represented relative hypotension from the fetal standpoint.

Case 6

This case illustrates the evolution of FHR changes to fetal death (Figs. 8.23 A, B, and C). The patient was at 34 weeks' gestation with amnionitis and meconium staining. No intervention occurred because of the perceived maternal risk of cesarean section in the face of an infected uterus and a fetus of only 34 weeks' gestation.

Figure 8.23A shows fetal tachycardia that may be due to the maternal fever with late decelerations beginning in the lower panel. The variability is moderately decreased by the end of the lower panel. Figure 8.23B shows persistence of late deceleration with progressive loss of variability and progressively shorter latent periods between the onset of the contractions and the onset of the late decelerations. Figure 8.23C shows continuation of late decelerations, tachycardia, and no variability.

At the end of the middle panel, rather deep decelerations are seen that progress to a disorganized pattern in the lower panel and fetal death occurs at the end of the lower panel. This tracing represents 3 hr of tracing and it would be reasonable to expect that fetal salvage could have occurred with earlier intervention.

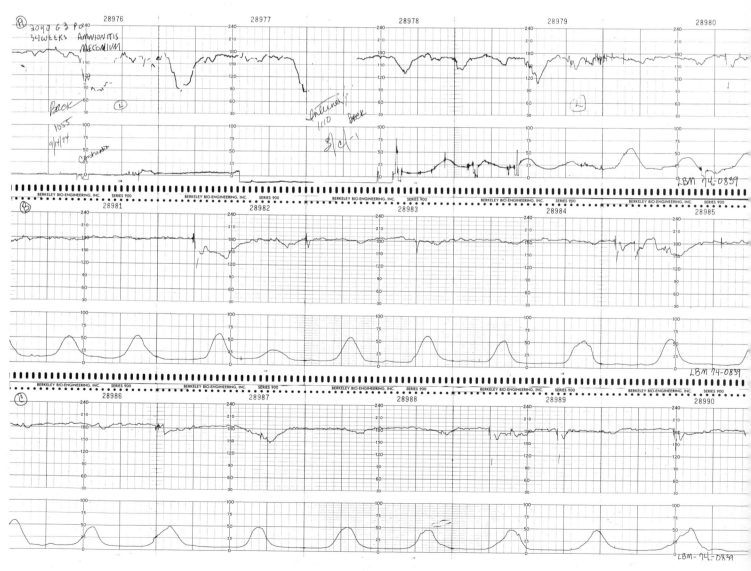

Figure 8.23. *A*, Case 6.

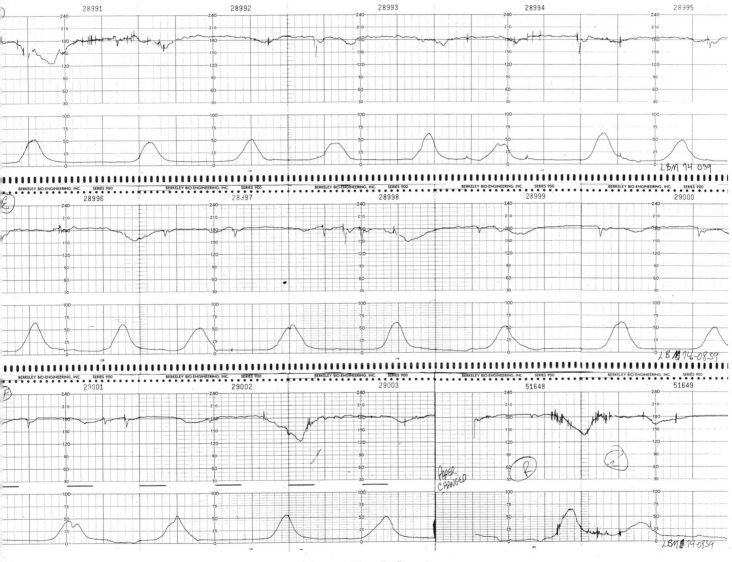

Figure 8.23.   *B*, Case 6.

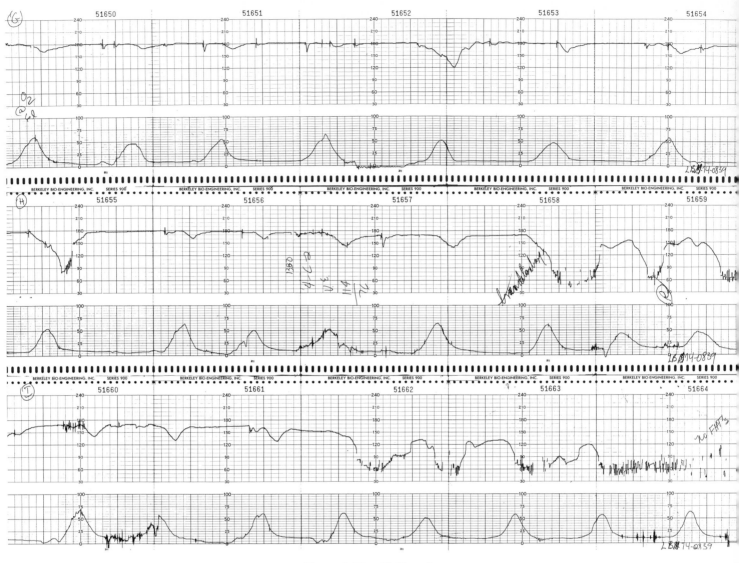

Figure 8.23. *C*, Case 6.

Case 7

This case represents an example of progressive uteroplacental insufficiency in a patient with a prolonged pregnancy with premature rupture of membranes (Figs. 8.24 A, B, and C). This tracing is from an internal fetal scalp electrode and an internal pressure catheter. The scaling factors on the monitor are 20 BPM/cm vertical scale and 3 cm/min horizontal scale. Therefore, the depth of decelerations appear accentuated as compared with a 30 BPM/cm vertical scale which is customary in the United States.

The upper panel in Figure 8.24A reveals fetal tachycardia with decreased variability, but late decelerations are not present until the middle of the center panel. Oxygen is started at the beginning of the lower panel. At the end of the lower panel and in the upper part of Figure 24B there are mild variable decelerations seen but late decelerations are persistent as is the loss of variability and the tachycardia. At this

point the patient is 7 cm dilated, fully effaced, and at 0 station. It was elected to do a fetal scalp blood sample, which revealed a fetal pH of 7.08 at the end of the lower panel of Figure 24B. At this point, the patient has been receiving O_2 by mask and has been on her side or in the Trendelenberg position except for the time of sampling in lithotomy position. She was now 8 cm dilated and was taken to the operating room, as shown in Figure 8.23C. At cesarean section, a neonate with Apgar scores of 3 at 1 min and 6 at 5 min was delivered. The cord blood pH was 6.9 on the artery and 7.1 on the vein.

It is possible that some delay occurred here because the patient was well dilated and the clinician was hoping for a vaginal delivery. It is our general philosphy that with uncorrectable late decelerations, absent variability, and fetal tachycardia, fetal pH sampling may only serve to delay intervention. This pattern would have justified earlier intervention without pH sampling.

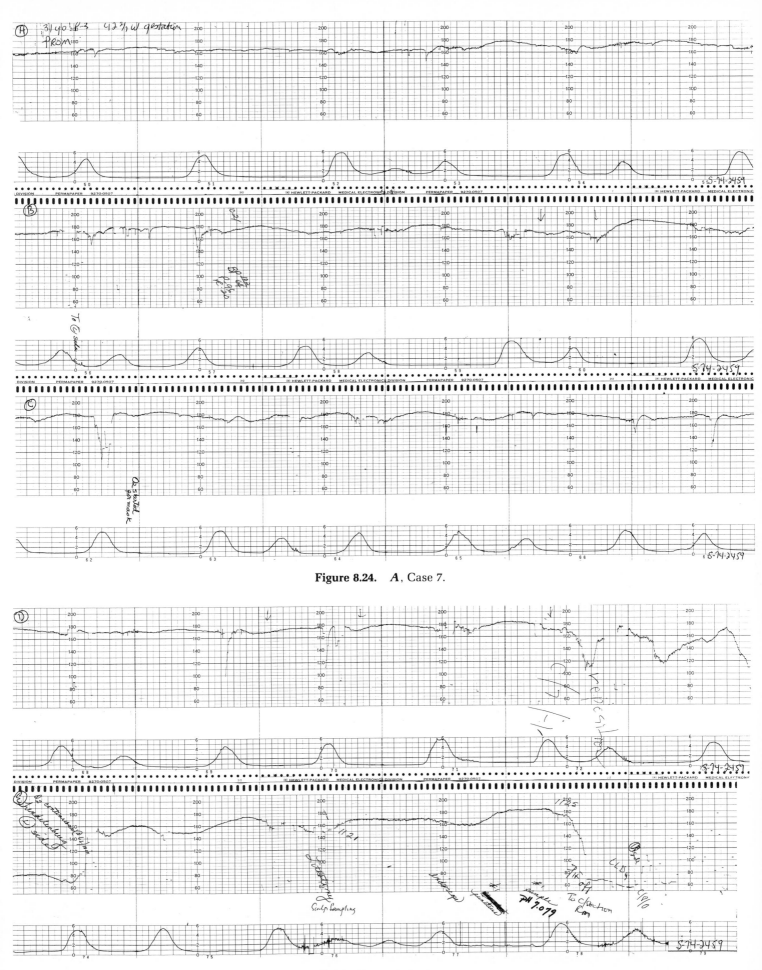

Figure 8.24. *A*, Case 7.

Figure 8.24. *B*, Case 7.

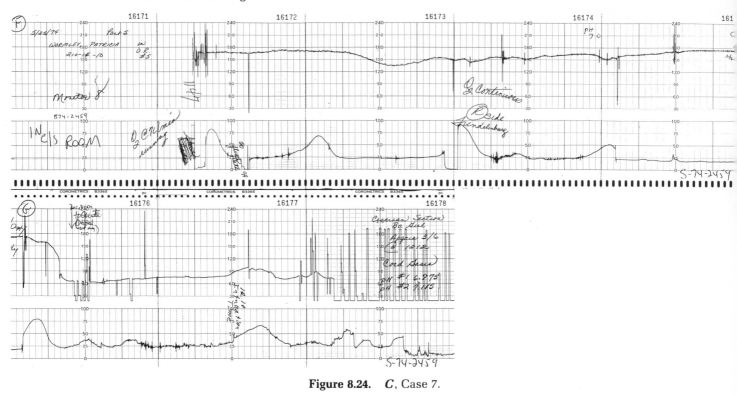

Figure 8.24.   *C*, Case 7.

Case 8

This case illustrates prolonged decelerations and an unusual fetal response resembling a sinusoidal FHR pattern (Fig. 8.25). The patient was at 42 weeks' gestation and was being monitored with external Doppler and toco. In the upper panel the patient vomited and a sudden prolonged deceleration occurred after a previously perfectly normal FHR tracing. She was put on her left side and oxygen was started. The cervix was 4 cm dilated and membranes were intact. At the end of the middle panel, membranes were ruptured, 4+ meconium was noted and an internal scalp electrode was inserted. At this time another profound deceleration occurred and it was followed by an FHR pattern characterized by exaggerated uniform long-term variability that would qualify as a sinusoidal pattern. The patient was delivered by cesarean section within 15 min and Apgar scores of 3 at 1 min and 7 at 5 min were observed. There was a tight nuchal cord, no amniotic fluid, and thick meconium, and the stigmata of postmaturity were noted. The neonate suffered meconium aspiration syndrome, despite adequate tracheal suctioning.

This probably represents a case of intrauterine meconium aspiration occurring as a result of a profound vagal stimulus related to umbilical cord compression. The sinusoidal pattern is rare but can be seen with acute intrapartum asphyxia as was noted here.

Case 9

This case illustrates the value of FHR monitoring during the initial evaluation of a severe preeclamptic (Fig. 8.26). It also shows the difficulty sometimes encountered in detecting uterine activity from a small uterus. The patient was a severe preeclamptic admitted at 28 weeks' gestation with evidence of liver dysfunction and thrombocytopenia. It was decided to deliver her for maternal indications. Oxytocin was started and she was monitored with Doppler and external toco. The upper panel of Figure 8.26 reveals no evidence of uterine activity despite several attempts to adjust the toco. The FHR is smooth and there are several decelerations characteristic in shape for late deceleration. The patient was moderately obese and the uterus measured only 22 cm, but good dates with sonographic confirmation revealed a 28 weeks' gestation with probable fetal growth retardation and oligohydramnios accounting for the small uterus. The FHR pattern was considered to represent late deceleration with decreased or absent variability and a cesarean section was performed that resulted in a moderately depressed 740-g growth-retarded neonate that did well in the nursery.

Even though one cannot record contractions sometimes, the FHR changes should be observed closely and if the clinical picture fits as in this case, one should be willing to interpret such changes as ominous.

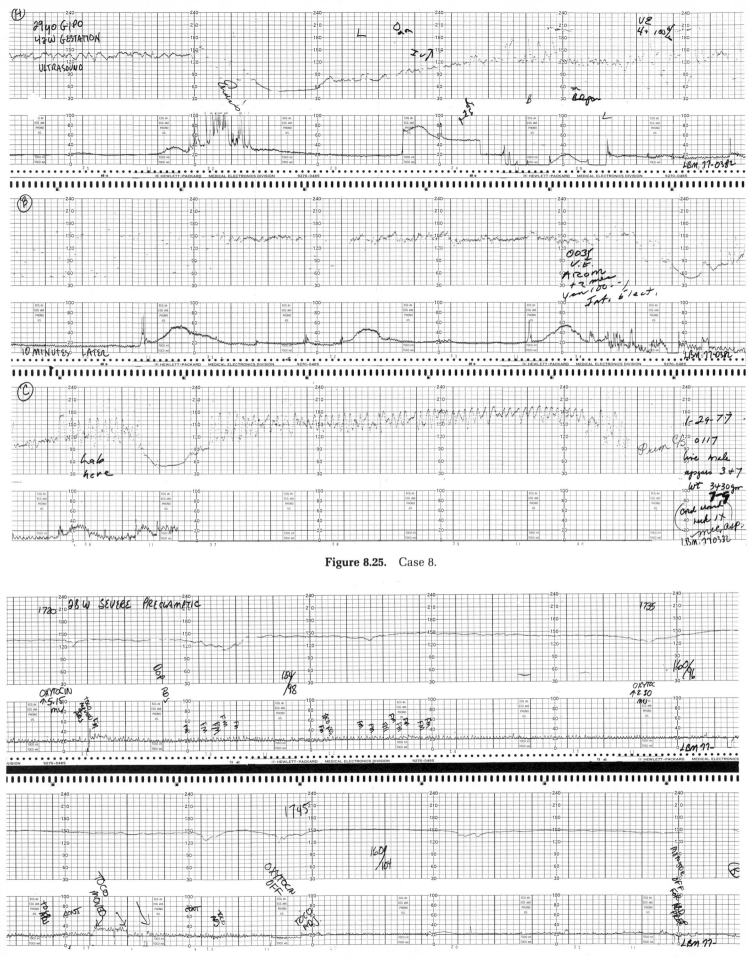

Figure 8.25. Case 8.

Figure 8.26. Case 9.

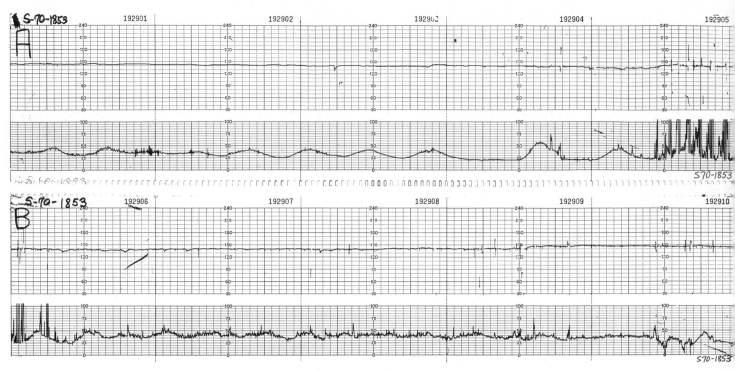

Figure 8.27. Case 10.

Case 10

This case represents an example of complete loss of variability without periodic changes (Fig. 8.27). The neonate was severely depressed with a questionable neurologic potential. Complete absence of variability without periodic changes may represent a very severely damaged fetus that is either currently hypoxic or that may have suffered brain damage from a previous insult. It also may represent a CNS malformation. It is our approach in such instances to do a fetal scalp blood sample, and if the pH is normal, intervention would not seem advisable. However, one cannot reassure the parents as there may have been a previous insult or structural defect of the CNS that will result in severe developmental problems, but operative intervention would not appear to offer any advantage if the pH is normal. If the pH is low, intervention may be indicated but the prognosis should remain guarded. (Reproduced with permission from Paul R. Freeman R: Selected Records of Intrapartum Fetal Monitoring with Self Instruction. USC Publishers, 1971.)

REFERENCES

1. Kubli FW, Hon EH: Observations on heart rate and pH in the human fetus during labor. Am J Obstet Gynecol 104:1190, 1969
2. Hon EH, Khazin AF: Biochemical studies of the fetus II. Fetal pH and Apgar scores. Obstet Gynecol 33:237, 1969
3. Schifrin B, Dame L: Fetal heart rate pattern of Apgar score. JAMA 219:322, 1973
4. Martin CB, De Haan J, Wilot BVD, et al: Mechanisms of late decelerations in the fetal heart rate. A study with autonomic blocking agents in fetal lambs. Eur J Obstet Gynecol Reprod Biol 9:361, 1979
5. Tejani N, Mann L, Bhakthavathsalan A: Correlation of fetal heart rate patterns and fetal pH with neonatal outcome. Obstet Gynecol 48:460, 1976
6. Greiss FC Jr, Crandell DL: Therapy for hypotension induced by spinal anesthesia during pregnancy. JAMA 191:793, 1965
7. Garite TJ, Linzey EM, Freeman RK, et al: Fetal heart rate patterns and fetal distress in fetuses with congenital anomalies. Obstet Gynecol 53:716, 1979

CHAPTER 9

Antepartum Fetal Monitoring

Since more than two-thirds of fetal deaths occur before the onset of labor,[1] it would be natural to extend the principles of intrapartum fetal heart rate (FHR) monitoring to the antepartum period in an effort to prevent these fetal deaths. A substantial number of antepartum deaths occur in women with risk factors for uteroplacental insufficiency (UPI).[2] Other causes include hydrops fetalis, intrauterine infections, cord accidents, congenital anomalies, and a number of unknowns. The development of an effective test for assessing the antepartum fetus, could allow intervention before fetal death or asphyxic damage. Before the availability of such tests, the only method for attacking this problem was to prematurely deliver such fetuses based on empirical risk data as in the method proposed by Priscilla White for managing diabetics.[3] The problem with such an approach is two-fold: the majority of such prematurely delivered fetuses were not really in jeopardy; and often the morbidity and mortality from premature intervention exceeded that of the original risk factor. Ideally it would be preferable to treat the disease and allow the fetus to go to term; however, we have made few advances in treating UPI.

Several biochemical tests have been developed to evaluate the antepartum fetus. These include estriol, human placental lactogen, diamine oxidase, heat stable alkaline phosphatase, and others. These have proven variably useful, but none is alone a satisfactory answer. Other forms of testing before antepartum electronic fetal heart rate monitoring were essentially limited to evaluation for the presence or absence of meconium using amnioscopy or amniocentesis.

PHYSIOLOGY AND PATHOPHYSIOLOGY

UPI is a term that implies inadequate delivery of nutritive and/or respiratory substances to appropriate fetal tissues. The term, UPI, may be applied specifically to inadequate exchange within the placenta due to decreased blood flow, decreased surface area, or increased membrane thickness. UPI may also be applied more generally to problems of inadequate maternal delivery of nutrients or oxygen to the placenta as in starvation or cyanotic cardiac disease, or to problems of inadequate fetal uptake as in fetal anemia. Kubli et al.[4] suggested that UPI be divided into nutritive and respiratory components; nutritive deficiency leading to intrauterine growth retardation (IUGR) and respiratory insufficiency leading to asphyxic damage and subsequent fetal death. Parer[5] has suggested that fetal nutritive function generally precedes fetal respiratory compromise (except in diabetics). Figure 9.1 is a theoretical scheme through which a fetus might pass with declining placental function. The rapidity with which this occurs may vary, being gradual in some cases such as chronic hypertension, or happening very abruptly as in abruption. Other conditions, perhaps including diabetes, might bypass the stage of nutritive insufficiency completely.

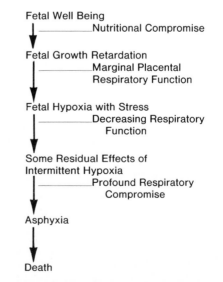

Fetal Well Being
    ⟶ Nutritional Compromise

Fetal Growth Retardation
    ⟶ Marginal Placental
        Respiratory Function

Fetal Hypoxia with Stress
    ⟶ Decreasing Respiratory
        Function

Some Residual Effects of
Intermittent Hypoxia
    ⟶ Profound Respiratory
        Compromise

Asphyxia

Death

Figure 9.1. Theoretical scheme of fetal deterioration with progressive uteroplacental insufficiency. (Reproduced with permission from Garite TJ, Freeman RK: Clin Obstet Gynecol 6:295, 1979.

Table 9.1.
Conditions Placing the Fetus at Risk for UPI

1. Preeclampsia/Ecclampsia
2. Chronic Hypertension
3. Collagen Vascular Disease
4. Diabetes Mellitus
5. Renal Disease
6. Anemia
7. Rh isoimmunization
8. Hyperthyroidism
9. Advanced Maternal Age
10. Cyanotic Heart Disease
11. Prolonged Pregnancy (>42 Wk)
12. Severe Rh isoimmunization

RISK IDENTIFICATION

To apply this knowledge to patient management, one must first identify the patients at risk who are to be evaluated. This risk identification must include data from the patient's history, physical examination, ongoing patient assessment (including uterine growth and blood pressure), and laboratory data. Those conditions which place the patient at risk for UPI are listed in Table 9.1. In addition, some obstetrical/fetal conditions apparently unrelated to maternal disease may also be associated with UPI. These include postmaturity, fetal anemia (of whatever cause), discordant twins, and idiopathic IUGR.

DEVELOPMENT OF ANTEPARTUM HEART RATE TESTING

It can be surmised that given a condition of borderline fetal oxygenation, a test that further stresses the fetus in terms of oxygen deprivation might produce some biophysical sign of such compromise and that this data might be prognostically important. Early tests attempting to accomplish this utilized the maternal exercise stress test and breathing gas mixtures with decreased oxygen concentrations.[6] It can be suggested from animal data that uterine contractions producing an intraamniotic pressure in excess of about 30 mm Hg create an intramyometrial pressure that exceeds mean intraarteriolar pressure, thereby, temporarily halting uterine blood flow.[7] A well-oxygenated fetus tolerates this limited period of intervillous stasis well. However, a hypoxic fetus will manifest late decelerations. It was therefore suggested that by inducing such contractions in the antepartum period one might be able to detect the compromised fetus before death (and possibly damage) occurred. In 1966, Hammacher[8] studied 207 pregnancies in the antepartum period and found late decelerations to correlate with lower Apgar scores at subsequent delivery and that 17 of 23 that resulted in stillbirth had manifested such late decelerations with spontaneous contractions in the antepartum period. Subsequently, Pose et al.,[9] Kubli et al.,[4] and Spurett[10] found late decelerations in the antepartum period to correlate with stillbirth, IUGR, and low Apgar scores.

Sanchez-Ramos et al.[11] found no fetal deaths within a week of testing when no late decelerations were seen.

The first systematic trial in this country was performed by Ray et al. in 1972.[12] They performed a prospective blinded trial on 66 patients. They defined criteria for adequate testing, frequency of testing, and results, all of which are in common use in this country today. Of the 66 patients, there were 15 with positive tests of which 3 had fetal deaths, and 6 had low Apgar scores. Furthermore, there were no deaths within a week of a negative test. Ray and Freeman called the test the oxytocin challenge test (OCT) and this has been the most frequently used name for the test. Other names include contraction stress test (CST) and antepartum stress cardiotocography.

PERFORMING THE OCT

Indications for testing and the gestational age for beginning testing are listed in Table 9.2. Many factors go into the decision as to when to begin testing. Single factors with minimally to moderately increased risk for antepartum death nearly all warrant surveillance starting at about 34 weeks (e.g., previous stillbirth, advanced maternal age). The highest risk factors are chronic hypertension with preeclampsia and the more severe classes of diabetes mellitus (D, F, and R); here testing should begin at 30 to 32 weeks. When these are combined (diabetes and hypertension), the risk is most severe. Should any of these be complicated by documented or suspected IUGR, then risk is extremely high, and in all these high risk situations, testing should begin when it is reasonable to expect a chance of neonatal viability (26 to 28 weeks). It should be a general rule with antepartum heart rate

Table 9.2.

Indication	Start Testing At:
Diabetes	
Class A (Uncomplicated)	40 Wk
Class A with Previous Stillbirth, Abnormal Fasting Blood Sugar, or Hypertension	34 Wk
Class B, C, D	34 Wk
Class F, R	28–32 Wk
Preeclampsia/Eclampsia	When Diagnosed after 26–28 Wk
Chronic Hypertension	34 Wk
Maternal Anemia	34 Wk
Rh Isoimmunization (Severe)	28–34 Wk
Previous Stillbirth	34 Wk
Suspected IUGR*	28 Wk or when Suspected
Post Dates	42 Wk
Cyanotic Heart Disease	34 Wk
Hyperthyroidism	34 Wk
Meconium-Stained Amniotic Fluid	When Diagnosed after 28 Wk

* Should IUGR be suspected earlier in any of these conditions, testing should begin as soon as neonatal viability would be reasonable to assume (26–28 wk).

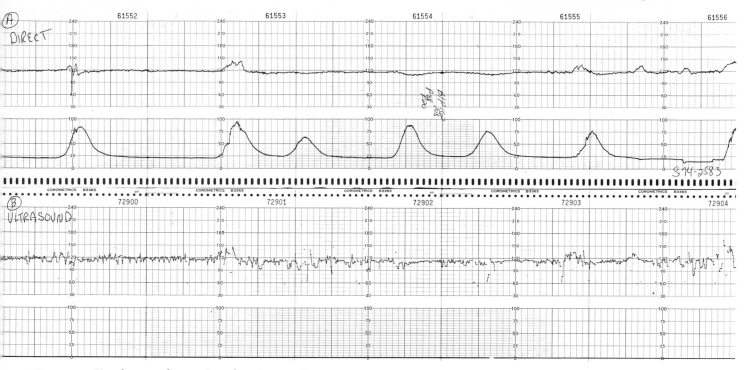

Figure 9.2. Simultaneously monitored patient with internal/direct FHR (***panel A***) and external/ultrasound FHR (***panel B***). A single, late deceleration seen on internal monitor is not easily seen externally because of the masking by the more noisy ultrasound modality.

testing, that one should not begin testing until it would be possible to intervene (i.e., deliver) when a clearly abnormal test is obtained.

To perform the test, external monitors for contractions and heart rate are placed on the patient. Contractions are monitored using a standard tocodynamometer. As pointed out in Chapter 5 on contraction monitoring with an external tocodynamometer, frequency is reliably measured, duration less so, and strength of contractions only relatively. The FHR is monitored by one of three means: phonocardiography, Doppler ultrasound, or abdominal fetus electrocardiography (ECG). Phonocardiography is not generally used because of frequent problems of artifact caused by outside noise, patient movement, etc. Doppler ultrasound is the most widely used and has become increasingly satisfactory with improved logic and bidirectional modes. Older ultrasound units are often undesirable for antepartum testing since artifactually increased variability may mask late decelerations which are often subtle (Fig. 9.2). Fetal ECG gives an excellent signal for antepartum testing. However, sometimes signals cannot be obtained from obese patients, rarely is abdominal fetal monitoring successful before 32 weeks, and after that only in about 70% (Fig. 9.3).

Experience is a key to obtaining quality tests in the shortest period of time. It is most desirable for nurses or technicians to specialize in antepartum testing. Optimally, a quiet, separate area should be used generally near the labor and delivery suite. The pa-

tient is placed in the semi-Fowler position to avoid the supine hypotension syndrome. Baseline blood pressure is recorded and repeated every 10 min for the duration of the test, again to be sure that supine hypotension does not occur as this may be a cause of decreased uteroplacental perfusion and falsely positive tests. Baseline contractions and FHR are recorded for a period of 20 min. The baseline heart rate and reactivity (to be discussed) are noted as is the background uterine activity. If there are three contractions in 10 min during this baseline period and heart rate recording is adequate, the test is concluded (Fig. 9.4). If not, oxytocin is begun by infusion pump at 0.5 munits/min. The rate is doubled every 15 min until three contractions lasting 40 to 60 sec occur in a 10-min period. Since it is not possible to quantitate the strength of contractions externally, the frequency and duration are used as the objective measurement of adequate stress. The only requirement of the contraction strength is that it be sufficiently strong to be palpable by the person performing the test. If late decelerations are persistent even before adequate contraction frequency is obtained, the test is positive and may be concluded. In either case, the patient is kept on the monitor until contractions have returned to baseline frequency. Should contractions persist after stopping the oxytocin, we sometimes administer oral alcohol which is generally successful in stopping contractions. Before the patient is allowed to leave, someone should review the test for adequate uterine contractions and adequacy of FHR recording. One

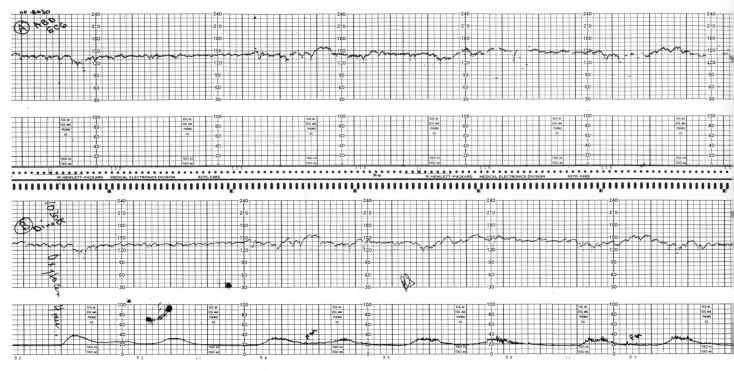

Figure 9.3. Simultaneously recorded FHR by abdominal fetal ECG (*panel A*) and direct electrode (*panel B*).

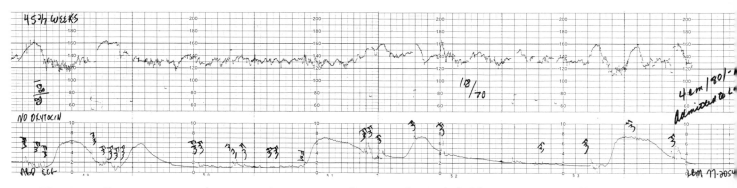

Figure 9.4. Spontaneous negative contraction stress test (no oxytocin needed). The patient is actually found to be in labor.

must be meticulous here; we have found unsatisfactory tracings to be a cause of a few of the rarely occurring "false negative" tests.

INTERPRETATION OF THE OCT

Negative

No late decelerations appearing anywhere on the strip. Adequate contraction frequency (3 in 10 min) and FHR recording must be obtained (Fig. 9.5).

Positive

Late decelerations present with the majority (greater than one half) of contractions during the period of maximum contraction stress without excessive uterine activity (see hyperstimulation). If persistent late decelerations are present before the contraction frequency is adequate, this is a positive test and may be concluded (Fig. 9.6).

Suspicious

Any late deceleration present on the strip but with less than half the contractions (Fig. 9.7).

Hyperstimulation

Decelerations after contractions lasting more than 90 sec or with contraction frequency greater than every 2 min constitutes hyperstimulation (Fig. 9.8). When such prolonged frequent contractions occur without late decelerations, it is not hyperstimulation (Fig. 9.9). Hyperstimulation may occur with either spontaneous or oxytocin induced contractions (Fig. 9.10).

Unsatisfactory

When adequate contraction frequency cannot be induced or when adequate recording of FHR is unattainable, the test is unsatisfactory (Fig. 9.11).

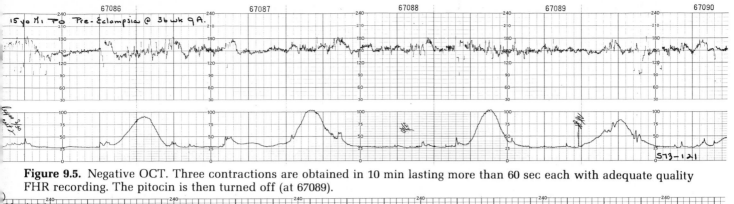

Figure 9.5. Negative OCT. Three contractions are obtained in 10 min lasting more than 60 sec each with adequate quality FHR recording. The pitocin is then turned off (at 67089).

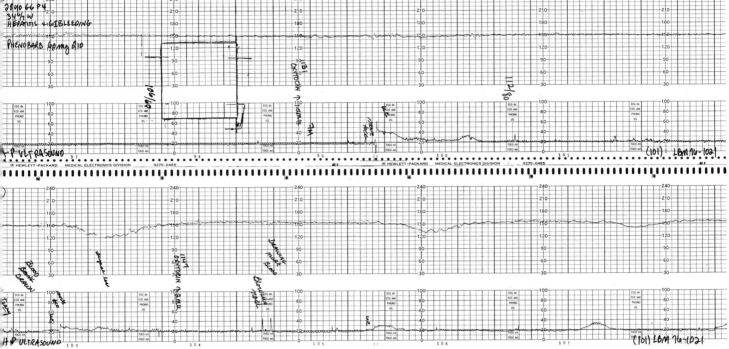

Figure 9.6. Positive OCT. Late decelerations are seen after all contractions. There is no need to increase contraction frequency since late decelerations are present with all contractions.

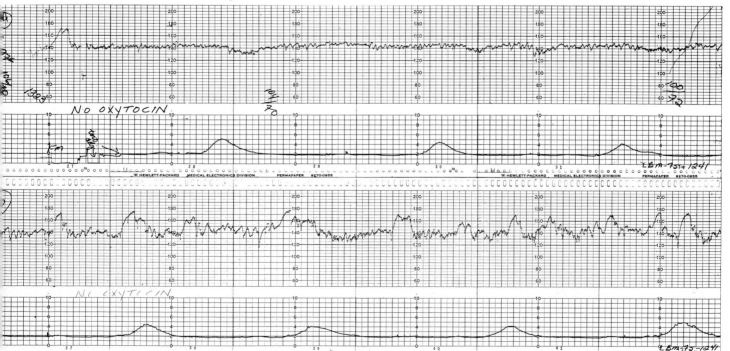

Figure 9.7. Suspicious OCT. Late decelerations are seen in **panel A** but disappear in **panel B.** As is often the case, the late decelerations are seen during a period of absent reactivity (no accelerations) but resolve when the fetus becomes reactive. The explanation for this is unclear.

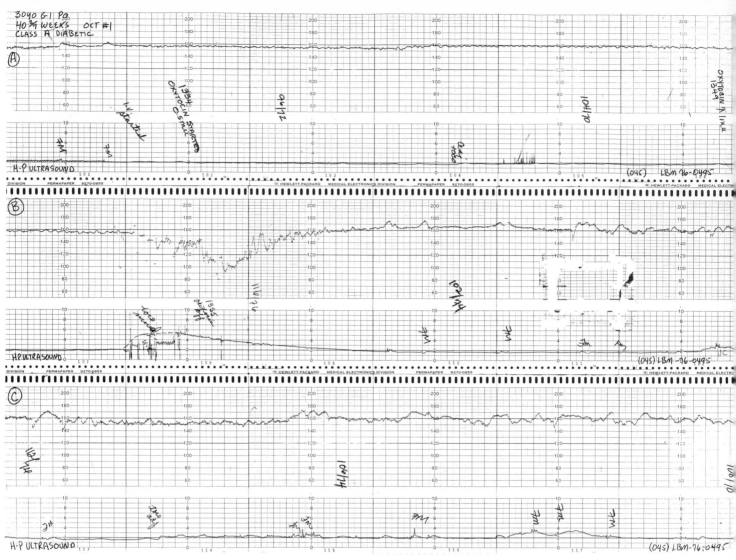

Figure 9.8. Hyperstimulation. A delayed deceleration is seen after a prolonged oxytocin-induced contraction. The test should be discontinued and repeated the next day.

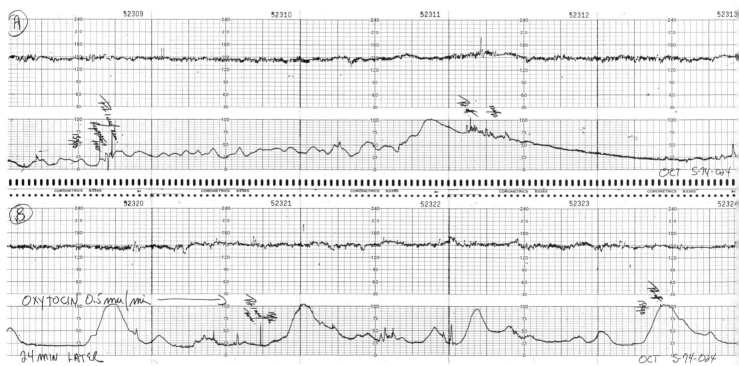

Figure 9.9 A prolonged contraction is seen in **panel A** but *no* FHR deceleration seen. The patient goes on to have a negative OCT in **panel B**. This would be interpreted as a negative OCT (*not* hyperstimulation).

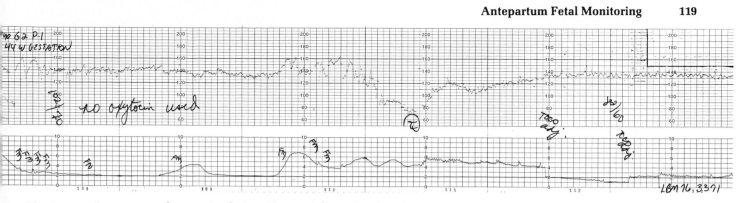

Figure 9.10. Spontaneous hyperstimulation. Here a prolonged contraction is seen with a resultant prolonged late deceleration. This occurs in this patient spontaneously (no oxytocin used). The test is discontinued and repeated the next day.

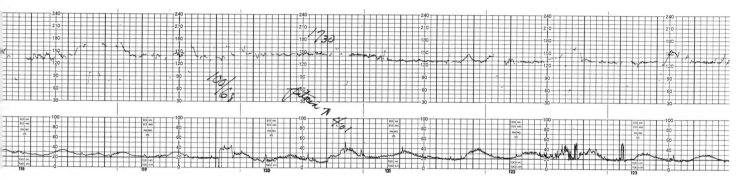

Figure 9.11. Unsatisfactory OCT. This OCT would be interpreted as unsatisfactory because the FHR is not consistently recorded sufficiently to interpret the tracing. Often the FHR data are lacking just at or after the contraction which is the critical time necessary to look for late deceleration.

OTHER PATTERNS

Variable decelerations are occasionally seen. Small frequent variable decelerations are suggestive of oligohydramnios (Fig. 9.12). More prolonged and deep variables may suggest cord entrapment, prospective data on such patterns have not been reported (Fig. 9.13). Such tests are considerably suspicious and should be repeated the next day. Variables associated with loss of variability and blunting of accelerations have been reported by Freeman and James[13] to be very ominous (Fig. 9.14). The final significant finding is the so-called sinusoidal pattern (Fig. 9.15). This consists of sine wave undulations of the FHR, with a cyclicity of about 4 to 6/min. What is actually occurring, it seems, is absence of short-term variability with increased uniform long-term variability. Late decelerations are commonly seen in association with sinusoidal patterns. They have been reported to be associated with severe fetal anemia as in Rh isoimmunization[14] or fetomaternal transfusion.[15] These patterns may also be seen in hypoxic fetal distress in the absence of fetal anemia. Generally, the sinusoidal pattern is ominous and has been associated with a high incidence of perinatal mortality. However, other tracings with increased long-term variability may be easily confused with sinusoidal patterns and might cause inappropriate intervention (Fig. 9.16). It is important to notice that sinusoidal patterns fluctuate above and below the baseline and are uniform.

Negative tests are repeated weekly. Unsatisfactory, suspicious, and hyperstimulation, are all equivocal results and require repeat testing the next day. Positive tests are acted upon only in context with the entire clinical condition including gestational age and maturity, maternal condition, and other corroborating indices of fetal well-being. Limitations of nonreassuring (positive) tests must be realized and will be discussed in the chapter on antepartum fetal management. Repeatedly equivocal tests present a difficult problem. Usually after the second or third equivocal test, we change to frequent nonstress testing and/or estriol monitoring.

Finally, it must be clearly emphasized that changing maternal status may demand more frequent test intervals. When preeclampsia worsens, when the diabetic gets significantly out of control or with any other aggravation of maternal condition which may further worsen placental perfusion or exchange, the test must be repeated immediately regardless of when the previous test was done.

CONTRAINDICATIONS

The only part of contraction stress testing that carries any potential risk is the administration of oxytocin and the resulting contractions. Therefore, patients who are at risk for uterine rupture or premature labor are those in whom stress testing would be generally precluded. These contraindications are

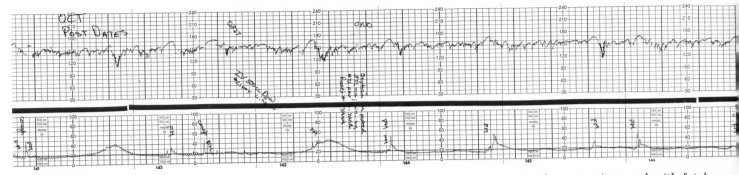

Figure 9.12. Small variable decelerations are seen in this antepartum tracing associated with contractions and with fetal movement. These may represent mild cord compression and are seen in association with oligohydramnios which may fit clinically with this postdates patient.

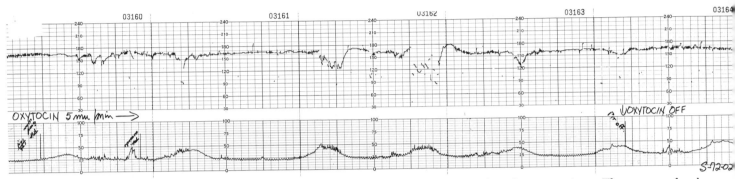

Figure 9.13. Somewhat larger variable decelerations on this OCT are associated with contractions. These may also be associated with decreased amniotic fluid volume or with cord entrapment. Their prognostic significance is not clear. Such a test would be interpreted as suspicious and repeated the next day.

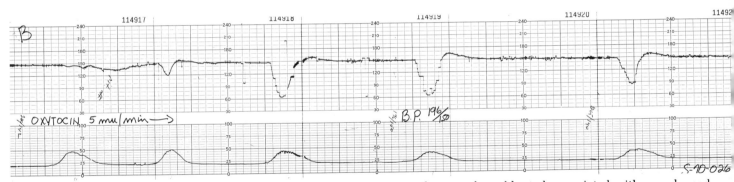

Figure 9.14. These variable decelerations are particularly ominous. They are deep, blunted, associated with a prolonged terminal acceleration (overshoot) and with a smooth nonreactive baseline. Such patterns have been associated with a high rate of fetal death and neonatal depression.

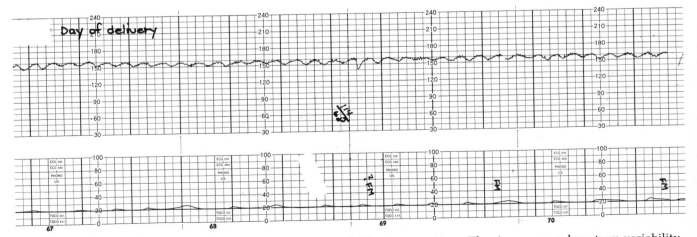

Figure 9.15. Sinusoidal pattern. This is an antepartum sinusoidal heart rate pattern. The sine wave, as long-term variability, may be seen to fluctuate above and below the baseline, is constant, and may be seen with late decelerations. This often represents severe fetal anemia or hypoxia.

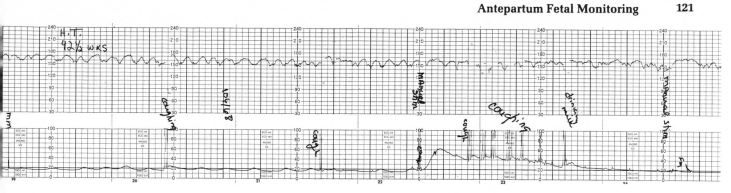

Figure 9.16. Pseudosinusoidal pattern. This is a more commonly seen pattern that may easily be confused with a sinusoidal FHR. Here is seen increased long-term variability in a healthy fetus. This differs from the true sinusoidal pattern in several ways. Notice the flattening at the low point or trough which is probably the baseline. Later on in the tracing, a more usual or normal appearing reactive FHR is seen which would not be seen if this was indeed sinusoidal.

Table 9.3.
Contraindications to the OCT

1. Premature Rupture of Membranes
2. Previous Classical Cesarean Section
3. Placenta Praevia
4. Multiple Gestation
5. Incompetent Cervix
6. History of Premature Labor

listed in Table 9.3. There are unusual situations where one might stress the patient even in the presence of such contraindications. Generally, these would be where all other indices suggest antepartum fetal distress and the only alternative to the OCT is intervention.

The authors are not aware of any cases of uterine rupture associated with the OCT. The risk of premature labor is also a theoretical one. Several studies have looked at this in their series of OCT's and found no increase in the incidence of premature labor.[10, 12, 16-18] Recently Braly et al.[19] have examined this problem in a retrospective review of 3000 OCT's where oxytocin was used (i.e., no spontaneous CST's). They found no increase in premature labor over reported incidences at various weeks of gestation. Furthermore, in the patients given oxytocin, there was no more labor in the first 72 hr after the test than in the subsequent 3 days.

EFFICACY OF THE TEST

For any antepartum test to be valuable, it must meet certain criteria. To demonstrate that the test is indeed selecting out fetuses significantly distressed, there must be correlation with signs of such distress. Freeman et al.[18] looked at a series of patients with positive OCT's and found highly significant correlation between a positive OCT and low 5-min Apgar scores, late decelerations in labor, low and falling estriols, and IUGR (Fig. 9.17). Such a test is designed to prevent antepartum fetal death so this index cannot be used to examine the tests specificity because of intervention. Freeman et al.[18] proposed that in a patient who had a positive OCT but subsequently

tolerated induction of labor without late decelerations that this was a false positive test. Using this criteria, several authors have reported incidences of false positive tests to be from 8 to 57%,[2, 10, 18, 20, 22] with an average of about 30%. Unfortunately this points out the main limitation of this test, which, like most other tests of antepartum well-being, is highly reliable when negative but much less so when positive. The explanation of these false positive tests is unclear. Perhaps since contraction strength is not measured externally, some patients are being hyperstimulated; perhaps some patients have locally decreased uteroplacental perfusion from hypotension not reflected in brachial blood pressure; or perhaps when amniotomy is performed and the patient is placed on her left side and given oxygen, the previously borderline placental compromise is reversed. This problem, however, with false positive tests can be improved upon. When a positive OCT is seen and there are no accelerations of the fetal heart rate, it is not likely to be a false positive test (Fig. 9.18).[17, 23] Conversely, when fetal reactivity (accelerations with fetal movement) is present, it is more likely to be falsely positive (about 50%)[17, 23] (Fig. 9.19). It is important to realize that assigning false positivity by virtue of absence of persistent late decelerations in labor does not totally prove that the fetus was not compromised. There most probably is a spectrum of loss of placental reserve; in addition, it must be realized that placental compromise is not a one way street. Positive tests may revert to negative if the condition which caused the inadequate placental oxygen exchange can be improved or corrected.

While there is a substantial problem with false positive tests, the converse is not true. False negative tests are extremely rare and herein lies the value of the test. Since the test is designed to predict and prevent antepartum fetal death, and since the frequency of testing is weekly, a false negative test is one after which there is a fetal death without apparent cause within a week of a negative test. Garite and Freeman[21] reviewed the literature on this point (Tables 9.4 and 9.5). The combined incidence from the literature was 3.6/1000 or 9 deaths in 2491 patients.

	Positive	No Positive	Significance
Low 5 Min. Apgar	21%	5%	p < .001
Late Decelerations in labor	76%	9%	P < .001
Low Estriols	47%	21%	p < .001
Falling Estriols	37%	10%	p < .001
IUGR	37%	10%	p < .001
Perinatal Mortality Rate	167/1000	40/1000	NS

Figure 9.17. Significance of a positive OCT. (Reproduced with permission from Reference 18.)

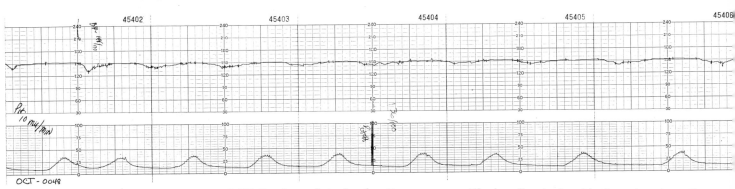

Figure 9.18. Nonreactive positive OCT. Persistent late decelerations are seen. The baseline is devoid of accelerations, (i.e., nonreactive). Such patterns are associated with more morbidity than are reactive positive OCT's.

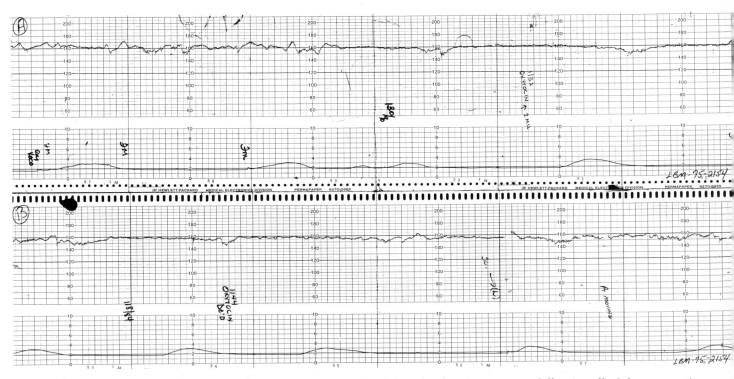

Figure 9.19. Reactive positive OCT. This is a positive OCT with late decelerations present following all of the contractions. Note, however, in contrast to Figure 9.18 that accelerations are present during at least part of this tracing.

Table 9.4.
Studies Using the CST as the Primary Means of Fetal Surveillance*

Author	Year	Total Number of Patients Studied	Number of Patients With Negative Tests	False Negatives
Spurett[10]	1971	193	170	0
Ray et al.[12]	1972	68	43	0
Christie and Cudmore[50]	1974	50	35	0
Boye et al.[16]	1974	41	36	1
Ewing et al.[41]	1974	58	49	0
Cooper et al.[42]	1975	89	66	0
Schifrin et al.[43]	1975	120	101	0
Gaziano et al.[44]	1975	72	64	0
Hayden et al.[45]	1975	105	97	0
Weingold et al.[22]	1975	154	109	0
Freeman et al.[18]	1976	390	324	2
Farahani et al.[20]	1976	333	288	1
Boehm et al.[46]	1976	152	137	2
Fox et al.[17]	1976	209	163	0
Bhakthavathsalan et al.[47]	1976	100	68	0
Garite et al.[2]	1978	430	403	0
Baskett†[48]	1975	Not Stated	205	2
Marcum†[49]	1977	Not Stated	140	1

False Negative Rate = 9/2498 patients with negative tests = 3.6/1000

* Reprinted with permission from Zuspan F, Christian D (editors) In: Reid's Controversies in Obstetrics and Gynecology (3rd ed). WB Saunders, Philadelphia, 1979.
† Studies published as case reports where total number of patients with negative tests are stated.

Table 9.5.
False Negative CST*

Apparent Cause	Time Interval between CST and Fetal Death
Thrombosis of Chorionic Vessels	Seven days
Tight Nuchal Cord—Several Loops	Not Specified
Multiple Congenital Anomalies	Not Specified
Multiple Congenital Anomalies†	Seven days
Abruptio Placenta	Five days
No Apparent Cause	Five days
No Apparent Cause	Seven days
No Apparent Cause (Associated with Acute Lowering of Blood Pressure with Hypotensive Agents)	Seven days
No Apparent Cause†	Thirteen hours

* Reproduced with permission from Zuspan F, Christian D (editors) In: Reid's Controversies in Obstetrics and Gynecology (3rd ed) WB Saunders, Philadelphia, 1979.
† Test probably suspicious in review.

However, in reviewing the cases more closely, there were only three deaths in which the likely cause was UPI and the test was indeed negative for a corrected false negative rate of 1.2/1000. Remember, the test can only be expected to detect antepartum compromise from UPI in conditions with at least some degree of chronicity. Other conditions such as cord accidents or abruptions are not likely to be predicted. Since the test is so sensitive, its value lies in allowing the clinician to keep his hands off when the OCT is reassuring rather than intervening on empirical bases such as risk scores.

NONSTRESS TESTING

The examination of characteristics of the baseline fetal heart rate unrelated to contractions and its application to the antepartum period came as a result of observations by Hammacher[8] in 1969, and by Kubli et al.[24] in the same year. They observed that "healthy" fetuses displayed normal oscillations and fluctuations of the baseline FHR and when these were absent there was an increased chance of depressed neonates and perinatal mortality. Freeman in 1974[25] pointed out that accelerations of the FHR during antepartum stress testing seemed to correlate with fetal well-being. Subsequently, several investigators[14, 26-31] have looked at accelerations of the FHR and other parameters of the nonstressed antepartum FHR as a means of evaluating the fetus at risk. These other parameters include baseline heart rate, apparent heart rate variability, and the presence or absence of spontaneously occurring decelerations.

Accelerations of the FHR occur in response to fetal movement, uterine contractions, or external stimuli such as sound or movement (Fig. 9.20). Since accelerations generally occur in response to such other events, the presence of such accelerations is often referred to as reactivity. Accelerations of the FHR seem to be an objective reflection of FHR variability which is not well-monitored externally. Fetal sleep-like states and central nervous system (CNS) depressant drugs depress both variability and reactivity. Accelerations may also be caused by partial occlusion of the umbilical cord resulting in venous occlusion and fetal hypotension without umbilical arterial occlusion. Therefore, FHR accelerations seem to be a reflection of CNS alertness and activity and their absence seems to depict CNS depression which can be caused by hypoxia/asphyxia, drugs, fetal sleep, or congenital anomalies. There is some question whether the inciting cause of the acceleration is or is

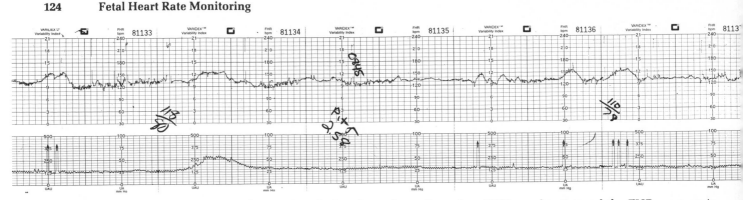

Figure 9.20. FHR Accelerations. On this tracing, during the early portion of an OCT, accelerations of the FHR are seen in association with both fetal movements (***arrows***) and with a contraction.

Table 9.6.

Studies Using NST as the Primary Means of Fetal Surveillance

Author	Year	End Point of NST	Frequency of Testing
Lee et al.[26]	1976	3–4 AFM*/15 Min	Weekly
Rochard et al.[14]	1976	HR ⟨120⟩160 6 BPM/LTV No AFM Scoring System	Not Stated
Kubli et al.[24] (Low-Risk Patients Only)	1977	Scoring System	Hr to Every 3 Wk
Visser and Huijes[40]	1977	Absent BL Irregularity or Deceleration	Hr to Weekly
Tushuizen et al.[27]	1977	HR ⟨120⟩160 Deceleration of 30 Sec + 30 BPM No BTB Variability and No AFM	Once or Twice/Weekly or Daily if Abnormal
Flynn and Kelly[28]	1977	4 AFM of 15 BPM in 20 Min	Weekly if Normal
Krebs and Petries[29]	1978	5 AFM of 10 BPM in 30 Min	Weekly if Normal 1 to 3 Days if Abnormal
Nochimson et al.[30]	1978	4 AFM of 15 BPM in 20 Min	Not Stated
Evertson et al.[31]	1979	2 AFM of 15 BPM in 20 Min	Weekly

* Abbreviations: AFM, accelerations with fetal movement; BL, baseline; HR, heart rate; LTV, long-term variability; BTB, beat-to-beat.

not important. Accelerations in response to fetal movement, uterine contractions or external stimuli all seem to be reassurring; however, whether there is a gradient here is open to question.

DEVELOPMENT OF THE NONSTRESS TEST (NST)

When baseline heart rate parameters are used as the primary means of fetal surveillance, the test is referred to as the NST or nonstressed antepartum cardiotocography. Between 1976 and 1978, a number of studies using nonstress testing for antepartum surveillance were published. The main problem with these studies is the wide variance of end points and frequency of testing (Table 9.6). Externally, FHR variability is not generally monitored accurately. Changes in the baseline rate of the fetal heart are generally not seen from hypoxia in antepartum fetuses except preterminally. However, fetal reactivity is easily measured with external systems and probably provides reliable information about fetal condition.

PERFORMING THE NST

In the United States, the most common method of nonstress testing is similar to that described for the OCT. The patient is placed in the semi-Fowler position, blood pressure is recorded, the external monitors are applied. The tocodynamometer is included for recording of spontaneous contractions and fetal movement. Fetal movement is recorded on the lower channel in one of two ways. Either the patient informs the nurse who writes the movement (FM) on the tracing (Fig. 9.21), or an event marker which is supplied with many monitors is given to the patient to push each time the fetus moves (Fig. 9.22). This is recorded on the lower channel usually with an arrow (Fig. 9.23). A 20-min period is recorded. According to the criteria of Evertson et al.[31] if there are two or more accelerations in 20 min, the test is interpreted as reactive and is concluded (Fig. 9.24). Accelerations are defined as an increase of at least 15 beats per minute (BPM) above the baseline lasting at least 15 sec. If there are insufficient accelerations (0 or 1) in 20 min (Fig. 9.25), the fetus is stimulated by 1 min of

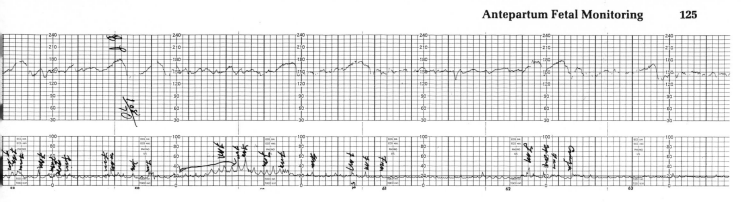

Figure 9.21. This is an NST. The nurse is recording "FM" for fetal movement on the lower channel when the patient informs her that she feels movement. Note that the tocodynamometer is often sensitive enough to record the fetal movement, though this is not always the case.

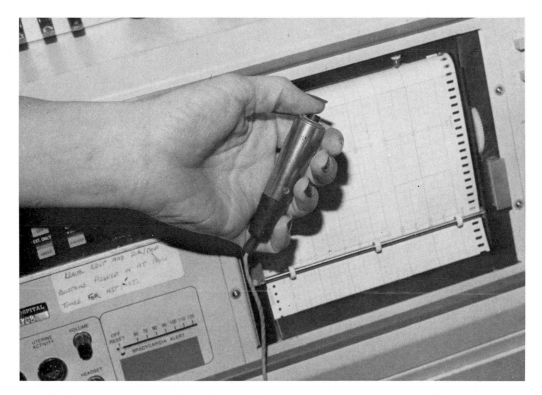

Figure 9.22. Event marker for recording fetal movement. When the patient presses the button an arrow is printed on the lower channel of the fetal monitor record (see Fig. 9.23).

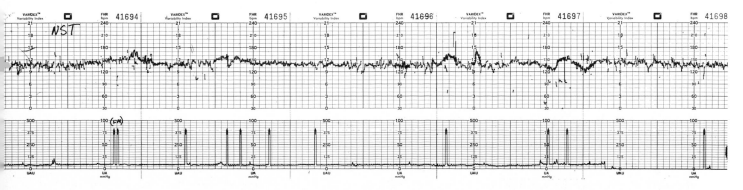

Figure 9.23. This monitor has an event marker whereby the patient may push a button (Fig. 9.22) when she feels fetal movement. This is then recorded on the lower channel with an **_arrow._**

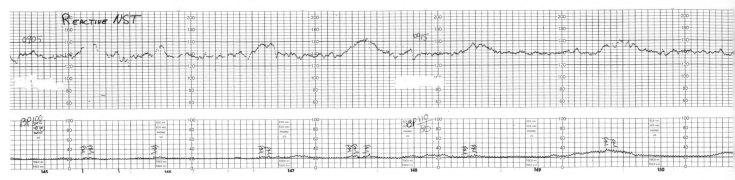

Figure 9.24. Reactive NST. This tracing shows six accelerations of the FHR during a 20-min recording. Each lasts greater than 15 sec and rises more than 15 BPM above baseline, therefore, all meet criteria for clear accelerations. Whenever there are two or more accelerations in 20 min the test may be interpreted as reactive.

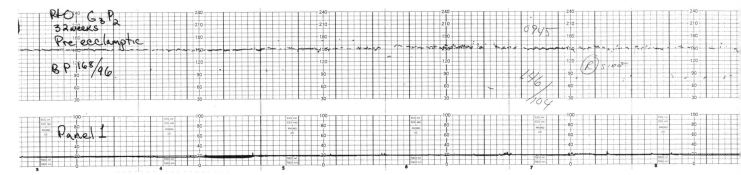

Figure 9.25. Nonreactive NST. Here is a 20-min FHR recording. No accelerations of the FHR are seen, therefore, this is a nonreactive NST.

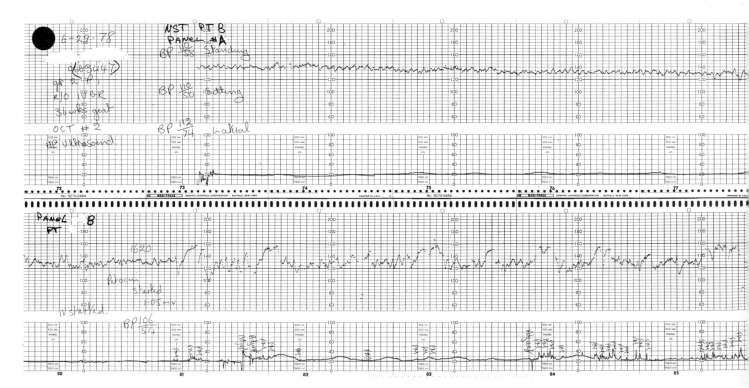

Figure 9.26. *Panel A* shows a baseline 20-min recording with no accelerations and no fetal movements. Therefore, in *panel B*, an IV was started in order to begin an OCT. Immediately the fetus became active as can be seen by the frequent "FM's", and many accelerations are seen.

manual manipulation of the uterus and fetus. Another 20-min period is then recorded. Such manipulation is utilized to arouse the fetus and avoid a nonreactive interpretation caused by a sleep-like state. Should the lack of accelerations (less than 2) in the next 20-min period persist, the test is interpreted as "nonreactive" and an OCT must be performed. Often even while starting the OCT, the FHR becomes reactive (Fig. 9.26); the OCT may be discontinued at any point when the FHR becomes reactive. Other proposals for arousing the fetus before proceeding with the OCT include acoustic stimulation[32] or bringing the patient back several hours later, especially after a meal.[33]

Some additional points should be made for clarification. First, accelerations of the FHR probably have the same significance and are counted as such whether they occur in response to fetal movement, contractions, or spontaneously. The chief values of recording fetal movement are to determine, first, if the fetus is active or inactive, which is another parameter of fetal well being; and second, to help judge whether the absence of accelerations is caused by fetal sleep.

As one can judge from Table 9.6, there has not been universal agreement, even in this country, on the number of accelerations required to call the test reactive. Evertson et al.[31] looked at this question specifically. They found that in NST's followed by OCT's there were no positive OCT's when two or more accelerations were seen in 20 min. This is the only objective data available and seems the most appropriate way of choosing this end point. However, in our extensive experience with OCT's, we have seen many positive OCT's with more than two accelerations in the prestress recording period.

It is most important to realize in doing an oxytocin challenge test that not only does the oxytocin challenge test give you the data regarding presence or absence of late decelerations, but one can look at accelerations of the FHR in addition, giving the clinician both parameters to evaluate. Therefore, in performing the oxytocin challenge test, fetal movement and FHR accelerations should be recorded as part of this test also.

EFFICACY OF THE NST

The NST is a very nonspecific test. Since fetal quiescence and drugs such as phenobarbital can cause nonreactivity,[34] there are many nonreactive tests in well fetuses. Roughly, 10 to 35% of tests (depending on definition) will be nonreactive and require backup with an OCT. Of course, since all nonreactive tests are followed with an OCT, the NST can be viewed as a screening test since no action is based on the NST alone. The more important question then is the sensitivity of the test. In a review of the literature[35] where the end points were accelerations specifically and the frequency of testing was weekly, the number of false negative tests or fetal death within a week of a reactive test, where the patients were high risk, reveals one death in 875 patients, a rate quite similar to OCT's

COMPARING THE OCT AND NST

The OCT clearly has disadvantages. It is time consuming and needs to be done by an experienced nurse who is patient and persistent. Oxytocin is required, thereby, requiring an IV and making the test contraindicated in certain patients. There are a number of equivocal tests requiring a repeat in 24 hr. Late decelerations, the end point of the test, are often subtle and difficult to interpret. The test is relatively expensive.

Most of these disadvantages are eliminated with the NST. It is less time consuming, requires less experience and patience to perform, has no contraindications, and is less expensive. Equivocal results are not usually a problem and accelerations are a more easily interpreted end point than late decelerations. Because of these considerations, many clinicians have turned to the NST as their primary means of fetal surveillance. However, there are certain factors that suggest that the OCT is an earlier sign of fetal jeopardy.

Myers et al.[36] and Martin et al.[37] have demonstrated in animals that hypoxia alone without acidosis can cause late decelerations. Druzin and associates[38] have found in animals that loss of variability seems to be a late sign of hypoxia and requires significant acidosis. Accelerations, a similar sign of CNS intactness, seem to go hand-in-hand with variability. Therefore, late decelerations would seem to precede loss of accelerations. Braly and Freeman,[23] Fox et al.,[17] and Farahani and Fenton,[39] and Evertson et al.[31] have shown that when the OCT is positive and nonreactive, that low Apgar scores and neonatal mortality are more frequent than when the positive OCT is reactive. This would seem to corroborate the animal data. It makes sense that a test that stresses the placental reserve (the OCT) might provide an earlier warning than a baseline test (the NST). In terms of the NST, the only time a positive OCT would be found is when the FHR is nonreactive since reactive NST's are never followed with an OCT. While there is no demonstrable proof that these assumptions are clinically valid except from inference, one must consider this possibility. A large comparative study is necessary. It should be appreciated that in reality, an OCT is a combination of a contraction stress test and a non-stress test. By this, it is meant that the OCT gives both important pieces of information on the fetal reactivity and late decelerations. Both aspects should be carefully evaluated during the OCT.

SUMMARY

The application of FHR monitoring to the antepartum period has proven to be useful. Observations of baseline heart rate and response to uterine contractions can show signs of fetal compromise from uteroplacental insufficiency. In using either the OCT or the NST, the clinician must be aware of the limitations of the tests. Their main value is in allowing the obstetrician to keep hands off and allow the patient to proceed to term or to intervene before term should clear signs of fetal compromise present before that time. In Chapter 10, the use of these tests in the antepartum management of the patient will be discussed.

REFERENCES

1. Predictors of fetal distress. In: Antenatal Diagnosis. United States Department of HEW/NIH. NIH Publ no 79-1973, 1979
2. Garite TJ, Freeman RK, Hochleutner I, et al: Oxytocin challenge test; achieving the desired goals. Obstet Gynecol 51:614, 1978
3. White P: Pregnancy and diabetes, medical aspects. Med Clin North Am 49:1015, 1965
4. Kubli FW, Kaeser O, Hinselmann M: Diagnostic management of chronic placental insufficiency. In: Pecile A, Finzi C (editors) The Foeto-Placental Unit. Excerpta Medica Foundation, Amsterdam, 1969, p 323
5. Parer JT: Normal and impaired placental exchange. Contemp Obstet Gynecol 7:117, 1976
6. Hon EH, Wohlgemuth R: The electronic evaluation of fetal heart rate IV. The effect of maternal exercise. Am J Obstet Gynecol 81:361, 1961
7. Hendricks CH: Amniotic fluid pressure recordings. Clin Obstet Gynecol 9:535, 1966
8. Hammacher K: Fruherkennung intrauterineo gefahrenzustande durch electrophonocardiographie und focographie. In: Elert R, Hates KA (editors), Prophylaxe Frunddkindicher Hirnschaden. Georg Theime Verlag, Stuttgart, 1966, p 120
9. Pose SV, Escarcena L: The influence of uterine contractions on the partial pressure of oxygen of the human fetus. In: Effects of Labour on the Foetus and Newborn. Pergamon Press, Oxford, 1967, p 48
10. Spurrett B: Stressed cardiotocography in late pregnancy. J Obstet Gynecol Br Commonw 78:894, 1971
11. Sanchez-Ramos J, Santisimo JL, Peman FC: La prueba del la oxitocina en el diagnostico del estado fetal anteparto. Acta Ginecol (Madrid) 22:697, 1971
12. Ray M, Freeman RK, Pine S, et al: Clinical experience with the oxytocin challenge test. Am J Obstet Gynecol 114:1, 1972
13. Freeman RK, James J: Clinical experience with the oxytocin challenge test II. An ominous atypical pattern. Obstet Gynecol 46:255, 1975
14. Rochard F, Schifrin BS, Goupil F, et al: Nonstressed fetal heart rate monitoring in the antepartum period. Am J Obstet Gynecol 126:699, 1976
15. Modanlou HD, Freeman RK, Ortiz O, et al: Sinusoidal fetal heart rate pattern and severe fetal anemia. Obstet Gynecol 49:537, 1977
16. Boyd IE, Chamberlain GVP, Ferguson ILC: The oxytocin stress test and the isoxsuprine placental transfer test in the management of suspected placental insufficiency. J Obstet Gynecol Br Commonw 81:120, 1974
17. Fox HE, Steinbrecher M, Ripton B: Antepartum fetal heart rate and uterine activity studies. Am J Obstet Gynecol 126:61, 1976
18. Freeman RK, Goelbelsmann U, Nochimson D, et al: An evaluation of the significance of a positive oxytocin challenge test. Obstet Gynecol 47:8, 1976
19. Braly PB, Freeman RK, Garite TJ, et al: Premature labor and the oxytocin challenge test. Am J Obstet Gynecol (in press)
20. Farahani G, Vasudeva K, Petrie R, et al: Oxytocin challenge test in high risk pregnancy. Obstet Gynecol 47:159, 1976
21. Garite TJ, Freeman RK: Antepartum stress test monitoring. Clin Obstet Gynecol 6:295, 1979
22. Weingold AB, DeJesus TPS, O'Keeffe J: Oxytocin challenge test. Am J Obstet Gynecol 123:466, 1975
23. Braly PB, Freeman RK: The significance of fetal heart rate activity with a positive oxytocin challenge test. Obstet Gynecol 50:689, 1977
24. Kubli F, Boos R, Ruttgers H, et al: Antepartum fetal heart rate monitoring. In: Bear R, Campbell S (editors) The Current Status of FHR Monitoring and Ultrasound in Obstetrics, Royal College of Obstetrics and Gynecology, London, 1977, p 28
25. Freeman RK: Oxytocin challenge test. Presented at the Symposium on Modern Perinatal Medicine, San Diego, California March 2-5, 1974
26. Lee CY, DiLoreto PC, Logrand B: Fetal activity acceleration determination for the evaluation of fetal reserve. Obstet Gynecol 48:19, 1976
27. Tushuizen PBT, Stoot JEGM, Ubachs JMH: Clinical experience in nonstressed antepartum cardiotocography. Am J Obstet Gynecol 128:507, 1977
28. Flynn AM, Kelly J: Evaluation of fetal well-being by antepartum fetal heart rate monitoring. Br Med J 1:936, 1977
29. Krebs HB, Petries RE: Clinical application of a scoring system for evaluation of antepartum fetal heart rate monitoring. Am J Obstet Gynecol 130:765, 1978
30. Nochimson DJ, Turbeville JS, Terry JE: The nonstress test. Obstet Gynecol 51:419, 1978
31. Evertson LR, Gauthier RJ, Schifrin BS, et al: Antepartum fetal heart rate testing I. Evaluation of the nonstress test. Am J Obstet Gynecol 133:29, 1979
32. Read JA, Milller FC: Fetal heart rate acceleration in response to acoustic stimulation as a measure of fetal well-being. Am J Obstet Gynecol 141:512, 1977
33. Keegan KA, Paul RH, Broussard PM, et al: Antepartum fetal heart rate testing V. The nonstress test—an outpatient approach. Am J Obstet Gynecol 136:81, 1980
34. Keegan KA, Paul RH, Broussard PM, et al: Antepartum fetal heart rate testing III. The effect of phenobarbital on the nonstress test. Am J Obstet Gynecol 133:579, 1979
35. Freeman RK, Garite TJ: Antepartum fetal monitoring; the optimum method and role. In: Zuspan F, Christina D (editors) Reid's Controversies in Obstetrics and Gynecology (3rd ed). WB Saunders, Philadelphia, 1979 (in press)
36. Myers RE, Mueller-Heubach E, Adamsons K: Predictability of the state of fetal oxygenation from a quantitative analysis of the components of late deceleration. Am J Obstet Gynecol 115:1083, 1973
37. Martin CB, deHaan J, van der Wildt B, et al: Mechanisms of late decelerations in the fetal heart rate. Eur J Obstet Gynecol Reprod Biol 9:361, 1979
38. Ikenouye T, Martin CB, Murata Y, et al: Effect of acute hypoxia and respiratory acidosis on the fetal heart rate in Rhesus monkeys. Presented at the Society for Gynecologic Investigation, San Diego, California, March 21-24, 1979
39. Farahani G, Fenton NF: Fetal heart rate acceleration in relation to the oxytocin challenge test. Obstet Gynecol 49:163, 1977
40. Visser GHA, Huisjes HJ: Diagnostic value of the unstressed antepartum cardiotocogram. Br J Obstet Gynecol 84:321, 1977

41. Ewing DE, Farina JR, Otterson WN: Clinical application of the oxytocin challenge test. Obstet Gynecol 43:563, 1974

42. Cooper JM, Soffronoff EC, Bolognese RJ: Oxytocin challenge test in monitoring high-risk pregnancies. Obstet Gynecol 45:27, 1975

43. Schifrin BS, Lapidus M, Doctor GS, et al: Contraction stress test for antepartum fetal evaluation

44. Gaziano EP, Hill DL, Freeman DW: The oxytocin challenge test in the management of high-risk pregnancies. Am J Obstet Gynecol 121:947, 1975

45. Hayden BL, Simpson JL, Ewing DE, et al: Can the oxytocin challenge test serve as the primary method for managing high-risk pregnancies? Obstet Gynecol 46:251, 1975

46. Boehm FH, Braun RD, Growdon JH, et al: The oxytocin challenge test. South Med J 69:884, 1976

47. Bhakthavathsalan A, Mann LI, Tejani NA, et al: Correlation of the oxytocin challenge test with perinatal outcome. Obstet Gynecol 48:552, 1976

48. Baskett TF, Sandy E: False negative oxytocin challenge tests. Am J Obstet Gynecol 123:106, 1975

49. Marcum RG: False negative oxytocin challenge test. Am J Obstet Gynecol 122:894, 1977

50. Christie GB, Cudmore DW: The oxytocin challenge test. Am J Obstet Gynecol 118:327, 1974

CHAPTER 10

Antepartum Management of the High Risk Patient

The previous Chapter was devoted to introducing antepartum fetal heart rate (FHR) testing, describing methodology, interpretation and understanding the limitations and pitfalls. With this understanding, we shall now proceed to applying this methodolgy to various clinical situations. Several specific questions arise for each different clinical problem. When do we start testing; what additional tests do we use; when do we deliver the patient; what route of delivery is best?

First we must decide what group of patients require antepartum FHR testing. It should be clear that this test is designed to warn the clinician of hypoxic uteroplacental insufficiency (UPI) only. Probably between 35 and 50% of antepartum deaths after 26 to 28 weeks (a potentially viable time) are caused by a form of UPI.[1, 2] Approximately 50% of antepartum fetal deaths without apparent cause occur in patients without risk factors; the other 50% occur in patients with risk factors and these comprise 10 to 20% of the general prenatal population.[1-3] Therefore, one may choose to apply this technology to the 10 to 20% of patients at risk and thereby potentially prevent one-half of fetal deaths, or test all patients to get at the remaining preventable deaths. This is a question currently being investigated; we shall limit discussion in this Chapter to testing patients at risk. However, there are two situations that occur in otherwise low risk patients which should cause one to consider testing and hopefully get at a portion of the fetal deaths in the low risk population. These include a lag in the uterine/fundal growth which should suggest possible intrauterine growth retardation (IUGR) and the patient who reports decreased fetal activity. The second fact that should be clear is that the testing should not be begun until the clinician, if faced with definitely ominous data, is ready to intervene (i.e., deliver).

WHICH PATIENTS TO TEST

Patients at risk for fetal hypoxia secondary to UPI should have antepartum FHR testing as a primary

Table 10.1.
Indications for the OCT/NST

Diabetes, Class B Through R
Diabetes—Class A; Only if:
  1. Abnormal Fasting Blood Sugar, or
  2. History of Previous Stillbirth, or
  3. Pregnancy Complicated by Hypertension or IUGR
Hypertension, Chronic or Pregnancy Induced
Postdates (More than 42 wk)
Elderly Gravida (More than 35 yr)
Previous Stillbirth
Cyanotic Maternal Cardiac Disease
Hemoglobinopathy/Severe Anemia
Rh Isoimmunization
Hyperthyroidism
Decreased Fetal Movement
Suspected IUGR
Discordant Twins

means of surveillance. Those indications for testing are listed in Table 10.1.

WHEN TO START TESTING

When one should begin testing a patient with a given risk factor will depend on several factors. First, when is the problem recognized? If a patient first shows signs of preeclampsia at 38 weeks, that is when to begin testing. Next, what is the relative risk of losing the fetus. Certain conditions such as advanced age or previous unexplained stillbirth are only moderate risk situations; whereas severe chronic hypertension or the more severe classes of diabetes are very high risk. The higher the risk situation, generally, the sooner one should start testing. In addition, estriol monitoring is advocated by many as a supplementary test in those higher risk situations.

ESTRIOL MONITORING

It is not within the scope of this text to describe the physiology, methodology, or limitations of estriol monitoring. The reader is referred to excellent available reviews.[4,5] We will assume a basic knowledge of estriol monitoring in proceeding with this Chapter.

Estriol is effectively measured either by using 24-hr urine collections or by analyzing serum for unconjugated ("free") estriol. The frequency of testing should depend on the clinical situation and will be discussed with these individual problems.

Reassuring estriol values generally fall within two standard deviations of the mean for a given week of gestation and should increase with advancing gestational age (Figure 10.1). Abnormal or nonassuring values may fall into one of three patterns. They may be chronically low, that is all values at or below the second standard deviation (Fig. 10.2). These are often seen in IUGR of any etiology. They may fall gradually (Fig. 10.3); this condition can be seen for example in a preeclamptic patient with declining placental function. Or, they may fall precipitously as can often be seen in diabetics (Fig. 10.4).

A significant fall in estriol is one in which there is a 35% fall from the mean of the three highest consecutive values (not necessarily the three previous values). An example of such a calculation is shown in Table 10.2.

Generally in chronic UPI, the fall in estriol precedes the development of a positive oxytocin challenge test (OCT) or truly nonreactive nonstress test (NST). This is because nutritive UPI (as reflected by estriol) generally precedes hypoxic UPI (as seen in a positive OCT) with declining placental function. One exception to this is in the diabetic (without IUGR) where the abrupt estriol fall is a late finding and may precede fetal death by only a day or two.

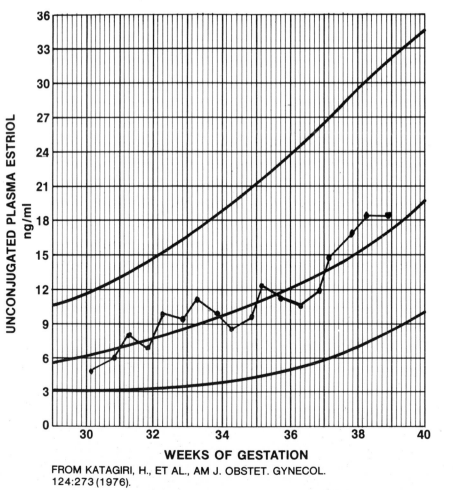

THIRD TRIMESTER UNCONJUGATED PLASMA ESTRIOL CONCENTRATIONS AND 95% CONFIDENCE LIMITS

FROM KATAGIRI, H., ET AL., AM J. OBSTET. GYNECOL. 124:273 (1976).

DATE	LEVEL NG/ML	TECHNOLOGIST
4/3	5.0	
4/7	6.1	
4/10	8.2	
4/14	7.1	
4/17	7.9	
4/21	9.3	
4/25	11.0	
4/28	10.2	
5/1	8.5	
5/5	9.7	
5/8	12.3	
5/12	11.2	
5/15	10.5	
5/19	11.8	
5/22	14.7	
5/26	17.0	
5/30	18.3	
6/2	18.3	

Figure 10.1. This is an example of a normal serum unconjugated estriol graph. The specimens being obtained twice weekly are in the normal range and rising appropriately. The center line represents the mean and the *upper* and *lower lines* are 95% confidence limits.

THIRD TRIMESTER UNCONJUGATED PLASMA ESTRIOL CONCENTRATIONS AND 95% CONFIDENCE LIMITS

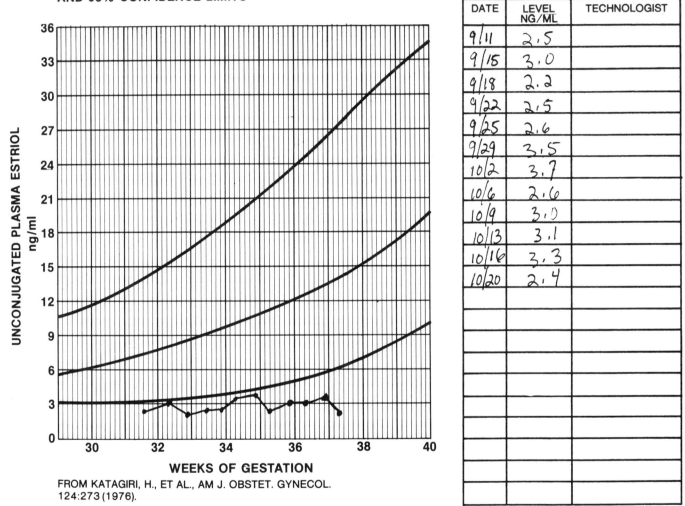

DATE	LEVEL NG/ML	TECHNOLOGIST
9/11	2.5	
9/15	3.0	
9/18	2.2	
9/22	2.5	
9/25	2.6	
9/29	3.5	
10/2	3.7	
10/6	2.6	
10/9	3.0	
10/13	3.1	
10/16	3.3	
10/20	2.4	

FROM KATAGIRI, H., ET AL., AM J. OBSTET. GYNECOL. 124:273 (1976).

Figure 10.2. Estriols are being drawn twice weekly. This represents a chronically low pattern and may often be seen with IUGR.

THIRD TRIMESTER UNCONJUGATED PLASMA ESTRIOL CONCENTRATIONS AND 95% CONFIDENCE LIMITS

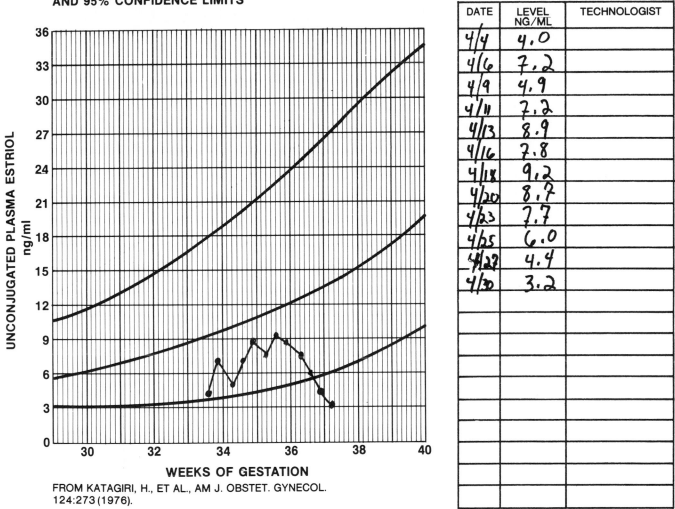

DATE	LEVEL NG/ML	TECHNOLOGIST
4/4	4.0	
4/6	7.2	
4/9	4.9	
4/11	7.2	
4/13	8.9	
4/16	7.8	
4/18	9.2	
4/20	8.7	
4/23	7.7	
4/25	6.0	
4/27	4.4	
4/30	3.2	

FROM KATAGIRI, H., ET AL., AM J. OBSTET. GYNECOL. 124:273 (1976).

Figure 10.3. Estriols are being drawn three times per week. At 35½ weeks a gradual fall in estriol begins. If one calculates falls from the three previous values rather than three highest consecutive values, a gradual fall might be missed.

THIRD TRIMESTER UNCONJUGATED PLASMA ESTRIOL CONCENTRATIONS AND 95% CONFIDENCE LIMITS

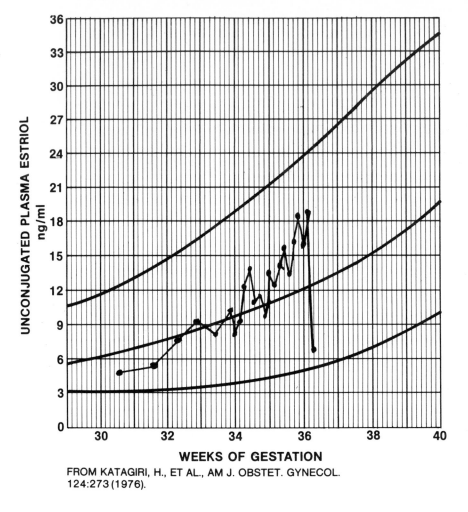

DATE	LEVEL NG/ML	TECHNOLOGIST
9/17	4.7	
9/24	5.3	
9/30	7.9	
10/3	9.3	
10/6	8.2	
10/9	10.6	
10/10	8.3	
10/11	9.3	
10/12	12.2	
10/13	13.8	
10/14	11.0	
10/15	11.5	
10/16	9.8	
10/17	13.6	
10/18	12.5	
10/19	14.2	
10/20	15.6	
10/21	13.8	
10/22	16.0	
10/23	18.3	
10/24	15.8	
10/25	18.5	
10/26	6.5	

FROM KATAGIRI, H., ET AL., AM J. OBSTET. GYNECOL. 124:273 (1976).

Figure 10.4. A sudden fall in estriol is seen at 36½ weeks. The patient had weekly specimens drawn at 30 to 31 weeks, twice weekly at 32 to 34 weeks and daily thereafter as would be done in a diabetic. Such significant precipitous falls would be most characteristic of a diabetic pregnancy.

Table 10.2.
Calculation of Falls in Estriol Values: Two Examples

Date	Estriol		Example 1
			January 8 = 9 ng/ml
January 1	14 ng/ml		Mean of Highest 3 Consecutive
January 3	16		$= 14 + 16 + 10 = 40/3 = 13.3$
January 5	10		
January 8	9		Fall $= \dfrac{13.3 - 9}{13.3} = \dfrac{4.3}{13.3} (100) = 32\%$
January 10	13		This *is not* a significant fall
January 12	10		
January 14	6		Example 2

January 14 = 6 ng/ml
Mean of Highest 3 Consecutive
$= 14 + 16 + 10 = 40/3 = 13.3$

Fall $= \dfrac{13.3 - 6}{13.3} = \dfrac{7.3}{13.3} (100) = 55\%$
This *is* a significant fall

TESTING PROTOCOL BY CLINICAL SITUATION

Certain clinical situations are conveniently categorized together in terms of an approach to antepartum testing. We shall present our approach to antepartum testing and use this format to provide case examples for illustration. It should be clear to the reader that there are many different approaches in terms of when to begin testing, when to intervene, ancillary tests, etc. The approach presented here is based on extensive clinical experience with antepartum testing in high risk patients, and on data which has been published by the authors and many others.[1, 6, 7]

Moderate Risk Groups

There are a group of conditions where the risk for fetal death from UPI is only moderately increased above that of the low risk population. Furthermore, in this group such fetal death tends to occur late in gestation. Clinical situations included in this group are: (1) advanced maternal age, (2) hyperthyroidism, (3) previous stillbirth.

Since these conditions are of only moderately increased risk, the OCT only (without estriols) is used, and since fetal death from UPI tends to occur late, we begin testing when intervention is reasonably likely to yield a healthy neonate. Therefore, the approach in this group is: (1) weekly OCT's beginning at 34 weeks, (2) allow gestation to carry to term; (3) no intervention unless a positive OCT is found.

At the conclusion of this Chapter, the management of the patient with the positive OCT will be discussed. Since this does not vary appreciably with different conditions, we can discuss these together (Fig. 10.5).

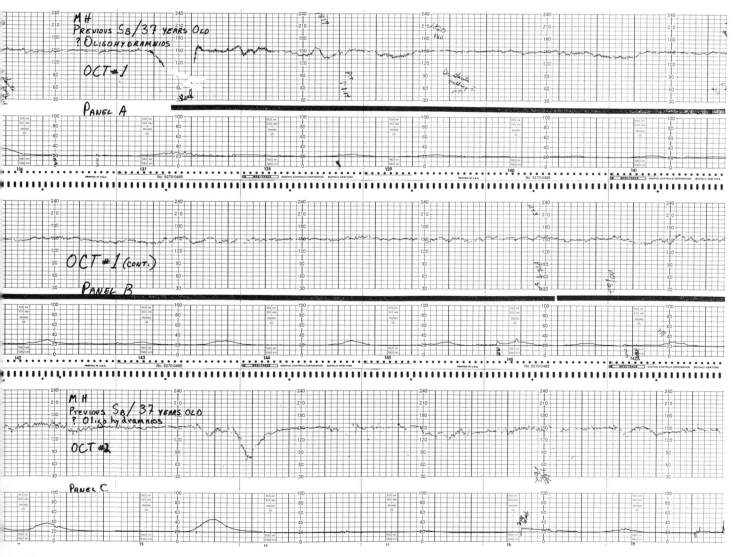

Figure 10.5. Patient MH is a G2 P1 sho was being tested for advanced maternal age and previous unexplained stillbirth. There was also a suspicion of oligohydramnios later confirmed by ultrasound. At 34½ weeks, the patient had her first OCT (**panels A** and **B**) which is suspicious because of the one variable deceleration. An estriol was drawn the next day and the value was 6.0 ng/ml (borderline low). An OCT was repeated the day after the suspicious test (**panel C**) which is positive and nonreactive. It was not possible to do an amniocentesis because of the severe oligohydramnios. Therefore, the patient was delivered by cesarean section. The baby had renal agenesis/Potter's syndrome and died shortly after birth.

Postdates

Postdate pregnancy is a condition that accounts for the majority of patients undergoing antepartum testing in most series. Primarily, this is because many patients have wrong dates. In the past, one approach to the postdate pregnancy was to evaluate for the presence or absence of meconium using amnioscopy or amniocentesis. The significance of meconium in the antepartum patient has been a controversial subject. A recent randomized study by Knox et al.[8] compared the OCT with amniocentesis for the management of post dates pregnancy, and showed the OCT to be superior in that intervention was less often required in the OCT group than in the meconium group (12 vs. 32%) without a difference in morbidity or mortality. Since this is also only a moderately increased risk group, we choose the OCT only, without estriol monitoring. The approach in this group is (with reasonably good dates): At 42 weeks (1) ripe cervix → induction of labor, (2) unripe cervix → weekly OCT's beginning at 42 weeks, (3) deliver when cervix is ripe or when OCT is positive.

Since 30% of all positive OCT's are false positive, it could be argued that further testing should be necessary before intervening. This is generally true for other clinical situations. However, with postdates patients with an unripe cervix, the OCT allows us to keep hands off in 90% of patients; therefore, only about 3% (30% of 10%) are unnecessarily intervened upon. Furthermore, there is virtually no risk of premature morbidity when intervening at 42 weeks (generally one is no more than 4 weeks off in dates which would be 38 weeks) and the only risk of induction with an unripe cervix is that of an unnecessary cesarean section. The OCT, therefore, can reduce these unnecessary cesarean sections to only that portion of the 3% with failed inductions (Fig. 10.6).

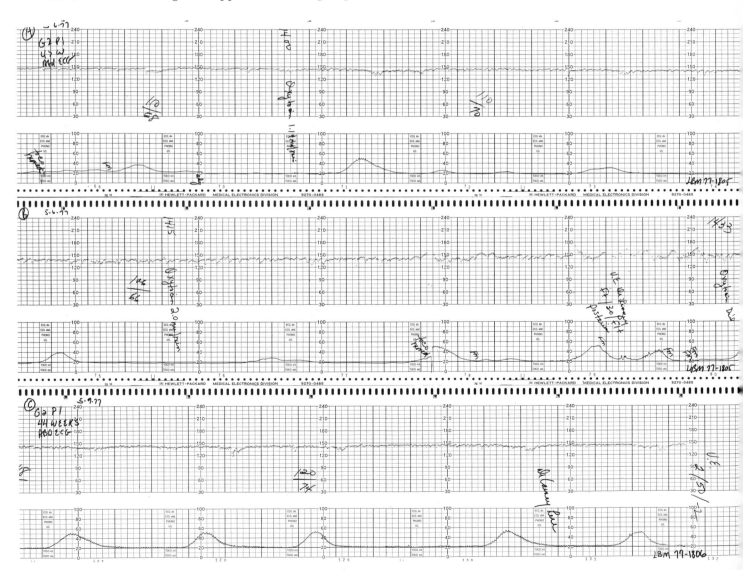

Figure 10.6. This is a postdates patient. An OCT at 42 weeks was negative. On 5/6 (*panel A* and *B*) a suspicious OCT was found. Note the late decelerations in *panel A* which disappear in *panel B*. Since the cervix was unfavorable for induction, the OCT was repeated on 5/7 and 5/8 which were again both mildly suspicious (not shown). On 5/9 (*panel C*) a positive OCT was obtained. The patient underwent a cesarean section and delivered an Apgar 6/8 meconium-stained newborn with stigmata of postmaturity.

Preeclampsia

Preeclampsia or pregnancy induced hypertension (PIH) is a disease for which it is difficult to outline a routine for antepartum evaluation. This is because management is usually guided more by maternal condition than by fetal condition. Furthermore, the conservative treatment of the maternal disease, i.e., bedrest, may also improve fetal condition, and conversely deterioration of maternal condition can also be associated with aggravation of UPI. Finally, Gant et al.[9,10] have data that strongly suggest that UPI may precede the clinical manifestations of the disease by 1 to 3 months, and the IUGR that can be seen in patients who develop PIH without other previous manifestations corroborates this data. Therefore, antepartum testing should be conducted with the following basic rules in mind.

1. Fetal jeopardy may exist even in the patient whose blood pressure normalizes at bedrest.

2. This condition may change rapidly. Changing maternal condition necessitates retesting the fetus regardless of when the previous test was done. Severely affected patients require continuous FHR monitoring.

3. Fetal condition is but one variable in the equation necessary to evaluate and manage these patients.

4. Occasionally, nonreassuring antepartum heart rate patterns may improve if maternal condition significantly changes for the better.

Antepartum fetal monitoring is begun at 28 weeks or any time thereafter when the disease is first recognized. Weekly OCT's and twice to thrice weekly estriols are generally used in the patient being managed expectantly even if blood pressure normalizes at bedrest. Should maternal condition deteriorate in any way, the OCT must be repeated immediately since fetal compromise may result from the deterioration of the maternal condition. In severe cases

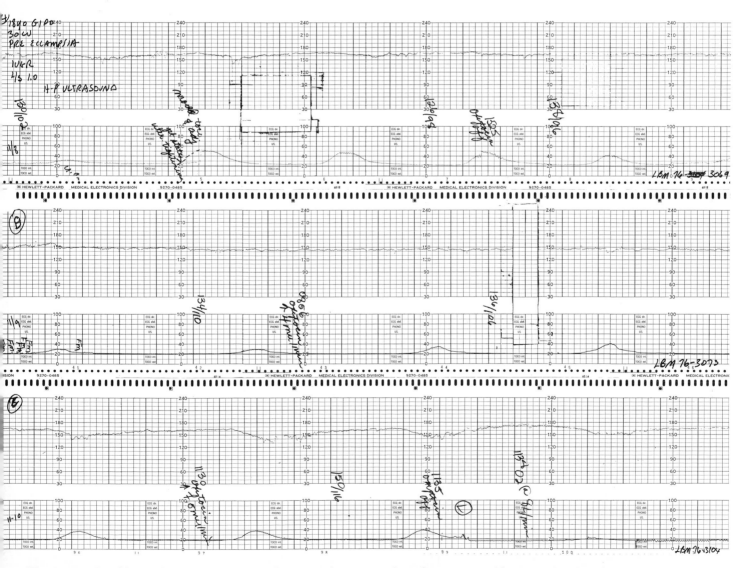

Figure 10.7. A mild preeclamptic was admitted at 30 weeks. Maternal condition was stable except for elevated blood pressure and proteinuria. An OCT was performed on 11/8 (***panel A***) and was interpreted as suspicious. Estriols were low. An L:S ratio was done and was immature (1.0:1). On 11/9, the OCT was again suspicious (***panel B***). The patient was on phenobarbital which may explain the absence of accelerations. The next day a positive OCT was obtained. Note the lack of accelerations and tachycardia. A 900-g baby was delivered by cesarean section with Apgar 4/6. The baby did well in the newborn period.

where there is *any* delay in delivery such as for stablization or when corticosteriods are used to accelerate fetal pulmonary maturity, continuous FHR monitoring is warranted. With mild preeclampsia, the patient is delivered at or after 38 weeks if the fetus is mature by the lecithin:sphingomyelin ratio. Should blood pressure or other parameters of multisystem disease remain abnormal but not severe, the patient is delivered as soon as the fetus is mature. Should maternal or fetal condition deteriorate sooner, earlier intervention is warranted. As with other conditions, we will discuss management with positive OCT's collectively (Fig. 10.7).

Chronic Hypertension

In terms of fetal jeopardy from UPI, chronic hypertension and diabetes are the most significant antepartum risk factors except for perhaps 3rd trimester hemorrhage which is generally a more acute problem. More severe cases of hypertension are also often associated with IUGR. In these latter cases risk is especially high and fetal death may occur early in the 3rd trimester. Therefore estriol monitoring is begun on a twice weekly basis at 28 weeks. If estriols are normal and rising, weekly OCT's are begun at 34 weeks. If estriol values are chronically low and/or IUGR is suspected by other parameters such as oligohydramnios, lag in fundal growth or ultrasound, then weekly OCT's are begun as early as 28 weeks. Some have questioned the validity of such early antepartum FHR testing, but Gabbe et al.[11] studied this question and found positive OCT's to correlate with other outcome criteria as significantly in early gestations as near term, and negative tests to be of similar value. Patients with negative OCT's and normal estriol patterns are delivered at or after 38 weeks. Should estriol values be chronically low (or IUGR otherwise confirmed), but OCT's remain reassuring, the patient is delivered when the L:S ratio is mature. Many of these patients will have preeclampsia de-

velop in addition to their chronic hypertension. These patients would then be managed as would preeclamptics. Patients with chronic hypertension are also at risk for placental abruption; this can rarely be predicted but vaginal bleeding or premature uterine activity should prompt immediate fetal evaluation. Finally, many of these patients require medications to lower blood pressure. Acute lowering of blood pressure places the already at risk patient in significant jeopardy. Such change therefore warrants intense monitoring such as daily or more frequent NST's during the period of blood pressure reduction (Fig. 10.8).

Diabetes

Diabetes mellitus is a clinical example where the combination of antepartum testing and maturity studies have definitely made an impact in improving perinatal outcome. Now in many centers the perinatal mortality from diabetes has been reduced to nearly that of nondiabetics when corrected for congenital abnormalities.[12, 13] Data suggest that uncomplicated Class A diabetics have no increase in antenatal fetal mortality over the general population.[14] This is only with a Class A diabetic who has a normal fasting blood sugar (not on insulin), is not preeclamptic and has not had a previous stillbirth. Therefore, these uncomplicated Class A diabetics do not get antepartum testing and are allowed to go to term. However, these patients are begun on weekly OCT's if they go beyond 40 weeks. The remainder of diabetics, both complicated Class A (previous stillbirth, abnormal fasting blood sugar, or preeclampsia) and all insulin dependent diabetics are managed similarly. The only important modifiers for this collective group is the presence of hypertension, IUGR, or renal disease.

Estriol monitoring is begun on a weekly basis at 28 to 30 weeks, then biweekly until 34 weeks. At 34 weeks, the patient is begun on weekly OCT's and daily estriol monitoring. Should these remain normal,

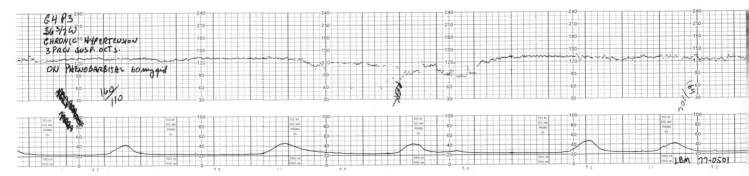

Figure 10.8. This is a 34-year-old G_4P_3 chronic hypertensive on no medications except phenobarbital. Twice weekly estriol determinations had been started at 30 weeks and had remained normal. OCT's were done weekly starting at 34 weeks and were negative until 36 weeks. At this time, the patient had a suspicious OCT which was repeated the next 2 days and the tests were suspicious on each of these occasions. The next day, the OCT was positive which is shown. Normally we would change to NST's after the second suspicious test, but all were nonreactive as is this positive OCT, probably related to phenobarbital administration. An L:S ratio was mature and a cesarean section was done delivering a 2500-g nondepressed healthy male.

the patient is taken to 38 weeks and delivered if the L:S ratio is mature. Occasionally if the cervix is unripe and OCT's and daily estriol values are continuously reassuring, the patient is allowed to go beyond 38 weeks.

Daily estriol monitoring is indeed necessary if one is to use estriol at all in the diabetic. The fall in estriol in diabetics is abrupt, as opposed to most other cases, and tends to be a late sign of fetal compromise and may precede fetal death by 24 hours or less. Goebelsmann et al.[15] studied this question in 60 diabetic pregnancies monitored with daily urinary estriols. There were 14 significant falls in estriol; 9 (64%) of these would have been missed if the patient was monitored with only biweekly estriol; and 6 (43%) would have been missed with estriol monitored only 3 times a week. Therefore, it is necessary to monitor these daily, 7 days a week. Furthermore, a system must be developed to check the results the same day the estriol is run (which must be the same day the specimen is collected) and previous values must be available for comparison. Chronically low estriol values between 28 and 34 weeks mandate beginning OCT's earlier.

In diabetic pregnancies additionally complicated by IUGR, proteinuria and/or hypertension, antepartum surveillance is stepped up even further. Daily estriol monitoring and weekly OCT's are begun in these cases at 28 to 30 weeks. These patients may also be taken to 38 weeks if tests are continuously reassuring. However, if estriol values remain chronically below the second standard deviation, consideration for delivery should begin as soon after 34 weeks as one is confident of fetal lung maturity (Figs. 10.9–10.11).

Third Trimester Bleeding

Patients with acute 3rd trimester bleeding are of course a difficult problem in antepartum management and must be individualized. In and around an acute episode of bleeding, fetal condition may be an important modifier in the decision regarding immediate delivery or expectant management. When bleeding is not excessive and there is no coagulopathy or premature labor, then fetal condition becomes the main concern. At and around the acute episode continuous fetal monitoring and fetal maturity studies

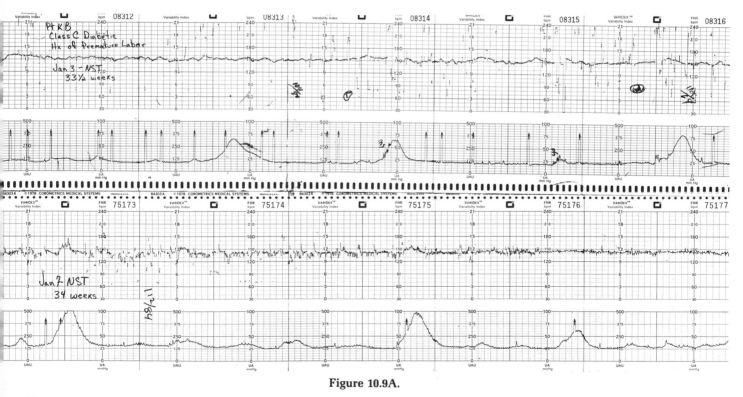

Figure 10.9A.

Figure 10.9. KB is a 25-year-old G_1 Class C diabetic. During this pregnancy at 31 weeks the patient was transferred in premature labor and tocolysis was successful with $MgSO_4$. Estriols were begun biweekly at that time and increased to daily at 34 weeks. Because of the history of premature labor, biweekly NST's were used rather than OCT's. On January 3, the NST is reactive and there are no decelerations present with spontaneous contractions. (Fig. 10.9*A top*). On January 7, the test is again reactive with no decelerations (Fig. 10.9*A bottom*). On January 11, the test is reactive but late decelerations are seen after the first and possibly the second contractions on Figure 10.9*B*. There are no further late decelerations with the remainder of the spontaneous contractions. Therefore, the test was repeated the next day (Fig. 10.9*C*). January 12 (at 35 weeks) the patient had a spontaneous positive CST with no reactivity. Efforts at manual stimulation failed to increase reactivity. That same day, the estriol fell by 61% (Fig. 10.9*D*). The patient was delivered by cesarean section without a trial of labor because of a nonreactive positive CST and an unfavorable cervix (either of which would be a reason). A 3570-g Apgar 8/9 baby was delivered which did well except for hypoglycemia. (See pages 140–141 for parts 9B–9D).

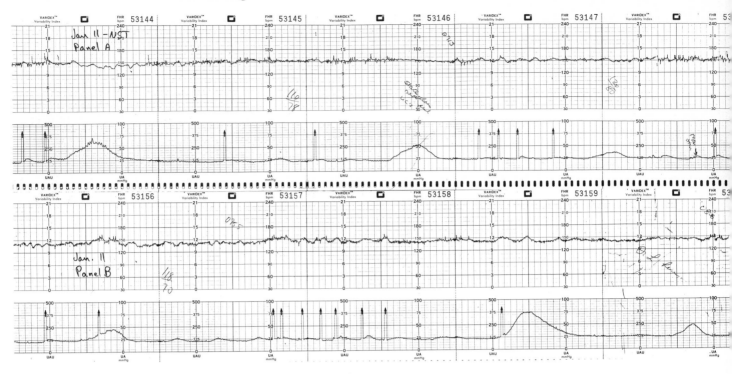

Figure 10.9B.

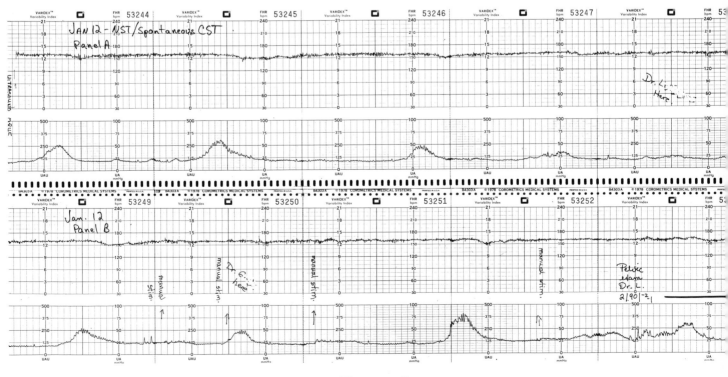

Figure 10.9C.

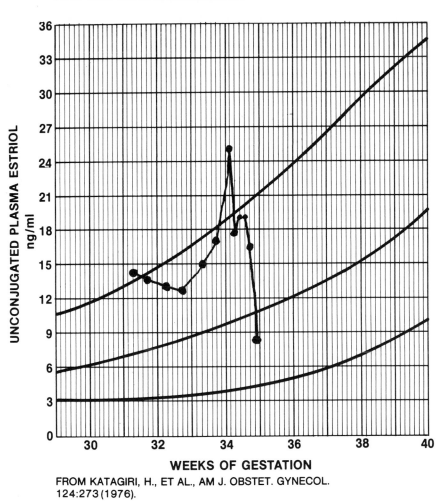

THIRD TRIMESTER UNCONJUGATED PLASMA ESTRIOL CONCENTRATIONS AND 95% CONFIDENCE LIMITS

DATE	LEVEL NG/ML
12/17	14.0
12/20	13.6
12/24	13.1
12/27	12.6
12/31	15.0
1/3	16.9
1/7	25.1
1/8	17.6
1/9	19.1
1/10	19.6
1/11	16.4
1/12	8.4

FROM KATAGIRI, H., ET AL., AM J. OBSTET. GYNECOL. 124:273 (1976).

Figure 10.9D.

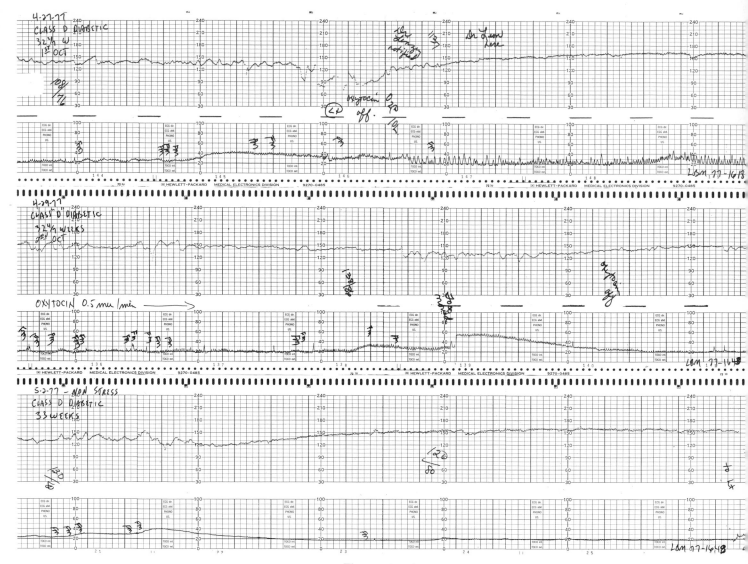

Figure 10.10A.

Figure 10.10. This is a 28-year-old Class D diabetic with a fibroid uterus and polyhydramnios. Plasma unconjugated estriols were begun at 31 weeks. The patient developed mild preeclampsia at 32½ weeks and OCT's were begun. On 4/27 and 4/29 hyperstimulation occurred with oxytocin. Note the rebound tachycardia and loss of variability seen after hyperstimulation on 4/27. The patient was therefore changed to NST's done three times weekly. Esteriols continued to rise in excess of 2 SD of the mean, consistent with macrosomia, which the patient had both clinically and by ultrasound. On 5/2, the test is minimally reactive. There is a late deceleration following a normal contraction (**A**) and a prolonged contraction (**B**). An amniocentesis was done which showed an L:S ratio of 1.3. Since the estriols were normal, the patient was not delivered. NST's on 5/3, 5/5, and 5/9 were reactive but on 5/11 there was a spontaneous hyperstimulation. On 5/13, the NST was minimally reactive; there are no decelerations after the spontaneous uterine activity. On 5/16, a spontaneous OCT was positive with late decelerations following each contraction. In addition, this test is nonreactive. Attempts at stimulation fail to increase reactivity. That same day, the estriol fell by 55%. A cesarean section was done and a 9 lb 8 oz LGA depressed newborn was delivered that day. The baby did well in the nursery except for hypoglycemia. This case illustrates that the loss of fetal reactivity and the fall in esteriol in the diabetic are rather late events. One probably would have seen earlier signs of decreasing reserve if contraction stress tests had been performed, but because of the tetanic contractions occurring in this patient (both with oxytocin and spontaneously) nonstress testing was necessary. Ideally one should strive to intervene when the fetus is still reactive and waiting for the complete loss of reactivity as we see in this case may be longer than ideal. (See pages 143–145 for parts B–F).

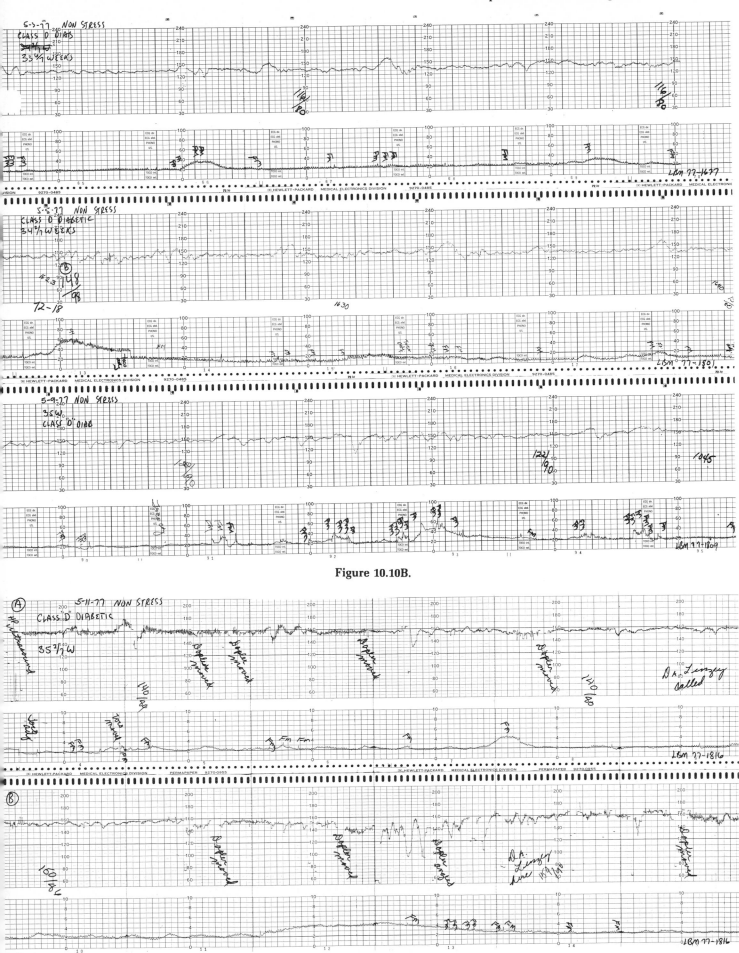

Figure 10.10B.

Figure 10.10C.

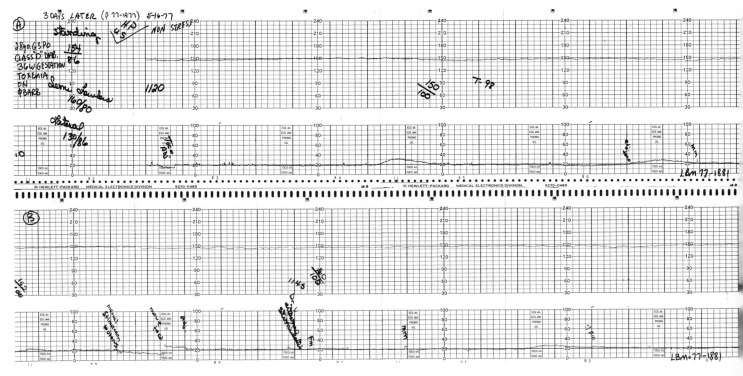

Figure 10.10D.

Figure 10.10E.

THIRD TRIMESTER UNCONJUGATED PLASMA ESTRIOL CONCENTRATIONS AND 95% CONFIDENCE LIMITS

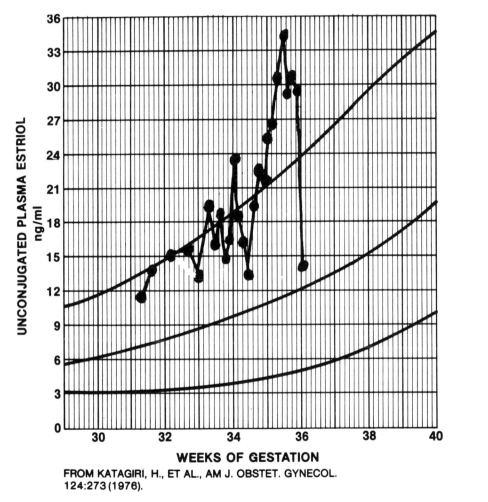

FROM KATAGIRI, H., ET AL., AM J. OBSTET. GYNECOL. 124:273 (1976).

Figure 10.10F.

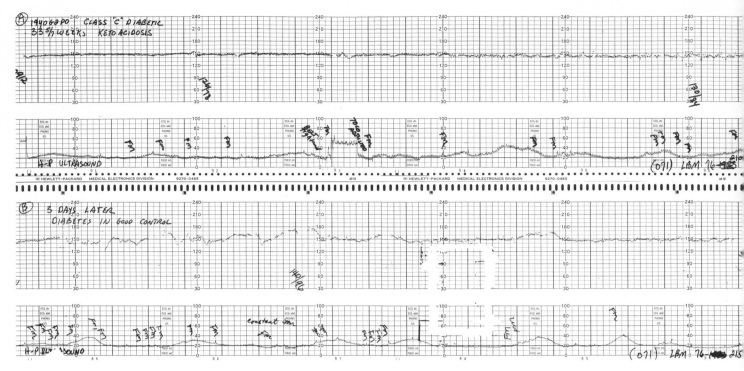

Figure 10.11. This case illustrates the effect of ketoacidosis on the fetus. *Panel A* is the FHR tracing of a diabetic admitted in ketoacidosis at 33½ weeks. Note the nonreactive pattern. Three days later (*panel B*) with the patient euglycemic and nonketotic a normally reactive negative spontaneous CST is seen. This illustrates the potential reversibility of FHR patterns when treatable conditions exist.

are necessary. Occasionally, even with only minimal bleeding and minimal uterine activity, late decelerations will alert the physician to a significant abruption. Alternatively, in the face of a significant bleeding episode, a normal FHR tracing is an essential variable in the decision to delay delivery. Generally, uterine bleeding prior to term is a factor that contraindicates oxytocin challenge testing. Many of these patients will have sufficient uterine activity, however, for a spontaneous contraction stress test. The mainstay of testing in these cases is the NST and the response to spontaneous uterine contractions. After the initial episode of bleeding, degrees of chronic abruption may lead to UPI and therefore we follow these patients with twice weekly NST's. Given a patient with significant 3rd trimester bleeding, we would attempt to deliver this patient after 36 to 37 weeks with fetal maturity (Figs. 10.12 and 10.13).

Hemoglobinopathy/Severe Anemia/Cyanotic Cardiac and Pulmonary Disease

Patients with decreased numbers of effective oxygen-carrying red blood cells or other reasons for decreased oxygen delivery to the placenta such as cyanotic maternal cardiac disease or pulmonary disease can indeed have a form of preplacental UPI. Such UPI can lead to growth retardation and/or hypoxic compromise. There is, however, potential in these cases for reversal of compromise and therefore this is an important group of patients to monitor.

Patients with sickle cell disease, severe anemia (hematocrit less than 25), or significant hypoxia should be followed with twice weekly estriol determinations starting at 28 to 30 weeks. If these are normal, OCT's may be started at 34 weeks. Significant deterioration in maternal status necessitates immediate FHR testing (NST or OCT). At this point, treatment of the immediate condition by oxygen therapy or transfusion may cause the FHR pattern to revert to normal. If the clinical condition is stable and antepartum tests remain normal, these patients may be delivered after 36 to 38 weeks, (depending on the individual problem) if the L:S ratio is mature (Fig. 10.14).

Suspected IUGR

In patients without other significant risk factors a lag in fundal growth, or ultrasound may suggest IUGR. This is a subject of some controversy. One aspect of this controversy is, given nutritional UPI with resultant IUGR, is it better to deliver the fetus at that point (or as early as extrauterine survival is likely and safe) or should one wait for signs of hypoxic (respiratory) UPI to mandate delivery. A second point of contention is the question of whether it is indeed absolutely necessary to have ultrasound confirmation of IUGR. Since the following approach to management is the same whether or not ultrasound confirms IUGR, ultrasound does not really change management.

Once the condition of IUGR is suspected (not be-

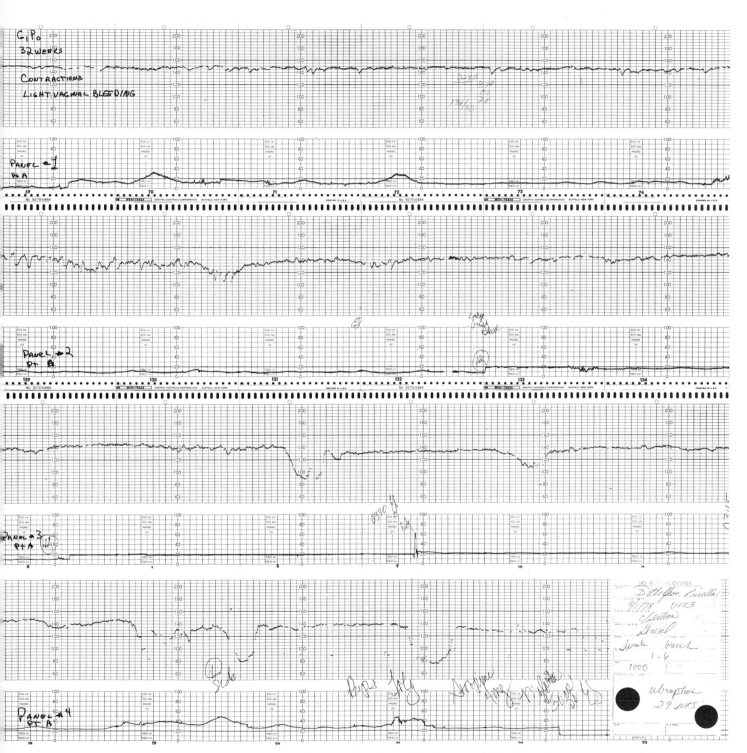

Figure 10.12. A G₁ is admitted at 32 weeks with mild uterine activity and light vaginal bleeding. The uterus was soft between contractions and nontender. Vital signs were normal. External monitoring revealed irregular uterine contractions which were difficult to record. At the ***second panel***, the patient has a large gush of blood. Late decelerations are seen on the ***second, third***, and ***fourth panels***. Immediate cesarean section produced a 1000-g Apgar 1/6 female which had moderate respiratory distress syndrome but subsequently did well. A 30 to 40% placental abruption was found. This case illustrates how fetal monitoring may be a sensitive indication of significant abruption.

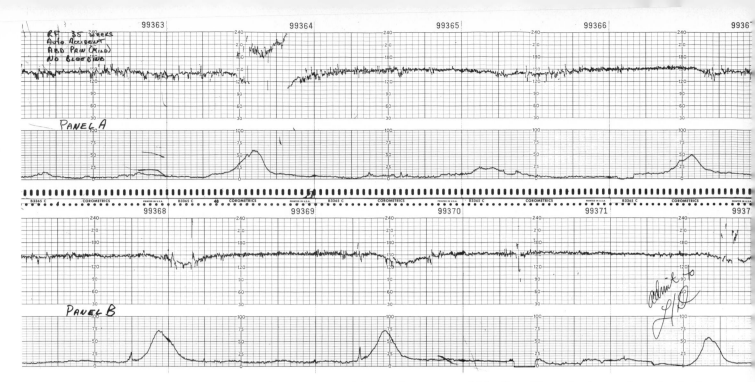

Figure 10.13. Often patients are admitted in premature labor without external bleeding. The only clue to abruption in these patients may be late decelerations in which case any attempt at inhibiting preterm labor might be unwise. This patient was admitted at 35 weeks after being in an auto accident. She was having mild abdominal pain but no bleeding. The external monitor shows contractions occurring every 6 min each followed by a late deceleration. The apparent acceleration after the first contraction in panel A is artifactual doubling by the ultrasound external monitor and is in reality a late deceleration. The patient was taken for cesarean section and a vigorous 2200-g baby was delivered. An occult 30% abruption was found. Mother and baby did well.

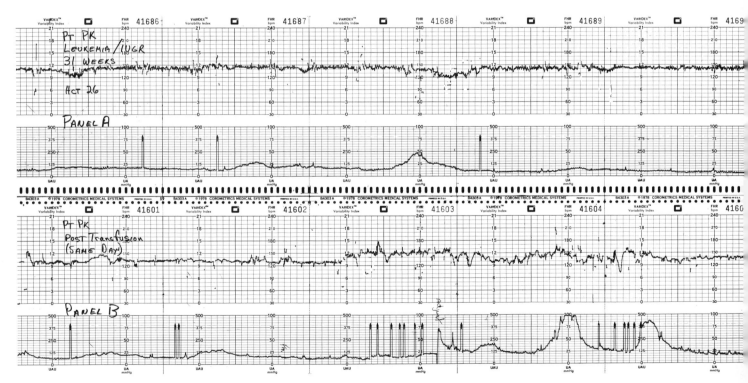

Figure 10.14. PK is a 25-year-old G_1P_0 with acute lymphocytic leukemia and suspected IUGR. The patient was on maintenance chemotherapy at the time of her conception. At 16 weeks the leukemia exacerbated and full chemotherapy again achieved remission, however, she became septic associated with the bone marrow depression. Subsequently, uterine growth after 20 weeks was lagging considerably. The patient was also markedly anemic. Estriol monitoring was begun at 30 weeks and the values were below the second standard deviation line. An OCT was done at 31 weeks (***panel A***). There is no reactivity and late decelerations are seen after three of the four contractions. In view of the low hematocrit, it was elected to transfuse the patient and repeat the test before deciding on intervention. The patient was transfused with two units of packed cells and later that day the OCT was repeated (***panel B***). Note the normal reactivity and negative OCT. The patient was kept at bed rest and OCT's were repeated weekly. At 37 weeks, the OCT again became positive. The cervix at that time was unripe and cesarean section was performed. A mildly growth-retarded, nondepressed, apparently normal baby was delivered. The baby had polycythemia and hyperbilirubinemia. Mother and baby are both doing well now 6 months after delivery. This case illustrates how some conditions such as anemia are potentially reversible and fetal conditions at least temporarily may be improved.

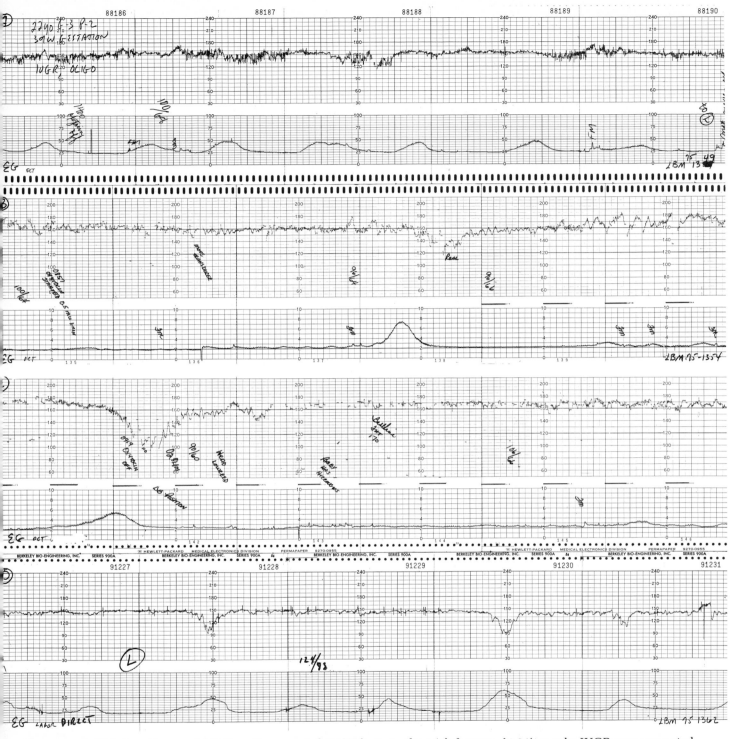

Figure 10.15. This is a 22-year-old G₃P₂ with suspected IUGR but no other risk factors. At 34½ weeks IUGR was suspected based on lagging uterine growth. Also the patient had oligohydramnios clinically. Estriols were started at twice weekly intervals and were low to low normal. OCT's were begun at 35 weeks and were reactive and negative until 39 weeks (**panel A**). **Panel A**, day 1—suspicious, reactive, tachycardia; **panel B** and **C**, day 2—suspicious, reactive, tachycardia **panel D**—spontaneous labor (internal electrode). Suspicious tests were seen on day 1 (**panel A**) and the next day (**panel B** and **C**). It should be noted that during the two OCT's there was mild maternal hypotension observed. This may have accounted for the fetal tachycardia which was seen in labor when the mother was on her side with normal blood pressure. The deep decelerations seen on the second stress test and during labor are commonly seen with oligohydramnios as are variable decelerations during labor which this patient had. An Apgar 9 growth-retarded baby was delivered without apparent etiology.

fore 28 weeks) estriol monitoring is begun on a bi-weekly basis. Plasma unconjugated estriol determinations seem best for this purpose.[5] If the estriol values are within the normal range and rising, this is all that is done. If they are chronically low or falling, weekly OCT's are begun immediately and the patient is delivered after 36 weeks with a mature L:S ratio as long as the OCT's do not become positive (Fig. 10.15).

Discordant Twins

Twin to twin transfusion occuring in monozygotic twins is a form of growth retardation. Ultrasound is currently the best indication of such a problem in the antepartum period. Should such a condition be present, twice weekly NST's are begun as early as the condition is suspected (no sooner than 28 weeks). While OCT's are generally contraindicated in twins because of the potential risk of premature labor,

should the NST be nonreactive, an OCT should be considered. If the NST remains reassuring, these patients may be allowed to procede to term. Estriol monitoring is generally of no value in twin gestation. This is also the general approach to managing twin gestations complicated by other risk factors such as diabetes or hypertension (Fig. 10.16).

Decreased Fetal Movement

A condition where patients without other risk factors might benefit from antepartum FHR testing is when the patient complains of decreased fetal movement. This may be the only sign of impending fetal death in an otherwise low risk patient. Often this may be a transient phenomenon, so the first step should be to ask the patient to lie down for 1 hr and count movements. If she feels three or more movements in that hour, she can be reassured, but she

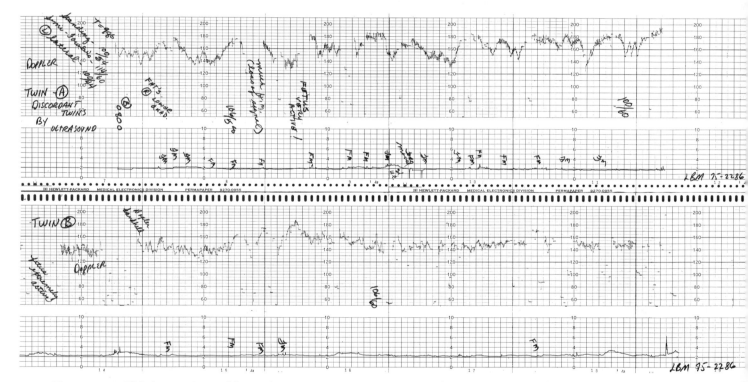

Figure 10.16. This is a patient with a twin gestation. A sonogram was done at 33 weeks when the patient was noted to be large for dates. Twins were found whose biparietal diameters differed by more than 1.0 cm. The patient was started on twice weekly NST's. Both twins remained reactive. Spontaneous vaginal delivery followed spontaneous labor at 36½ weeks. Vertex/vertex male twins were delivered with birth weights of 2230 and 1580 g. The babies were typical of twin/twin transfusion (i.e., one plethoric and one anemic) but had no other complications and were both Apgar 9 at 1 min. The placenta was monochorionic/diamniotic with bridging vessels. The figure is an example of one of the NST's. Only ultrasound can be used. One must be sure the FHR's of both fetuses are obtained. Criteria for reactivity (i.e., 2 accelerations in 20 min) must be met; therefore a full NST is done on each twin.

Figure 10.17. Decreased fetal movement. This is a patient who had been having OCT's for mild chronic hypertension. An OCT had been done 4 days prior which was reactive and negative. At 34 weeks, the patient called reporting minimal fetal movement for 2 days. She was told to lie down for an hour and count movements but none was felt. She was therefore brought in immediately for an NST. The NST revealed a sinusoidal FHR pattern (*panels A* and *B*). An OCT (*panels C, D,* and *E*) was done and late decelerations are seen following most of the contractions. A cesarean section was performed and a 1950-g infant was delivered with an Apgar score of 1 at 1 min. The baby was resuscitated. Peripheral hematocrit and hemoglobin were 9.7 and 3.1 g/100 ml, respectively. The baby was transfused and subsequently did well. Kleihauer-Betke on maternal blood revealed a large fetal-maternal transfusion calculated at 275 ml. This case illustrates how a decrease in fetal movement may help detect sudden unexpected changes in fetal condition and further testing may allow intervention before death or damage.

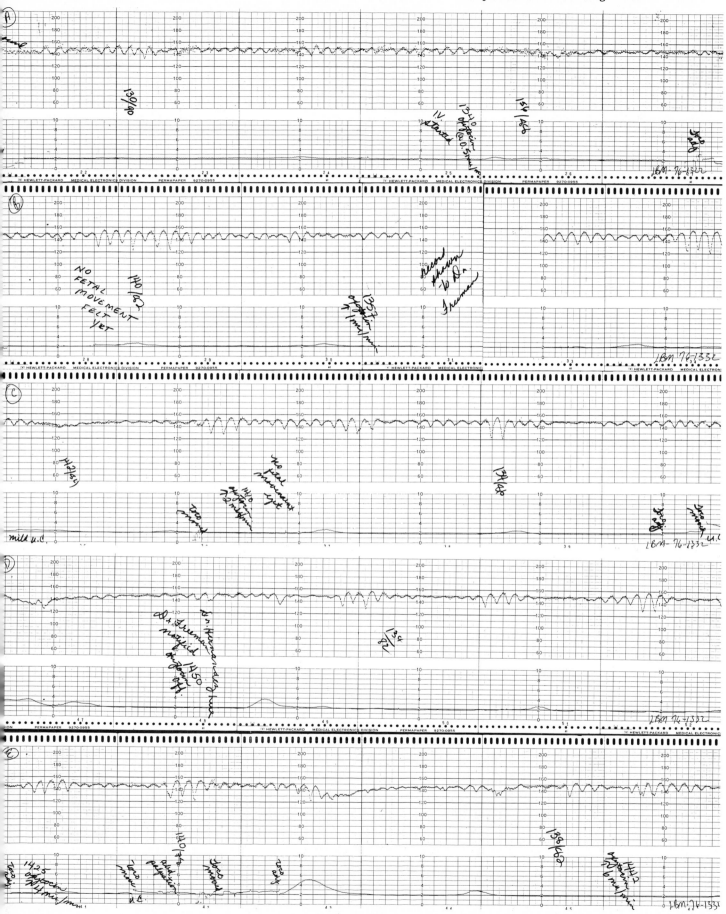

Figure 10.17

should be warned to continue to be aware of this and repeat the hourly observations should the problem continue or recur. Two or less movements should prompt an immediate NST in these patients (at or after 28 weeks). If the NST is reactive, no further testing is warranted in the absence of other risk factors. Nonreactive NST's as in other situations are followed by an immediate OCT.

Monitoring fetal movement daily by high risk patients is also an important adjunct to the other tests that are being used. Should a high risk patient report decreased fetal movement, the same policy as described above is followed regardless of when the preceding OCT or NST was done (Fig. 10.17).

MANAGEMENT OF NONREASSURRING TESTS

Equivocal Tests

About 10% of OCT's are equivocal (unsatisfactory, suspicious, or hyperstimulation). These test results should have little or no place in the decision to alter management. They mean only that the test cannot be used to prognostically state that the fetus is safely left alone for 1 week. The test must be repeated the next day. In using NST's rather than OCT's primarily, a late deceleration seen after a spontaneous contraction should not be ignored simply because the test is reactive, this patient should be stressed if there is no contraindication. Alternatively, when OCT's are repeatedly equivocal (two on sequential days), it would be reasonable at that point to change to frequent NST's (two to three per week) and/or estriol monitoring. Should these then become less reactive, the patient should then be stressed again.

Positive OCT's

As previously stated, positive OCT's have a high correlation with fetal and neonatal morbidity and even with fetal mortality, if ignored. However, there is a relatively high rate of false positive tests (about 30%). One would not want to deliver a premature baby on this basis alone. However, a mature fetus with a positive OCT on a statistical basis is definitely better off in the nursery. While a mature L:S ratio does not insure that the newborn will not have other complications of prematurity, lung maturity is generally the limiting factor in survival of the premature neonate. Furthermore, if the hypoxic placental insufficiency is allowed to persist and a depressed newborn is delivered, many complications of prematurity are more likely including respiratory distress syndrome even in the face of a mature L:S ratio.[16] Therefore, a positive OCT with or without reactivity is an indication for delivery if the L:S ratio is mature. For this reason a positive OCT is generally an indication for an amniocentesis (Fig. 10.18). An exception to this

is when other tests of fetal well-being including loss of reactivity and a fall in estriol indicate delivery even in the face of an immature L:S ratio.

In the face of an immature L:S ratio, a reactive positive OCT requires further evidence of fetal jeopardy before intervention is warranted. Assuming maternal condition is not heavily entering into the decision, fetal reactivity and estriol determinations are useful. If estriols have been chronically low or have fallen and the baseline FHR is completely nonreactive (no accelerations), the patient should be delivered regardless of the immaturity (Fig. 19). With a positive OCT, however, which is reactive, and where estriol values are reassurring, then estriol values and NST's are looked at more frequently, such as daily to three times a week. A particularly difficult problem with the immature fetus and a positive OCT, is when the NST is nonreactive and the estriol is reassurring or vice versa. A normal estriol value measured at appropriate intervals is very reassurring as is a negative OCT. Both tests have many falsely abnormal results. Therefore, it is generally best to rely on the normal test when fetal maturity is not present. Fetal reactivity is only reassurring at the time it is observed but may not have future predictive value.

When one has a patient with a reactive positive OCT, one can individualize looking for the presence of accelerations and comparing present FHR tracings with previous ones. This may be a rather hard concept to understand, perhaps the upcoming case example (Fig. 10.20) will help to clarify this approach. In the face of low estriol values and a reactive positive OCT, where accelerations are still present and the fetus is immature, there are two alternatives of management. One is to administer corticosteriools to accelerate fetal pulmonary maturity as described by Liggins and others[17] and then deliver the fetus in 48 hr. During this time period, the fetus should be monitored continuously; should accelerations be lost while waiting,[18] intervention is accomplished immediately. Alternatively, especially with a very premature fetus (i.e., 28 to 30 weeks), daily NST's, using the preceding tests for comparison, and daily fetal movement counting by the patient may buy a significant amount of time. Intervention is then indicated when reactivity is clearly decreasing or when the fetus is judged sufficiently mature for delivery. While such an approach is clearly expensive and time consuming, it is certainly less so than neonatal intensive care.

Falls in Estriol Values

An isolated 35% fall in estriol is much more likely to be a false positive test than is a positive OCT. Goebelsmann[5] suggests that any one estriol value has a 0.35% chance of falling without clinical significance, so many patients with multiple estriols will have a fall in estriol which is not really fetal compromise.

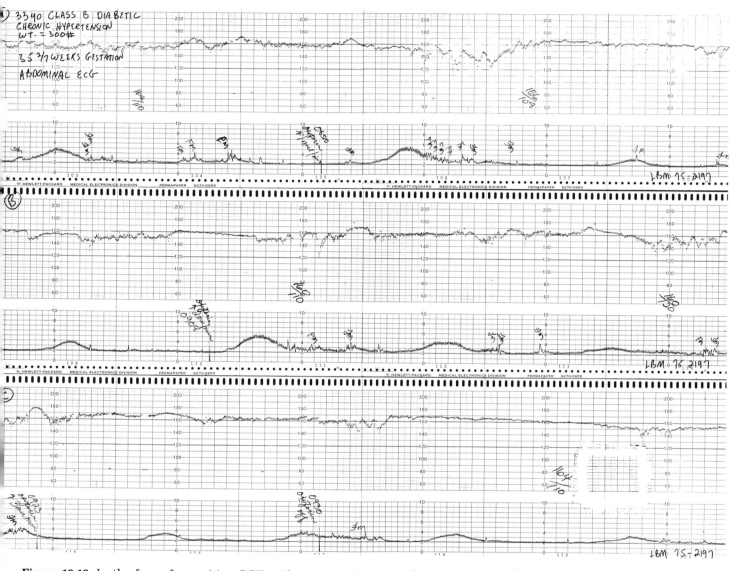

Figure 10.18. In the face of a positive OCT with a mature L:S ratio, the patient is usually delivered even if the FHR is reactive and estriol values are normal. Here a 300-lb Class B diabetic with chronic hypertension has an OCT at 35½ weeks. This OCT is clearly positive but reactive. Daily estriol values were consistently normal and rising. An amniocentesis revealed an L:S ratio of 2:3. The patient was given a trial of induced labor after artificial rupture of membranes and O₂ administration. However, the internal monitor recording revealed persistent late decelerations. A cesarean section was done and an Apgar 7/9 AGA baby was delivered which had no complications except mild hypoglycemia.

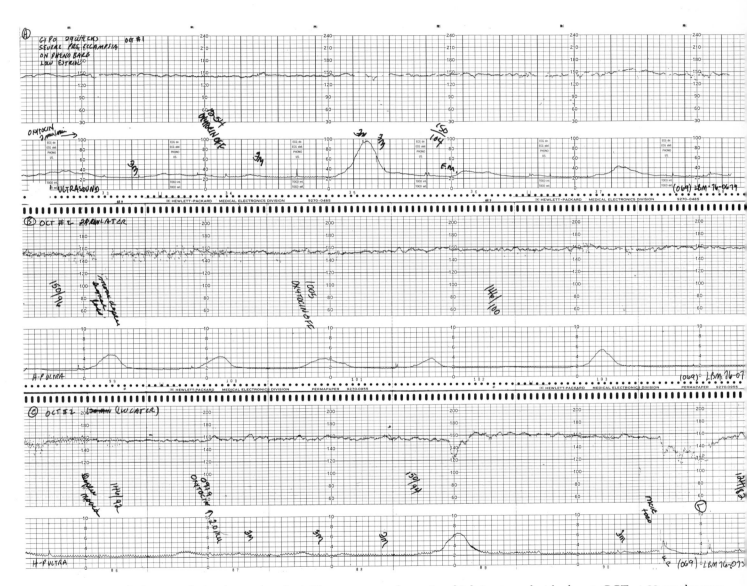

Figure 10.19. A G₁ was admitted at 28 weeks with severe preeclampsia which improved at bed rest. OCT at 29 weeks was negative but nonreactive probably because of phenobarbitol. Estriols remained low at less than 3.0 ng/ml. An OCT was repeated one week later (***panel B and C***). Six days later, the patient reported no fetal movement. BP was also worsening at this time. An OCT was done (***panels A, B and C***, p. 155) which was nonreactive and positive. No amniocentesis was done since delivery was planned in the face of a nonreactive positive OCT and low estriol values regardless of maturity.

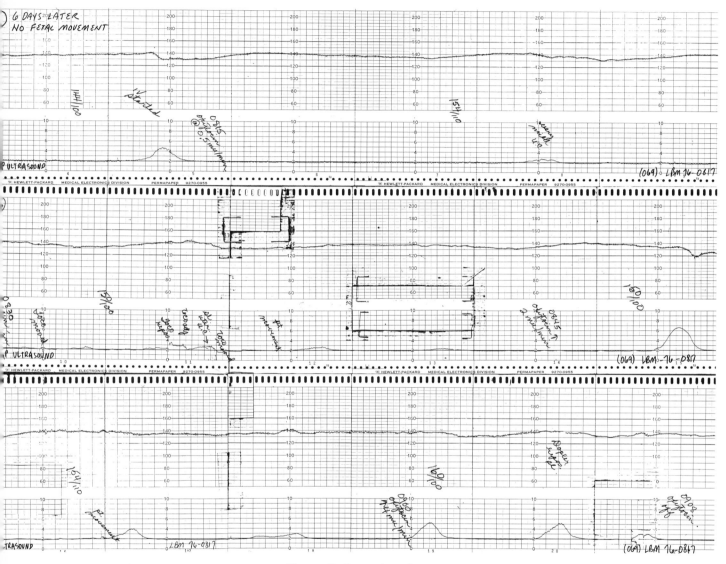

Figure 10.19 *continued*

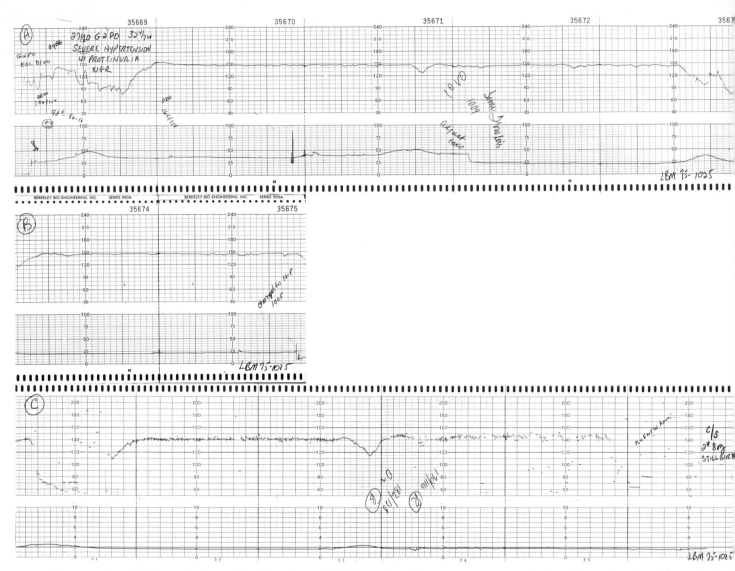

Figure 10.20. *A*, This patient was first transferred at 32½ weeks with severe pregnancy-induced hypertension. The patient was placed on the monitor. The FHR is smooth, nonreactive and there are late decelerations after each contraction. Fetal heart tones were lost at the end of *panel C* while preparations were being made for cesarean section—immediate cesarean section delivered a 2 lb 8 oz stillborn without anomalies. Figure 10.20 *B*, The patient was cared for in her next pregnancy 1 year later and was normotensive until 26 weeks when BP rose to 140/100. The patient was hospitalized with improvement in blood pressure. Antepartum testing was done as follows:

Panel	Date	Gestational Age	Type Test	Test Result
A	6–13	26 Wk	NST—	minimally reactive
B	6–13	26 Wk	NST—	reactive
C	6–16	27 Wk	NST—	reactive
D/E	6–20	27 Wk	OCT—	positive/reactive
F	6–21 (Daily NST's Done— Not All Shown)	28 Wk	NST—	reactive
G	6–24	28 Wk	NST—	reactive
H	6–27	28 Wk	OCT—	positive/minimally reactive
I	6–28	29 Wk	NST—	minimally reactive
J	6–29	29 Wk	NST—	minimally reactive
K	6–30	29 Wk	NST—	reactive
L/M/N	7-5	30 Wk	OCT—	positive/reactive
O	7-6	30 Wk	NST—	reactive
P	7-13	31 Wk	NST—	minimally reactive
Q	7-16	31 Wk	NST—	minimally reactive
R/S	7-18	31 Wk	NST—	nonreactive

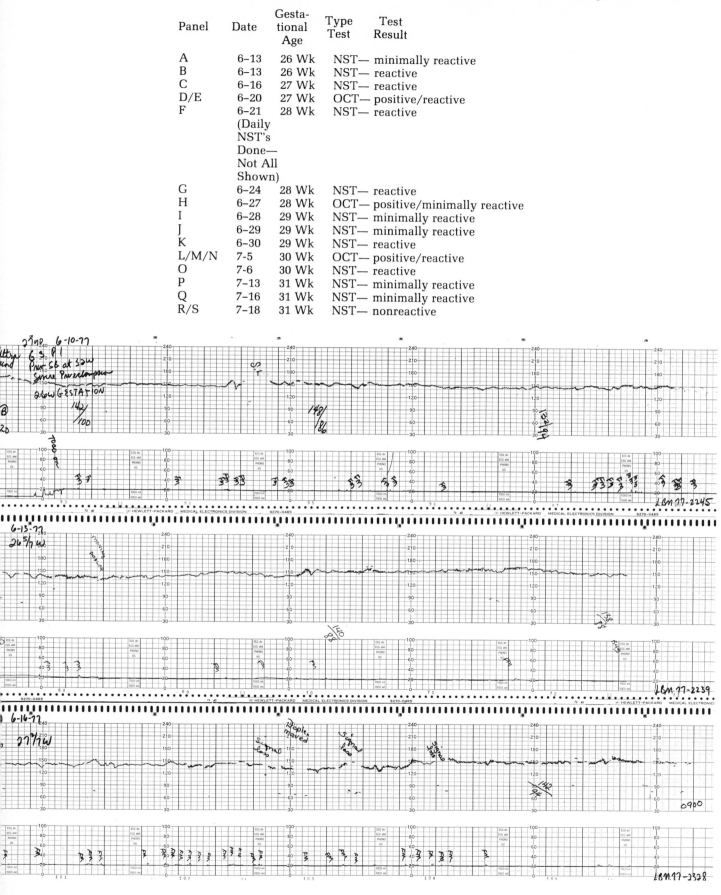

Figure 10.20 panels A–C.

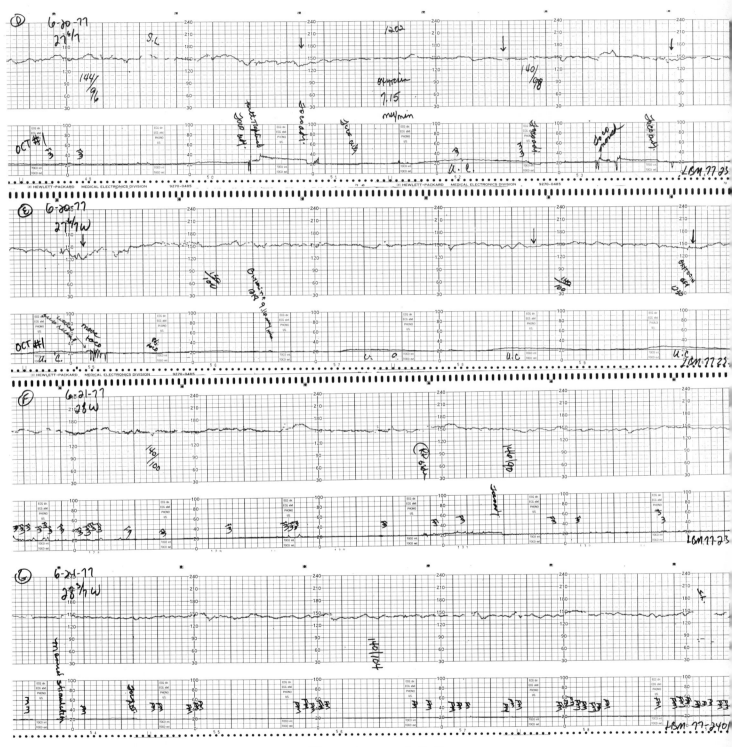

Figure 10.20 panels D–G.

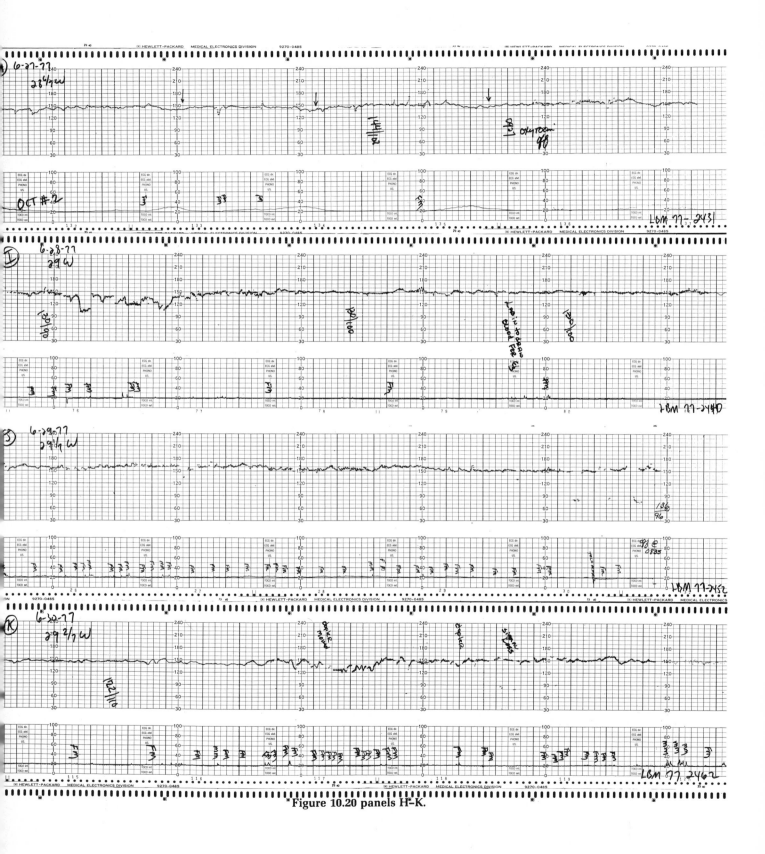

*Figure 10.20 panels H–K.

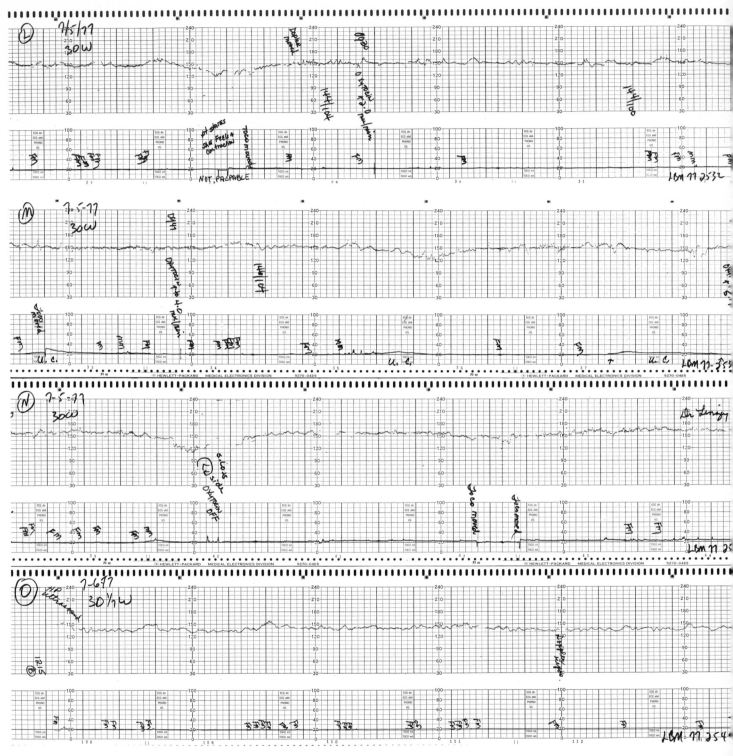

Figure 10.20 panels L–O.

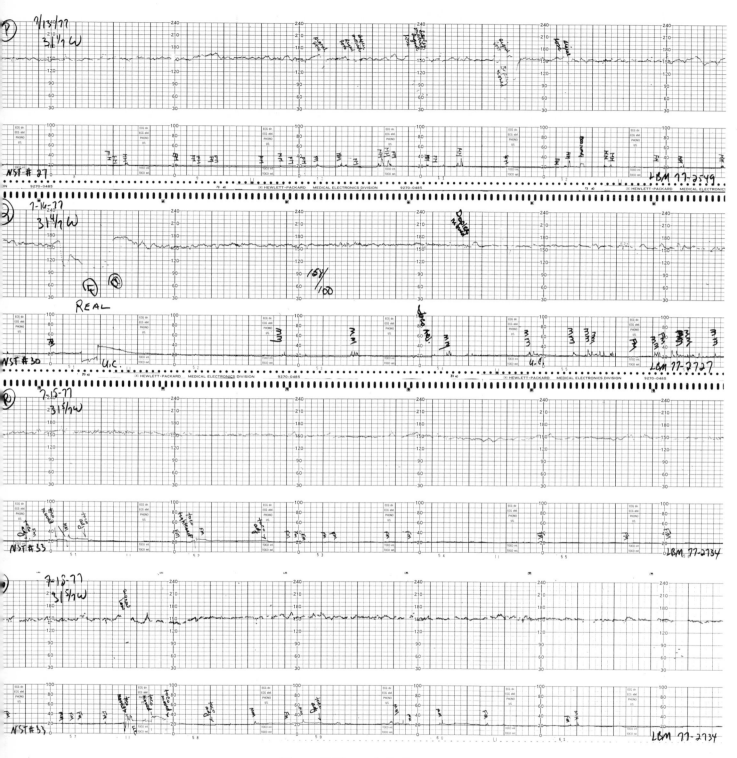

Figure 10.20 panels P–S.

THIRD TRIMESTER UNCONJUGATED PLASMA ESTRIOL CONCENTRATIONS AND 95% CONFIDENCE LIMITS

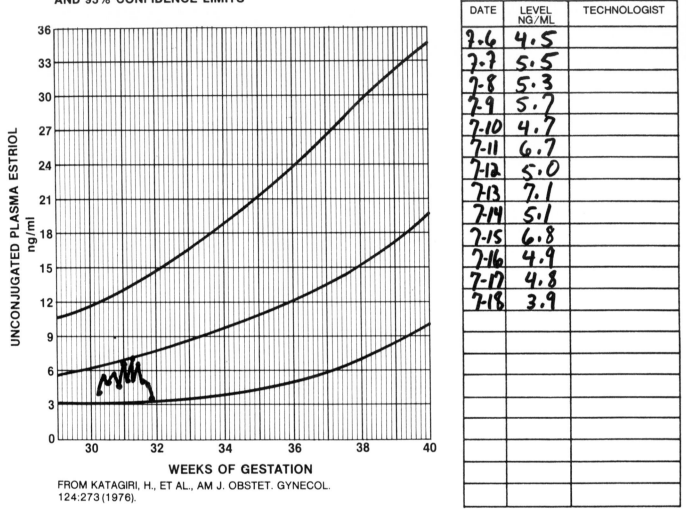

DATE	LEVEL NG/ML	TECHNOLOGIST
7-6	4.5	
7-7	5.5	
7-8	5.3	
7-9	5.7	
7-10	4.7	
7-11	6.7	
7-12	5.0	
7-13	7.1	
7-14	5.1	
7-15	6.8	
7-16	4.9	
7-17	4.8	
7-18	3.9	

FROM KATAGIRI, H., ET AL., AM J. OBSTET. GYNECOL. 124:273 (1976).

Figure 10.20 *continued.*

Since the patient had normal estriols, it was decided to follow the patient with daily NST's after the first positive OCT on 6/20. No L:S ratio was done at this time since it was so unlikely to be mature. The OCT's were intermittently repeated; since maternal condition improved, it was possible the OCT might have reverted to negative. On 7/5 and 7/6 L:S ratios were done and were 1.1 and 1.6, respectively. On 7/18 with the reactivity essentially lost and with the fall in estriol to 3.9 (38%) the patient was delivered by repeat cesarean section. The baby was a 1080-g Apgar 5/7 growth retarded female. The baby did well without significant newborn complications and is developing normally at 2½ years of age.

However, one virtually never sees a fetal death occur without low or falling estriols preceding demise. Therefore, our approach to a significant (35%) fall in estriol, is to call the patient in for an immediate NST and if it is fully reactive, repeat the estriol the next day (Fig. 10.21). If the estriol is back up to normal, previous monitoring methods and intervals are resumed. If the estriol remains down, an OCT is done. If it is negative, an amniocentesis is done and if the L:S ratio is mature, unless the fetus is very premature, delivery is strongly considered.

The Nonreactive NST

The NST should be viewed as a screening test when used as the primary means of antepartum testing. Nonreactive patterns may be caused by fetal sleep states or by central nervous system depressant drugs. In performing the NST, when a nonreactive 20-min period (0 to 1 acceleration) is found, the first step should be to stimulate the fetus by uterine manipulation for 30 sec to 1 min (Fig. 10.22). Another 20-min period is then monitored and if the fetus is still nonreactive, an OCT must be done immediately (Fig. 10.23). Should the fetus become reactive during the OCT, the OCT may be discontinued. Another way to obviate the nonreactive NST due to fetal quiescence is to do the test shortly after the mother has eaten. Sugar tends to heighten fetal arousal. When a nonreactive NST is followed by a negative OCT, the test is reassurring and may be repeated in 1 week. This combination is relatively unusual and may be more likely to be associated with an eventual positive test or with neonatal morbidity (Fig. 10.24). Therefore, the patient should be alerted to monitor fetal movement. A nonreactive positive OCT is handled as has been previously detailed in the section on the positive OCT. Management using the NST and the OCT is outlined graphically in Figures 10.25 and 10.26.

Choosing the Route of Delivery

Once the decision has been made to intervene on behalf of the fetus, one must decide whether to proceed directly to cesarean section or to give the patient a trial of labor. If one could be certain that the test was a true positive, then there would be no need for a trial of labor. One way to determine this is to evaluate reactivity. Braly and Freeman[19] retrospectively reviewed positive OCT's in patients given a trial of labor. They found when there were no accelerations present, there were no false positive tests, i.e., all patients had persistent late decelerations in labor. When accelerations were present, 50% of patients were able to be induced, and labored without further persistent late decelerations. There is one other method recently described by Bisonette et al.[20] to predict which patients will or will not tolerate labor. The interval between the onset of the contraction and the onset of the late deceleration is called the "latency period" (Fig. 10.27). Myers et al.[21] showed in the monkey that the more profound the hypoxia,

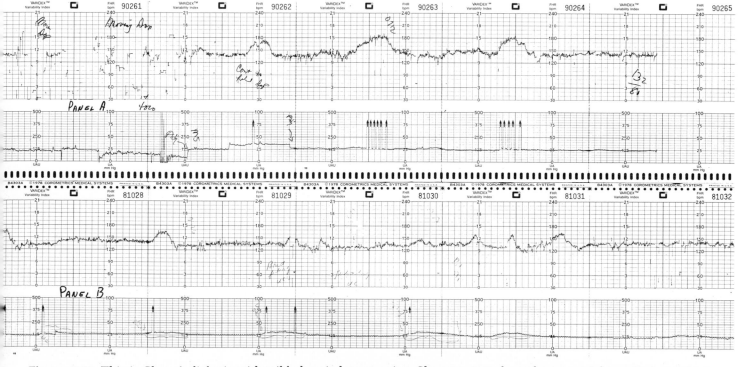

Figure 10.21. This is Class A diabetic with mild chronic hypertension. She was started on plasma estriol monitoring at 32 weeks when she was transferred for care. OCT's were scheduled to be started at 34 weeks. On 1/1 at 33½ weeks the estriol value fell to 3.3 ng/ml. Previous values were 6.6, 4.4, and 7.3. This represents a 46% fall. Therefore, that evening the patient was called in for a NST (***panel A***) which is clearly reactive. The next day the estriol was 4.7 and subsequent values continued to rise. OCT's were begun on schedule (***panel B***, negative) and the patient continued to term without problems.

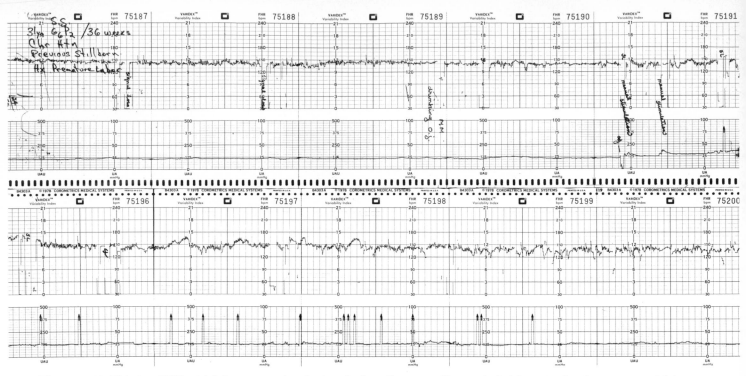

Figure 10.22. This is a NST which is nonreactive during the baseline recording period. After 20 min, the uterus and fetus are manually stimulated. The FHR immediately becomes reactive and the fetus begins to move as indicated by the **arrows** on the lower channel.

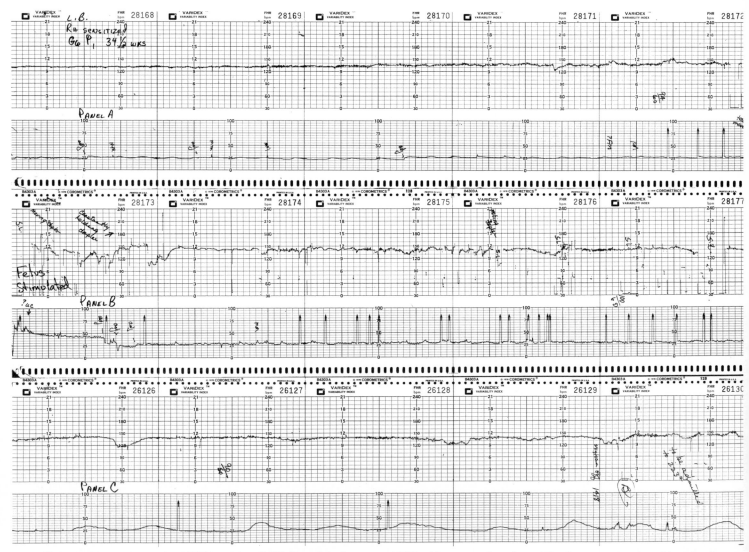

Figure 10.23. Nonreactive NST/positive OCT. **Panel A** shows an NST with no accelerations. The fetus is stimulated in **panel B** but there are still no accelerations despite an increase in fetal movement (**arrows**). An OCT is therefore done (**panel C**) which is positive and remains nonreactive.

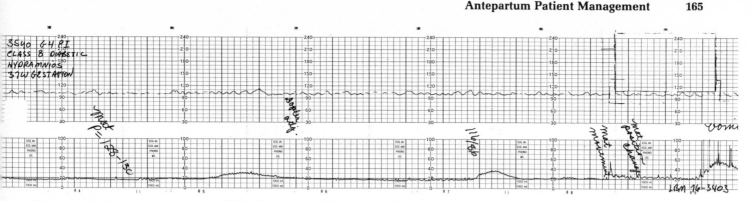

Figure 10.24. Nonreactive negative OCT. This is an OCT done in a diabetic with hydramnios. There is a baseline bradycardia of 100 BPM. No late decelerations are seen but no accelerations are seen. This unusual pattern was seen in a patient who later delivered a baby with multiple congenital anomalies including congenital heart disease, meningomyelocele, and hydrocephaly.

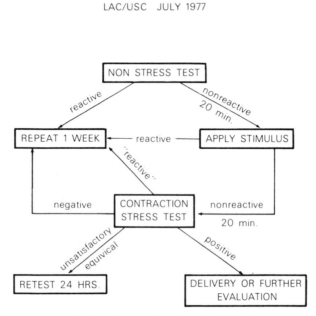

Figure 10.25. Outline for conducting the NST. (Reproduced with permission from Evertson LR, Gauthier RJ, Schifrin BS, et al: Antepartum fetal heart rate testing I. Evolution of the nonstress test. Am J Obstet Gynecol 133:31, 1979.)

the shorter the interval. Bisonette et al.[20] used this information in patients with positive OCT's and in a small series found that when the latency period was less than 45 sec, there were no false positives.

One must also consider cervical ripeness in the decision to allow a trial of labor. Obviously one does not want a long induction, so only those patients with ripe cervices are reasonable candidates for induction.

In performing the induction, the patient should be placed on her left side to maximize uterine perfusion. Oxygen should be administered by mask or nasal canula. Membranes should be artificially ruptured from the start of the induction and FHR should be monitored by scalp electrode. Oxytocin is administered with special care to avoid uterine hyperstimulation. Should late decelerations persist despite all these measures, the patient should be delivered by cesarean section.

All patients who have unripe cervices and/or nonvertex presentations should be delivered by cesarean section without a trial of labor. Patients with positive OCT's with no accelerations present and/or latency periods of less than 45 sec should be delivered by cesarean sections without a trial of labor as it is very unlikely that these fetuses will tolerate labor.

Finally, a note that is partly philosophy and partly good practice. Once the decision has been made to

OCT MANAGEMENT PROTOCOL

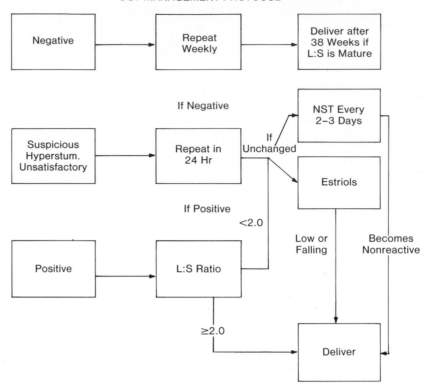

Figure 10.26.

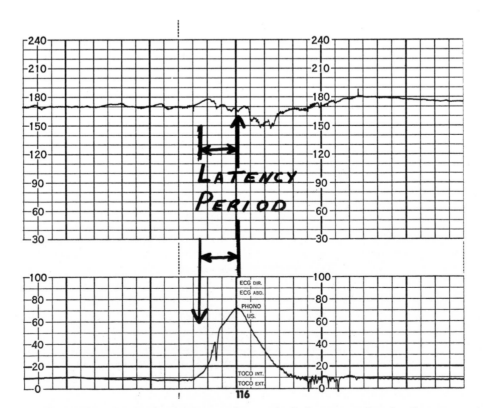

Figure 10.27. This Figure demonstrates the method for measuring the "latency period".

intervene, it is important to procede immediately. This is not a delivery reasonably delayed until the next day. In preparing for cesarean section with delay for blood cross-match or whatever reason, the fetus should be continually monitored until taken to the delivery/operating room.

Managing the antepartum patient is a difficult and challenging problem. Decisions to intervene or not have potentially grave consequences and should never be made on one parameter alone without knowledge of gestational age and maturity, or of maternal condition. The goal should be to deliver a healthy baby as near term as possible by the safest route for mother and fetus. Antepartum heart rate monitoring can contribute significantly toward this goal if understood well and used appropriately.

REFERENCES

1. Garite TJ, Freeman RK, Hochleutner I, et al: Oxytocin challenge test: achieving the desired goals. Obstet Gynecol 15:614, 1978
2. Nesbitt REL, Aubry RH: High risk obstetrics, II. Value of semi-objective grading system in evaluating the vulnerable group. Am J Obstet Gynecol 103:972, 1969
3. Hobel CJ, Hyvarinen MA, Okada DM, et al: Prenatal and intrapartum high risk screening. I. Prediction of the high risk neonate. Am J Obstet Gynecol 117:1, 1973
4. Ostergard DR: Estriol in pregnancy. Obstet Gynecol Surv 28:215, 1973
5. Goebelsmann U: The use of oestriol as a monitoring tool. In: Quilligan EJ (editor) Clinics in Obstetrics and Gynecology, Vol 6. W. B. Saunders, London, 1979, p 223–244
6. Freeman RK: The use of the oxytocin challenge test for antepartum clinical evaluation of uteroplacental respiratory function. Am J Obstet Gynecol 121:481, 1975
7. Freeman RK, Goelbelsmann U, Nochimson D, et al: An evaluation of the significance of a positive oxytocin challenge test. Obstet Gynecol 47:8, 1976
8. Knox GE, Huddleston JF, Flowers CE Jr, et al: Management of

prolonged pregnancy: Results of a randomized prospective trial. Am J Obstet Gynecol 134:376, 1979
9. Gant NF, Daley GL, Chand S, et al: A study of angiotensin II pressor response throughout primagravid pregnancy. J Clin Invest 52:2682, 1973
10. Gant NF, Chand S, Worley RJ, et al: A clinical useful test for predicting the development of acute hypertension in pregnancy. Am J Obstet Gynecol 120:1, 1974
11. Gabbe SG, Freeman RK, Goebelsmann U: Evaluation of contraction stress test before 33 weeks gestation. Obstet Gynecol 52:649, 1978
12. Gabbe SG, Mestman JH, Freeman RK, et al: Management and outcome of pregnancy in diabetes mellitus, classes B to R. Am J Obstet Gynecol 129:723, 1977
13. Goldstein AI, Cronk DA, Garite TJ, et al: Perinatal outcome in the diabetic pregnancy: A retrospective analysis. J Reprod Med 20:61, 1978
14. Gabbe SG, Freeman RK, Mestman JH, et al: Management and outcome of Class A diabetes mellitus. Am J Obstet Gynecol 127:465, 1977
15. Goebelsmann U, Freeman RK, Mestman JH, et al: Estriol in pregnancy II. Daily urinary estriol assays in the management of the pregnant diabetic woman. Am J Obstet Gynecol 115:795, 1973
16. Cruz AC, Buhi WC, Birk SA, et al: Respiratory distress syndrome with mature lecithin/sphingomyelin ratios: Diabetes mellitus and low Apgar scores. Am J Obstet Gynecol 126:78, 1976
17. Shields JR, Resnik R: Fetal lung maturation and the antenatal use of glucocorticoids to prevent the respiratory distress syndrome. Obstet Gynecol Surv 34:343, 1979
18. Ricke PS, Elliott JP, Freeman RK: The use of corticosteroids in the presence of pregnancy induced hypertensive states. Obstet Gynecol 55:206, 1980
19. Braly, PB, Freeman RK: The significance of fetal heart rate reactivity with a positive oxytocin challenge test. Obstet Gynecol 50:689, 1977
20. Bisonette JM, Johnson K, Toomey C: The role of a trial of labor with a positive contraction stress test. Am J Obstet Gynecol 135:292, 1979
21. Myers RE, Mueller-Huebach E, Adamsons K: Predictability of the state of fetal oxygenation from a qualitative analysis of the components of late decelerations. Am J Obstet Gynecol 115:1083, 1973

CHAPTER 11

The Risks and Benefits of Electronic Fetal Monitoring

The introduction of intrapartum electronic fetal heart rate (FHR) monitoring (EFM) as common clinical practice began about 1970. At that time it was rarely used except in high risk pregnancies. Because of the poor quality of external monitoring systems available at that time, practically all patients were monitored internally, and the use of external techniques has gradually increased since then with the improvement of technology. The use of EFM was originally validated by numerous studies that showed correlations between FHR patterns and outcome measures, such as Apgar scores and fetal and neonatal acid-base status.[1-6] Now, 10 years later, there is developing a very skeptical attitude regarding the actual value of EFM. Some have said that the technology was accepted without proof of its value or serious questioning of its risks.[7] As is the case with most medical diagnostic technology, the acceptance of the technique makes the evaluation of its risks and benefits very difficult or impossible, after the fact. It is especially difficult to evaluate such a method as EFM in a setting where the health professionals are already convinced of its value.

This chapter will attempt to briefly review available data on this subject, but the reader who is interested in a more detailed presentation is referred to NIH publication no. 79-1973 (April 1979) entitled *Antenatal Diagnosis*. This is a report of a consensus development conference sponsored by the National Institute of Child Health and Human Development.

THE EFFECT OF EFM ON PERINATAL MORBIDITY AND MORTALITY

Intrapartum fetal death is a clear end point but only occurs between 1 and 4/1000 in most obstetric populations. For this reason, a rather large study population would be required to determine the effect of EFM on the intrapartum death rate. If we examine those reports referred to in the NIH consensus report on antenatal diagnosis, they are divided into two groups. The first group consists of the retrospective noncontrolled studies which now include over 135,000 patients, about one-third of whom had EFM. In these studies, the intrapartum death rate was 1.76/1000 in patients followed with auscultation during labor, and 0.54/1000 in patients followed with EFM during labor. This difference is significant at the P = <0.001 level. This is an intrapartum fetal death ratio of 3.26:1 of auscultated patients to those followed with EFM (see Table 11.1). These data were restricted to infants who weighed over 1500 g at birth and were corrected for congenital anomalies.

These studies can certainly be criticized on several bases, including different time frames in the EFM vs the auscultated group. It should also be pointed out that most of the studies had all or most of their high risk patients in the EFM group and still showed significantly less intrapartum fetal death in the higher risk EFM group.

More recently, there have been four randomized controlled trials (RCT) comparing EFM to auscultation in both high risk[8-10] and low risk[11] patients. This is clearly a better study design but there are only about 1000 patients in the EFM and about the same number in the auscultated group (see Table 11.2). They have shown no difference in intrapartum fetal death between the two groups, although the single intrapartum death did occur in the auscultated group. Table 11.1 shows that it would take approximately 18,000 patients in an RCT to prove no difference between the EFM and auscultated groups at P = <0.05 level of significance. Because of the very small numbers and the expected low intrapartum death rate, these RCT's are not sufficient to answer this question. It should also be pointed out that in each of these RCT's both groups had a dedicated one-on-one nurse assigned to the patient, and the auscultated groups were followed much more frequently than is commonly practiced in hospitals, even under ideal circumstances where fluctuations in the numbers of deliveries makes consistent nurse staffing impossible.

Table 11.1.
Intrapartum Fetal Death and Electronic Fetal Monitoring*

Primary Author	Year	No EFM	IFD†	EFM	IFD	Ratio
Chan[21]	1973	5,427	17	1,162	2	
Kelly[59]	1973	17,000	15	150	0	
Tutera[60]	1975	6,179	37	608	1	
Edington[61]	1975	991	4	1,024	0	
Koh[62]	1975	1,161	4	1,080	5	
Shenker[63]	1975	11,599	14	1,950	1	
Lee[64]	1976	4,323	15	3,529	1	
Paul[65]	1977	36,724	34	13,344	6	
Amato[66]	1977	2,981	12	4,226	1	
Johnstone[67]	1978	9,099	13	7,313	3	
Hamilton[68]	1978	4,353	11	4,399	1	
Total		99,842	176	38,785	21	
Rate		1.76/1000		0.54/1000		3.26 (P < 0.001)
		Critical No. of Subjects for P < 0.05 = 18,046				

* From Reference 32.
† Abbreviations: IFD, intrapartum fetal death.

Table 11.2.
Intrapartum Death and Electronic Fetal Monitoring from RCT* reports†

Primary Author	Year	No EFM	IFD*	EFM	IFD	Ratio
Havercamp	1976	241	0	242	0	
Havercamp	1978	232	0	463	0	
Renou	1976	175	1	169	0	
Kelso	1978	253	0	251	0	
Total		901	1	1,125	0	
Rate		1.1/1000				

* Abbreviations: RCT, randomized controlled trial; IFD, intrapartum fetal death.
† Reference 32.

Clearly, where this one-on-one nursing care is not available, EFM is preferable to "catch as catch can" nurse surveillance.

If one simply looks at the intrapartum death rates, one might argue that neonatal death rates may increase as the compromised fetus is rescued and converted to a compromised neonate. Again, if we turn to the retrospective studies referred to above, we can see that among about 140,000 patients studied, the neonatal death rate above 1,500 g (corrected for congenital anomalies) was 15.2/1000 in auscultated patients and 4.4/1000 in EFM patients. This ratio is 3.45 to 1. (P = < 0.001) (Table 11.3). In the RCT's there was no significant difference between the EFM and auscultated groups, but their numbers were again much too small to answer this question (Table 11.4). Because there are so many variables involved in neonatal survival, Neutra et al.[12] studied this problem, using a retrospective multivariate analysis technique on 16,000 deliveries at the Beth Israel Hospital in Boston, calculated a death rate ratio of 1:7 favoring EFM for the overall population, but when the lowest risk patients were analyzed separately, there was no benefit to EFM on neonatal death risk seen in this lowest risk group. It would thus appear that when large enough populations are studied, the perinatal mortality rate may be significantly decreased, due to both a reduction in intrapartum death and neonatal death. When studying the lowest risk populations, however, the benefit of EFM is difficult to show.

The effect of EFM on Apgar scores again has been generally shown to be positive among the retrospective studies, but no benefit was seen in the RCT's. Of course, this is a much less clear end point than perinatal death, and it is affected by many things other than fetal oxygenation which is what EFM should measure. The NIH consensus report referred to unpublished work by Sokol et al. from Cleveland that shows significant correlation between Apgar scores at 1 and 5 min and EFM, suggesting that as the fetal risk group increases, the benefit of EFM on Apgar scores becomes more significant. There were some questions raised by the NIH consensus task force about the data handling of this study.

There is very little data on the neurologic sequelae in infants from EFM and auscultated labors. The RCT's do not show any significant differences in the immediate neonatal neurological complication rate

Table 11.3.
Neonatal Death and Electronic Fetal Monitoring*

Primary Author	Year	No EFM	NND	EFM	NND	Ratio
Chan[21]	1973	5,427	15	1,162	5	
Kelly[59]	1973	17,000	238	150	1	
Tutera[60]	1975	6,179	48	608	1	
Edington[61]	1975	962	13	1,012	3	
Koh[62]	1975	787	4	285	1	
Lee[64]	1976	4,275	56	3,498	31	
Paul[65]	1977	36,071	184	13,151	72	
Amatos[66]	1977	2,923	24	4,210	4	
Hughey[69]	1977	3,431	14	3,826	9	
Neutra[70]	1978	8,764	48	7,182	23	
Hamilton[68]	1978	4,302	38	4,375	38	
Weinraub[71]	1978	692	9	554	1	
Total		90,713	1,382	40,013	179	
Rate		15.2/1000		4.4/1000		3.45 (P = < 0.001)
		Critical No. of Subjects for P 0.05 = 1,881				

* From Reference 32.

Table 11.4.
Neonatal Death and Electronic Fetal Monitoring from RCT Reports*

Primary Author	Year	No EFM	NND	EFM	NND	Ratio
Havercamp[8]	1976	241	0	242	1	
Havercamp[9]	1978	232	0	463	3	
Renou[10]	1976	176	0	169	1	
Kelso[11]	1978	253	1	251	0	
Total		901	1	1,125	5	
Rate		1.11/1000		4.44/1000		4.0

* From Reference 32.

except in Renou's study[10] where there were several neonates with seizures in the auscultated group, but these may have been due to difficult midforceps operations.[13] A recent study by Painter et al.[14] showed an increased incidence of neurologic abnormalities at 1 year of age in infants who had severe variable or late deceleration during labor. They found no neurologic abnormalities at 1 year of age in a control group selected for normal FHR patterns. These numbers were very small, however, and further studies on larger numbers are indicated. Borgstedt et al.[15] looked at four variables, including fetal EEG, FHR patterns, Apgar scores, and neonatal examination, and found that neurological abnormalities at 1 year of age were best identified if all four variables were used. However, using FHR data alone, more than half of the damaged infants could be identified prospectively.

What are the Risks of EFM?

There has been much written about the risk of invasive EFM and infection of the fetus and/or the mother. Fetal infections have consisted almost exclu-

sively of small scalp infections characterized by erythema and induration requiring no more than local medication. Occasionally there is a small abcess requiring drainage and there are isolated reports of more serious infection. Fetal scalp infections are reported in from 0.3%[16] to 4.5%[15] of internally monitored labors. In Okada's study[17] there were 35 infants treated with local measures alone, 7 required systemic antibiotics, and there were no systemic infections, sepsis, osteomyelitis, or subgaleal abcesses. His prospective study indicated that with careful examination and close follow-up, there may be more infections than previously thought.

Maternal infection in patients with internal EFM during labor has been said to be increased in several studies,[8, 18-20] and other studies have indicated no increased risk of maternal infection.[10, 20, 21] When one examines the reports, it becomes obvious that infection is most pronounced if the patient is monitored and then delivered by cesarean section as opposed to the patient who is monitored and then delivered vaginally. Closer scrutiny of the data will reveal that the patient with long labor, many vaginal examinations, prolonged ruptured membranes, and obstructed labor requiring cesarean section is also the most likely patient to be internally monitored for a prolonged time. This association is probably responsible for the presumed cause-effect relationship between EFM and infection following Cesarean section. Recently, Gibbs et al.[22] looked at all associated factors with post-cesarean infection and found that invasive EFM had little or no effect on infection as an independent variable. It is hard to believe, however, that invasive EFM does not contribute in some way to infection, but probably this contribution is minimal.

There have been many other isolated reports of risks from internal monitoring, including leakage of cerebrospinal fluid from the puncture site,[23] arterial scalp bleeding,[24] an eyelid lesion,[25] scalp hematoma,[26] a second degree scalp burn,[27] injury to the umbilical vessels from the catheter,[28] and uterine perforation with the catheter guide.[29]

Effect of EFM on the Cesarean Section Rate (CSR)

At Women's Hospital in Long Beach we essentially monitor all patients in labor. Over the last 4 years with total monitoring, we have had only one intrapartum fetal death among about 12,000 deliveries, excluding an occasional very immature fetus where fetal distress was diagnosed but intervention was not carried out. In this setting, we have a cesarean section rate for fetal distress that is under 2%. The one fetal death that did occur was in a monitored patient with unrecognized late decelerations that were present for several hours before fetal death. We have had an active policy that includes weekly ongoing monitor record review sessions with the labor and delivery nurses as well as periodic sessions with the private staff and the house staff. With a high level of understanding of fetal monitor data among our staff, there does not appear to be an excessive number of cesarean sections and the low number of intrapartum fetal deaths supports the value of this approach.

On the contrary, it is not uncommon to observe overreaction to benign monitor patterns in hospitals where the staff is not well trained in monitor interpretation. Frequently we see cesarean sections done for mild variable deceleration or for baseline heart rates in the range of 110 beats per minute, when the staff is insecure about reading monitor tracings. However, shallow, subtle, late deceleration may be missed by inexperienced observers and several instances have resulted in intrapartum death. Thus, some of the criticism that has been leveled by the government and by some lay groups may well be justified when EFM is done in settings where the personnel are not well trained in interpreting FHR tracings. For this reason, we recommend that any hospital that plans to use EFM should simultaneously introduce an education and on-going review program for their nursing and medical staffs, preferably together in the same setting so they develop common understanding and policies. It is only with a major effort in education that we can prevent the inappropriate use of monitoring and that we can avoid the risk of excessive cesarean sections resulting from EFM.

Perhaps the most discussed risk of EFM is this rise in the CSR that some have attributed to EFM (Table 11.5). Determining the exact contribution, if any, that EFM makes to the overall CSR is complicated by the fact that many other practices have changed during the same period that EFM has been on the increase. For example, difficult forceps operations have been largely abandoned, breeches are more commonly delivered by cesarean section, extended oxytocin augmentation has decreased, and premature fetuses are not written off when they present with complications for which they formerly would not have had a cesarean section. Of course, this increase is then compounded by the fact that most patients with previous cesarean sections are not given a trial of labor in this country.

Table 11.5.
Cesarean Section and Perinatal Mortality in California, 1966 to 1977*

Year	Total Births	Cesarean Sections	CSR	Annual Percentage Increase in CSR	Percentage Increase in CSR since 1965	Perinatal Mortality Rate (per 1000)
1966	343,092	17,978	5.2	2	2	27.1
1967	342,077	18,438	5.4	3	5	26.0
1968	344,716	19,373	5.6	4	10	25.7
1969	358,208	22,316	6.2	10	21	24.9
1970	357,991	25,298	6.9	9	34	23.6
1971	334,379	25,529	7.6	10	49	22.3
1972	310,628	27,028	8.7	12	69	21.4
1973	301,943	29,883	9.9	12	93	20.2
1974	316,020	35,661	11.3	12	120	19.5
1975	321,464	40,995	12.8	12	149	18.6
1976	336,384	47,089	14.0	9	173	17.9
1977	351,575	54,006	15.4	10	202	16.5

* From Reference 31.

Interestingly, when EFM was introduced at Yale University,[30] the cesarean section rate for fetal distress declined when compared with previous years. Clearly, there are patients who are allowed to labor because of the fetal monitor, whereas before EFM they would not have even been given a trial of labor. In our practice, this has been best demonstrated in diabetics, patients with clinical abruptions, elderly gravidas, and certain patients with previous intrapartum fetal death where the monitor reassures both the patient and the physician.

Recently, Williams and Hawes[31] looked at the impact of EFM and the CSR in California during 1977. They determined that about half the patients in California had electronically monitored labors during that year in which they surveyed 324,085 births. They determined the expected perinatal mortality rates for each hospital, based on the risk of the population served. They then determined those medical care factors that favorably or unfavorably affected those mortality rates. The most significant two medical care factors that favorably affected perinatal mortality were a high CSR and a high incidence of fetal monitoring. Other factors favorable to an improved perinatal outcome included a neonatal intensive care unit in the hospital, delivery by a trained obstetrician, a perinatal study committee in the hospital, and the birth occurring in a nonprofit community hospital with teaching. The data, which include a large number of deliveries over a 1-year period from all types of hospitals, suggest that the overall impact of high technology with its probable higher rate of intervention would seem to be justified on the basis of perinatal mortality.

The current state of the art is that the value of EFM is unquestioned by most practitioners who use fetal monitoring in the management of their high risk patients on a daily basis. The nonrandomized studies to date suggest the intrapartum death rate is diminished by EFM and that there is a corresponding reduction in neonatal death rate.

According to the NIH consensus development report[32] it would also appear that the value of EFM increases as the risk of the patient increases and as the gestational age decreases. There is currently no clearly demonstrated benefit to low risk patients.

The randomized controlled trials do not support this value of EFM but they lack sufficient numbers to refute the benefit demonstrated in the retrospective and nonrandomized concurrent trials. The CSR has clearly increased concomittantly with the increase in EFM, but the actual contribution of EFM to this increased rate cannot be measured because of the other changes that have taken place in obstetrical practice during the same time period. Other than the possibility of increasing the CSR, the risks of EFM appear to be minimal in relation to the benefits.

RISKS AND BENEFITS OF ANTEPARTUM FHR MONITORING

While there has been considerable discussion and debate over the risks and benefits of intrapartum FHR monitoring, antepartum monitoring has received little attention in this regard. This is true despite the fact that the potential for benefit is probably greater with respect to the antepartum period since over 70% of fetal deaths occur before the onset of labor.[32] Furthermore, the potential for doing harm, i.e., premature intervention, is more serious than the possible risk of unnecessary cesarean section that may be associated with intrapartum monitoring.

BENEFITS OF ANTEPARTUM FHR MONITORING

Prevention of Fetal Death

This is the most obvious potential benefit of antepartum FHR monitoring. In 1976, the rate of fetal death in the United States was 10.5/1000.[32] Approximately 20% of these deaths occurred intrapartum. Between 25 and 50% of antepartum fetal deaths occur in women with risk factors that would make them candidates for antepartum testing.[33, 34] Therefore, 2 to 4 fetal deaths per thousand births might be prevented if the 10 to 20% of women with risk factors were appropriately tested. While the above is hypothetical, there are at least two sources of data that suggest this might be at least partially true.

The first would be to look at the series thus far reported using oxytocin challenge tests (OCT's) as the primary means of surveillance (Table 11.6). These studies include 2496 patients and 6 fetal deaths. Since only high risk patients were tested, the expected fetal death rate would be 18/1000. (This number is based on the assumption that 50% of antenatal fetal deaths occur in the 20% of patients who are high risk and

Table 11.6
Studies Using the OCT as The Primary Means of Fetal Surveillance

Primary Author	Year	No. of Patients	Fetal Deaths
Spurett[35]	1971	193	0
Christie[36]	1974	50	0
Boyd[37]	1974	41	1
Ewing[38]	1974	58	0
Cooper[39]	1975	89	0
Schifrin[40]	1975	120	0
Gaziano[41]	1975	72	0
Hayden[42]	1975	105	0
Weingold[43]	1975	154	0
Freeman[44]	1976	390	2
Farahani[45]	1976	333	1
Boehm[46]	1976	152	2
Fox[47]	1976	209	0
Bhakthavathsalan[48]	1976	100	0
Garite[33]	1978	430	0

the overall antenatal death rate is 7/1000.) One would therefore expect about 46 fetal deaths in these 2496 reported cases instead of the 6 reported cases.

Garite et al.[33] examined this question more specifically. They reported on a 2-year series of 430 high risk patients using the OCT for primary fetal surveillance. There were a total of 5351 deliveries during that same time period. No fetal deaths occurred in patients appropriately tested. During that time, there were 31 antepartum fetal deaths in patients not tested. Eleven of these (35%) had risk factors that should have indicated antepartum testing, but these patients were not tested either because of no prenatal care or the patient was transferred from another institution after the fetus was found to have expired.

There are no randomized controlled series of OCT's or nonstress tests (NST's), but Ray and Freeman's original series[49] was blinded. Sixty-eight patients were tested; thirty-three had negative tests only and in this group there were no fetal deaths; fifteen had positive tests, and there were three antenatal deaths in this group. Our experience now includes over 3000 patients studied with OCT's and we have had no unexpected antepartum deaths from uteroplacental insufficiency in patients studied according to our protocol.

It is therefore reasonable to conclude that the OCT can prevent unexpected fetal death, from uteroplacental insufficiency in almost all cases.

Avoiding Unnecessary Premature Intervention

An underemphasized but most important objective of antepartum testing is that such testing allows the clinician to avoid intervention solely on empirical bases such as risk factors.

The best example of this is seen in insulin-dependent diabetics. Dr. Priscilla White[50] suggested that such fetal deaths might be avoided by premature delivery; the more severe or prolonged the diabetes, the earlier one was told to intervene. Such an approach is reasonable when one cannot precisely select which individual fetuses are actually in jeopardy. Many fetuses that were in no danger were delivered early and suffered morbidity and often mortality from prematurity. Such an approach obviously needs refinement. Recent series[51, 52] using intense antenatal FHR testing, estriols and maturity studies in addition to good clinical judgement have reported perinatal mortality for these diabetics reduced to nearly that of the low risk population while carrying the majority of these pregnancies beyond 38 weeks. Such a benefit not only prevents the morbidity of prematurity but is extremely cost effective, since even this intense antenatal testing does not compare in cost to neonatal intensive care.

Another example where antepartum FHR testing allows more specific identification of the fetus in

jeopardy is a study by Knox et al.[53] In a prospectively randomized series comparing amniocentesis for the detection of meconium with the OCT for management of postdates patients, the OCT was shown to reduce the necessity for intervention from 32% (in the amniocentesis for meconium group) to 12% (in the OCT group) without any difference in mortality or morbidity.

Risk identification only narrows a larger group to a smaller one which needs more attention. Once that smaller group has been identified, testing should identify which patients need intervention or further testing and which may be safely left alone. Only in this way can we be sure we are doing more good than harm.

Preventing Fetal Damage

Critics of intrapartum fetal monitoring say one of the reasons that such monitoring might not significantly reduce sublethal hypoxic/asphyxic damage is that much of this damage has occurred before the onset of labor. Indeed, we have seen many patients present in early labor with ominous heart rate patterns and absent FHR variability which may have been present for some time. Certainly, as was pointed out in earlier chapters, a goal of antepartum monitoring should not only be prevention of fetal death but prevention of hypoxic morbidity as well. There is no real data at this time to prove or disprove this point. Indeed, one might even argue theoretically that we are saving fetuses only to deliver babies damaged either from hypoxia or from prematurity.

Nevertheless, if fetal and neonatal hypoxic morbidity is to be effectively prevented, it seems reasonable that antepartum monitoring offers a means of rescuing a fetus early in the course of this disease process.

Other Benefits of Antepartum Testing

When patients have been informed adequately, the OCT can be a valuable source of reassurance. This is especially true in patients who have suffered previous fetal losses or who are very anxious about their risk of losing the baby. This is also true on a more short-term basis in the patient who calls complaining of decreased fetal movement. As pointed out in the previous section, this testing can also reassure the anxious physician and prevent premature or unnecessary intervention. In the case of the elderly gravida or the post dates patient, it may also prevent cesarean section by allowing the clinician to wait for cervical ripeness as well as fetal maturity.

Finally antepartum FHR monitoring can be a valuable tool in assessing response to therapy, either negatively or positively. The preeclamptic patient's fetus may improve with maternal bed rest. The response to antihypertensive medication can be indirectly assessed in regard to its effect on placental perfusion. For example, a recent study[54] suggests that diazoxide may be dangerous because of relative hypotension causing decreased placental blood flow detected by late decelerations observed with simultaneous FHR monitoring.

RISKS OF ANTEPARTUM FHR TESTING

The potential risks of antepartum monitoring fall into one of three general categories. These include the possible risks of Doppler ultrasound in external FHR monitoring, those risks that might be associated with the administration of oxytocin to the antepartum patient, and the potentially most significant risk of inappropriate or unnecessary intervention.

Risk of Ultrasound

When the FHR is monitored for antepartum testing, it must of course be done externally. The most common modality presently used for external FHR monitoring, both antepartum and intrapartum, is Doppler ultrasound. In terms of total energy, Doppler ultrasound transducers emit substantially more energy than do diagnostic ultrasound units. This is because the Doppler units emit continuous sound while diagnostic units are pulsed with greater proportions of time spent in the "listening" or off phase of the cycle. The average intensity of continuous output ultrasound systems (Doppler instruments) is 20 mw/cm^2 over the area of the transducer face and the peak intensity at the most concentrated point along the beam path is 50 mw/cm^2.[55] We will not review all the studies, but the reader is directed to an excellent review of the studies on the risks of obstetric ultrasound by Hobbins et al.[55] In 1978, the American Institute on Ultrasound in Medicine (AIUM) Committee on Bioeffects met for the second time to review the literature on the safety of ultrasound. They concluded, "In the low megahertz frequency range there have been as of October 1978, no independently confirmed significant biological effects of mammalian tissues exposed to intensities below 100 milliwatts/cm^2." While there may be subtle effects on human tissue not yet known, the present data would not suggest deleterious effects from ultrasound in FHR monitoring. One way to obviate even the fear of any yet to be found risk from Doppler ultrasound is to use the abdominal fetal ECG technique which may be successfully used, as experience is gained, in up to 70% of antepartum patients.

Risk of Oxytocin Administration

Since oxytocin is required for the majority of contraction stress tests, there are the theoretical risks of premature labor and uterine rupture. In addition, unrecognized hyperstimulation may overstress the fetus and as a result late decelerations may be seen in the noncompromised patient.

Premature labor as a potential risk has been a long discussed but never documented risk of the OCT. Several series on the OCT[35, 37, 44, 47, 49] have looked at the incidence of premature labor in patients tested and have reported no increase in the incidence of premature labor. To look at this question more specifically, Braly et al.[56] looked at the incidence of premature labor in 3000 patients from the OCT/NST Collaborative Study who had received oxytocin. They found no increase in the incidence of premature labor. Furthermore, there was no more labor on the day of the test and the next 2 days than in the subsequent 3 days. Therefore, there seems to be no increased risk of premature labor from the OCT. Since we do use oxytocin and cause frequent contractions, one might wonder why we have not seen even a slight increase in the occurrence of premature labor. There are probably several explanations. An important one is that patients of substantially increased risk for premature labor are excluded from the sample because the OCT has been said to be contraindicated in these patients. In addition, oxytocin is used at dilute concentrations and frequent contractions are maintained only for a short time period. As long as precautions are maintained, premature labor is probably not a cause for concern with the OCT.

Rupture of the uterus might also be a theoretical risk of oxytocin administration. We know of no reported cases of this complication. Certainly previous classical cesarean section is a contraindication to the OCT, and this precaution explains why the primary risk of uterine rupture has been excluded. We have, however, liberally performed OCT's in the presence of previous low transverse uterine scars without known complications.

There is one reported case of abruptio placenta[57] that followed an OCT not associated with uterine hyperactivity or other risk factors. The patient had the onset of symptoms 4 hr after conclusion of the test. An isolated case hardly suggests cause and effect, but since uterine hyperactivity may be associated with separation of the placenta, there is the possibility of a theoretical association.

External tocodynamometry has limitations in that contraction duration, and especially contraction strength, cannot be accurately monitored. Late decelerations, the end point of the OCT, can only be regarded as clinically significant if the fetoplacental unit has not been overstressed by excessive uterine activity. Since external monitoring does have this limitation, excessive stimulation may be, at least in part, an explanation for some of the false positive OCT's. Knowledge of such limitations and attention to this detail can, however, minimize this potential risk.

Table 11.7
Outcome Related to Intervention after a Positive OCT

Primary Author	Year	No. of Patients Tested	No. of Patients with Positive Tests	No. of Prematures Delivered (2500g)	No. of Babies with Stigmata of Compromise*	No. of Babies with Complications of Prematurity	No. of Neonatal Deaths	No. of Babies with Stigmata of Compromise* and Prematurity	No. of Premature Babies with No Stigmata of Compromise*
Ewing[38]	1974	58	8	4	5	2	1	3	0
Cooper[39]	1975	89	13	4	10	1	0	3	0
Gaziano[41]	1975	72	7	3	6	0	0	1	0
Bhakthavathsalan[48]	1976	100	10	4	9	2	1	3	1
Boehm[46]	1976	152	10	5	7	1	1	3	0
Garite[33]	1978	430	10	3	?	?	3	4	0

* Meconium, IUGR, low Apgar, low estriols, low pH, fetal distress in labor.

Inappropriate Intervention

This is the most serious potential risk of all antepartum testing. The lack of specificity of all available tests make the possibility of such a problem especially real. There are two possible consequences of intervention when the fetus is not really in jeopardy. In the term or mature fetus, there is the increased probability of unnecessary operative deliveries from either immediate cesarean section or from failed induction of labor. More importantly in the preterm fetus, there are the risks of morbidity and mortality from prematurity.

To what extent inappropriate intervention actually occurs is extremely difficult to assess in the absence of controlled prospective series. One way to answer this question is to review cases where intervention was based on a positive OCT and then attempt to determine which of these cases showed no other stigmata of fetal compromise especially in prematures. Table 11.7 shows a compiled series of 901 patients studied including 58 with positive OCT's. Overall, where the data can be analyzed, 17/58 or 29% of fetuses were delivered without other evidence of hypoxic compromise but only one of 58 patients with a positive OCT was delivered prematurely without other signs of compromise. There are six neonatal deaths in these series and most (four) of these babies were markedly depressed or there was significant maternal disease in three which dictated delivery. In addition, two of these deaths were associated with severe congenital anomalies.

Such series tend to be quite reassuring with respect to minimal apparently unnecessary premature intervention. The fact that 29% of the more mature babies were delivered without signs of compromise may or may not, however, be alarming. Perhaps the OCT is a sufficiently early warning sign of problems that we are able to deliver the fetus before other problems occur; if so, this would meet one of the goals of antepartum testing. Not all series are quite so positive however. Christie and Cudmore[36] reported on a series of 9 positive OCT's among 50 patients tested. All nine patients tolerated labor without fetal distress and none of the nine was depressed or had other reported signs of intrauterine hypoxic compromise. However, in this series extremely high doses of oxytocin to begin testing (10 munits/min) may have led to hyperstimulation. Furthermore, it must be admitted that most series come from university centers where the authors are generally well versed in the limitations and pitfalls of testing; what is not known is what the rate of inappropriate premature intervention is in most clinical situations.

Other Risks of Antepartum Monitoring

One particularly alarming fact is that fetuses with severe congenital anomalies have an increased rate of abnormal heart rate tracings that lead to intervention and often cesarean sections for fetal indications. Spurett[35] was the first to suggest this possibility when he noticed three patients with congenital anomalies among patients with abnormal OCT's. Garite et al.[58] studied this question and found a 27% incidence of antepartum and intrapartum fetal distress among babies born with severe congenital anomalies. Since many of these babies tend to be growth retarded, and diabetics have such an increased rate of anomalies, the rate of malformed fetuses may be high among patients who are candidates for antepartum testing. Since marked hydrocephaly and anencephaly are the only two detectable fetal anomalies that are clearly not salvageable, the clinician is forced to act on the result of abnormal tests even when the suspicion of major anomalies is high.

In summary, antepartum FHR testing as the primary means of fetal surveillance seems to be an effective method of preventing fetal death. A high proportion of fetuses destined to die come from patients with risk factors, so appropriate testing based on maternal risk can get at a substantial number of these fetuses. The OCT allows a clinician to keep "hands off" patients where the fetus is doing well and thereby one chief benefit is avoiding intervention based on risk factors alone. And possibly such antepartum FHR testing, especially the OCT, may be a sufficiently early warning to avoid permanent sublethal hypoxic fetal damage.

The risks of the administration of oxytocin, particularly premature labor, seem to be only theoretical and there is no data suggesting this is indeed a risk.

Ultrasound can be considered to be a theoretical risk to the fetus but at levels of energy in current use there is no data to suggest this. Finally, the risk of unnecessary premature intervention on the basis of a false positive test can be minimized by evaluating the whole clinical situation, watching fetal reactivity, and utilizing supporting data such as estriol assays.

REFERENCES

1. Hon EH, Khazin AF: Observations on fetal pH and fetal biochemistry. I. Base deficit. Am J Obstet Gynecol 105:721, 1969

2. Kubli EW, Hon EH, Khazin AF, et al: Observations on heart rate and pH in the human fetus during labor. Am J Obstet Gynecol 104:1190, 1969

3. Schifrin B, Dame L: Fetal heart rate patterns prediction of Apgar score. JAMA 219:322, 1973

4. Hon EH, Khazin AF: Biochemical studies of the fetus. I. The fetal pH monitoring system. Obstet Gynecol 33:219, 1968

5. Hon EH, Khazin AF: Biochemical studies of the fetus. II. Fetal pH and Apgar scores. Obstet Gynecol 33:237, 1969

6. Tejani N, Mann L, Bhakthavathsalan A, et al: Correlation of fetal heart rate—uterine contraction patterns with fetal scalp blood pH. Obstet Gynecol 46:392, 1975

7. Banta HD, Thacker SB: Costs and Benefits of Electronic Fetal Monitoring: A Review of the literature. Department of H.E.W. Publication no (PHS) 79-3245, Washington, DC

8. Haverkamp AD, Thompson HE, McFee JG, et al: The evaluation of continuous fetal heart rate monitoring in high risk pregnancy. Am J Obstet Gynecol 125:310, 1976

9. Haverkamp AD, Orleans M, Langendoerfer S, et al: A controlled trial of the differential effects of intrapartum fetal monitoring. Am J Obstet Gynecol 134:399, 1979

10. Renou P, Chang A, Anderson I, et al: Controlled trial of fetal intensive care. Am J Obstet Gynecol 126:470, 1976

11. Kelso IM, Parsons RJ, Lawrence GF, et al: An assessment of continuous fetal heart rate monitoring in labor: a randomized trial. Am J Obstet Gynecol 131:526, 1978

12. Neutra RR, Fienberg SE, Greenland, et al: Effect of fetal monitoring on neonatal death rates. N Engl J Med 299:324, 1978

13. Haverkamp AD: Personal communication

14. Painter MJ, Depp R, O'Donoghue PD: Fetal heart rate patterns and development in the first year of life. Am J Obstet Gynecol 132:271, 1978

15. Borgstedt AO, Rosen MG, Chik L, et al: Fetal electroencephalography. Relationship to neonatal and one-year developmental neurological examinations in high risk infants. Am J Dis Child 129:35, 1975

16. Cordero L, Hon EH: Scalp abscess: a rare complication of fetal monitoring. J Pediatr 78:533, 1971

17. Okada DM, Chow AW, Bruce VT: Neonatal scalp abscess and fetal monitoring: factors associated with infection. Am J Obstet Gynecol 129:185, 1977

18. Gassner CB, Ledger WJ: The relationship of hospital-acquired maternal infection to invasive intrapartum monitoring techniques. Am J Obstet Gynecol 126:33, 1976

19. Hagen D: Maternal febrile morbidity associated with fetal monitoring and cesarean section. Obstet Gynecol 46:260, 1975

20. Wiechetek WJ, Horiguchi T, Dillon TF: Puerperal morbidity and internal fetal monitoring. Am J Obstet Gynecol 119:230, 1974

21. Chan WH, Paul RH, Toews J: Intrapartum fetal monitoring maternal and fetal morbidity and perinatal mortality. Obstet Gynecol 41:7, 1973

22. Gibbs RS, Jones PM, Wilder CJY: Internal fetal monitoring and maternal infection following cesarean section: a prospective study. Obstet Gynecol 52:193, 1978

23. Goodlin RC, Harrod IR: Complications of fetal spiral electrodes. Lancet 1:559, 1973

24. Scanlon JW, Walkley EI: Neonatal blood loss as a complication of fetal monitoring. Pediatrics 50:934, 1972

25. Roux JF, Wilson R, Yeni-Komshian, et al: Labor monitoring: a practical experience. Obstet Gynecol 36:875, 1970

26. Chan WH:, Paul RH, Toews J: Intrapartum fetal monitoring maternal and fetal morbidity and perinatal mortality. Obstet Gynecol 41:7, 1973

27. Aktor MS: An unusual complication of intrapartum fetal monitoring. Am J Obstet Gynecol 124:756, 1976

28. Trudinger BJ, Pryse-Davies J: Fetal hazards of the intrauterine pressure catheter: five case reports. Br J Obstet Gynecol 85:567, 1978

29. Haverkamp A, Bowes WA: Uterine perforation: a complication of continuous fetal monitoring. Am J Obstet Gynecol 110:667, 1971

30. Paul RH: Clinical fetal monitoring: experience on a large clinical service. Am J Obstet Gynecol 113:573, 1972

31. Williams RL, Hawes W: Cesarean section, fetal monitoring and perinatal mortality in California. Am J Public Health 69:864, 1979

32. Antenatal Diagnosis. Report of a Consensus Development Conference. NIH Publication no. 79-1973, Bethesda, Maryland, April, 1979

33. Garite TJ, Freeman RK, Hoehleutner I, et al: Oxytocin challenge test; achieving the desired goals. Obstet Gynecol 51:614, 1978

34. Nesbitt RL, Aubry RH: High risk obstetrics II. Value of semiobjective grading system in identifying the vulnerable group. Am J Obstet Gynecol 103:972, 1969

35. Spurrett, B: Stressed cardiotocography in late pregnancy. J Obstet Gynecol Br Commonw 78:894, 1971

36. Christie GB, Cudmore DW: The oxytocin challenge test. Am J Obstet Gynecol 118:327, 1974

37. Boyd IE, Chamberlain GVP, Fergusson ILC: The oxytocin stress test and the isoxsuprine placental transfer test in the management of suspected placental insufficiency. J Obstet Gynecol Br Commonw 81:120, 1974

38. Ewing DE, Farina JR, Otterson WN: Clinical application of the oxytocin challenge test. Obstet Gynecol 43:563, 1974

39. Cooper JM, Sofforonoff EC, Bolognese RJ: Oxytocin challenge test in monitoring high risk pregnancies. Obstet Gynecol 45:27, 1975

40. Schifrin BS, Lapidus M, Doctor GS, et al: Contraction stress test for antepartum evaluation. Obstet Gynecol 45:433, 1975

41. Gaziano EP, Freeman RK, Hochleutner I, et al: Oxytocin challenge test: achieving the desired goals. Obstet Gynecol 51:614, 1978

42. Hayden BL, Simpson JL, Ewing DE, et al: Can the oxytocin challenge test serve as the primary method for managing high risk pregnancies? Obstet Gynecol 46:251, 1975

43. Weingold AB, DeJesus TPS, O'Keiffe J: Oxytocin challenge test. Am J Obstet Gynecol 123:466, 1975

44. Freeman RK, Goelbelsmann U, Nochimson D, et al: An evaluation of the significance of a positive oxytocin challenge test. Obstet Gynecol 47:8, 1976

45. Farahani G, Vasudeva K, Petrie R, et al: Oxytocin challenge test in high risk pregnancy. Obstet Gynecol 47:159, 1976

46. Boehm FH, Braun RD, Growden JH: The oxytocin challenge test. South Med J 69,884, 1976

47. Fox HE, Steinbrecher M, Ripton B: Antepartum fetal heart rate and uterine activity studies. Am J Obstet Gynecol 126:61, 1976

48. Bhakthavathsalan A, Mann LI, Tejani NA, et al: Correlation of the oxytocin challenge test with perinatal outcome. Obstet Gynecol 48:552, 1976

49. Ray M, Freeman RK, Pine S, et al: Clinical experience with the oxytocin challenge test. Am J Obstet Gynecol 123:206, 1972

50. White P: Pregnancy and diabetes medical aspects. Med Clin North Am 49:1015, 1965

51. Gabbe SG, Mestman JH, Freeman RK, et al: Management and outcome of diabetes mellitus, classes B-R. Am J Obstet Gynecol 129:723, 1977

52. Goldstein AL, Cronk DA, Garite TJ, et al: Perinatal outcome in the diabetic pregnancy: a retrospective analysis. J Reprod Med 20:61, 1978

53. Knox GE, Huddleston JF, Flowers CE Jr, et al: Management of prolonged pregnancy: a prospective randomized trial. Am J Obstet Gynecol 134:378, 1979

54. Neuman J, Weiss B, Rabello Y, et al: Diazoxide for the acute control of severe hypertension complicating pregnancy. Obstet Gynecol (Suppl) 53:50, 1979

55. Hobbins JC, Berkowitz RL, Hohler CW: How safe is ultrasound in obstetrics? Contemp Obstet Gynecol 14:63, 1979

56. Braly PB, Freeman RK, Garite TJ, et al: Premature labor and the oxytocin challenge test. (submitted for publication)

57. Seski JC, Compton AA: Abruptio placentae following a negative oxytocin challenge test. Am J Obstet Gynecol 125:276, 1976

58. Garite TJ, Linzey EM, Freeman RK, et al: Fetal heart rate patterns and fetal distress in fetuses with congenital anomalies. Obstet Gynecol 53:716, 1979

59. Kelly VC, Kulkarni D: Experiences with fetal monitoring in a community hospital. Obstet Gynecol 41:818, 1973

60. Tutera G, Newman RL: Fetal monitoring: Its effect on the perinatal mortality and cesarean section rates and its complications. Am J Obstet Gynecol 122:750, 1975

61. Edington PT, Sibanda J, Beard RW: Influence on clinical practice of routine intra-partum fetal monitoring. Br Med J 3:341, 1975

62. Koh KS, Greves D, Yung S, et al: Experience with fetal monitoring in a university teaching hospital. Canad Med Assoc J 112:455, 1975

63. Shenker L, Post RC, Seiler JS: Routine electronic monitoring of fetal heart rate and uterine activity during labor. Obstet Gynecol 46:185, 1975

64. Lee WK, Baggish MS: The effect of unselected intrapartum fetal monitoring. Obstet Gynecol 47:516, 1976

65. Paul RH, Huey JR, Yaeger CF: Clinical fetal monitoring—its effect on cesarean section rate and perinatal mortality: five-year trends. Postgrad Med 61:160, 1977

66. Amato JC: Fetal monitoring in a community hospital: a statistical analysis. Obstet Gynecol 50:269, 1977

67. Johnstone FD, Campbell DM, Hughes GJ: Antenatal care: Has continuous intrapartum monitoring made any impact on fetal outcome? Lancet 1:1298, 1978

68. Hamilton LA, Gottschalk W, Vidyasagar D, et al: Effects of monitoring high-risk pregnancies and intrapartum FHR monitoring on perinates. Int J Gynaecol Obstet 15:483, 1978

69. Hughey MJ, LaPata RE, McElin TW, et al: The effect of fetal monitoring on the incidence of cesarean section. Obstet Gynecol 49:513, 1977

70. Neutra RR, Fienberg SE, Greenland S, et al: Effect of fetal monitoring on neonatal death rates. N Eng J Med 299:324, 1978

71. Weinraub Z, Caspi E, Brook I, et al: Perinatal outcome in monitored and unmonitored high risk deliveries. Isr J Med Sci 14:249, 1978

Index